THE SENSES OF DEMOCRACY

THE WILLIAM & BETTYE NOWLIN SERIES
in Art, History, and Culture of the Western Hemisphere

The Senses of Democracy

Perception, Politics, and Culture in Latin America

FRANCINE R. MASIELLO

University of Texas Press
AUSTIN

Printed in the United States of America
First edition, 2018

Requests for permission to reproduce material from this work should be sent to:
Permissions
University of Texas Press
P.O. Box 7819
Austin, TX 78713-7819
utpress.utexas.edu/rp-form

♾ The paper used in this book meets the minimum requirements of ANSI/NISO Z39.48-1992 (R1997) (Permanence of Paper).

LIBRARY OF CONGRESS CATALOGING-IN-PUBLICATION DATA

Names: Masiello, Francine, author.
Title: The senses of democracy : perception, politics, and culture in Latin America / Francine R. Masiello.
Description: First edition. | Austin : University of Texas Press, 2018. | Includes bibliographical references and index.
Identifiers: LCCN 2017036467 | ISBN 978-1-4773-1503-3 (cloth : alk. paper) | ISBN 978-1-4773-1504-0 (pbk. : alk. paper) | ISBN 978-1-4773-1505-7 (library e-book) | ISBN 978-1-4773-1506-4 (nonlibrary e-book)
Subjects: LCSH: Latin America—Literatures—History and criticism. | Democracy in literature. | Senses and sensation—Social aspects. | Synesthesia—Social aspects. | Literature and society—Latin America. | Politics and culture—Latin America. | Social change—Latin America. | Democracy—Latin America.
Classification: LCC PN849.L29 M37 2018 | DDC 809/.933581—dc23
LC record available at https://lccn.loc.gov/2017036467

doi:10.7560/35033

In memory of
Tulio Halperin Donghi
and
Ricardo Piglia

Contents

Illustrations

Figures

Color Plates

Acknowledgments

Over the years I have been the fortunate recipient of the friendship and guidance of many talented individuals whom I met in my North/South travels. My training as an Argentinist began when Angela Dellepiane in New York pushed me toward graduate study. Years later, David Viñas in Minnesota invited me to audit his course on politics and literature; his brilliant claims about the materiality of texts have been a force that still keeps me going. When I began my career at Berkeley, I had the good luck to strike up a friendship with Tulio Halperin Donghi, not only a consummate historian and an insatiable reader of novels, but also my colleague and mentor for nearly forty years. He read an early draft of chapter 1 of this book, but I am indebted to him for much, much more.

A study trip to Argentina in order to check out the archives occurred at the end of my first year at Cal. There, in the storm of a terrible dictatorship, a group of young intellectuals came out to greet me and show me the lay of the land. Ricardo Piglia, Beatriz Sarlo, and Josefina Ludmer were my guides. Over the years and despite our disagreements, I have treasured their counsel and good words, and their willingness to engage with my work. On this last round and during his illness, Ricardo was alive with ideas, kept his good humor about politics and destiny, and even volunteered to be my writing coach for an all too sketchy novel; perhaps to my regret, I left the novel alone and finished this book instead. And then there has always been the irreplaceable Beba Eguía, leading me through the intricacies of Argentine life that I never could have seen on my own.

This book sparked many additional conversations, particularly among some of the writers and artists whose works are considered in these pages: thanks to Diamela Eltit, Guillermo Núñez, Nuno Ramos, Demian Schopf, and Raul Zurita, whose soaring talents in literature and the arts have inspired me to be a more demanding reader and to demand more of myself.

Adriana Amante has been a necessary and lively interlocutor regarding the Argentine archive and just about everything else. John King, my frequent e-mail pal, has shared with me a love for Latin American texts, avant-garde art, and gardens. His help at the last moment in locating some visual materials gave me a certain relief, but not as much as his reassuring words about more than a few of the pages here. Luis Cárcamo Huechante spent hours with me talking about the art of the voice so that sometimes we were left nearly speechless. Ksenija Bilbija, Nicole Caso, Tom McEnaney, Héctor Hoyos, and Ximena Briceño invited me to test my ideas through public lectures at their home institutions. Gwen Kirkpatrick and Diana Sorensen were implacable readers who generously went through the entire manuscript and gave thoughtful comments about ways to improve it. As always, I am in their debt for their intelligence and the long camaraderie that we share in the Latin American field.

In Argentina, Adriana Carreira and Silvina Marsimian kindly introduced me to the library collections of the Colegio Nacional; Juan Pablo Canala of the Biblioteca Nacional Mariano Moreno was generous with his time and materials. María Inés Lagos Pope gave me a venue for my work and allowed me to consult the Special Collections Division of the University of Virginia Library. UC Berkeley librarians Carlos Delgado and Claude Potts came to my rescue on multiple occasions. I also benefitted from the wonderful editors at the University of Texas Press: Theresa May, who encouraged this project from the start; Kerry Webb, who kept me on track; and Angelica López-Torres, who dealt patiently with my clumsy maneuvers through high-tech reproductions and pixels.

Finally, I am a beneficiary of the community that took shape around me at Berkeley. Several of my former students, now prominent scholars, read sections of this text and offered substantial comments: thanks to Munia Bhaumik, Anna Deeny, and Tom McEnaney at different stages of writing; to Chrissy Arce, Myrna García-Calderón, Victor Goldgel Carballo, Sarah Moody, Regina Root, Sergio Waisman, and Sarah Wells, who were always ready to jump into the conversation whenever I needed an ear. The late Humberto Cruz was a loyal friend with a tireless appetite for literature and the visual arts. Graduate students Sebastião Macedo and Ariel Wind were especially helpful as research assistants, but more important for me were our ongoing conversations about the craft of good writing. Mayra Bottaro was there from the start. I am in her debt for her observations on several chapters of this text, her endless company in the archives, and her unfailing devotion to scholarship of the kind that we desperately need. And then there are my colleagues to whom I am always grateful: Victoria Kahn, for her intellectual rigor and adamant good cheer; Robert Kaufman, for his relentless faith in the critical power of poetry; Daylet Domínguez, whose passion for nineteenth-century Cuba rekindled my own love for that field; Dru Dougherty, for his eye for detail while he read through chapter 3; Catherine Gallagher and Martin Jay, who were generous readers of draft material underlying chapter 1; and Teresa Stojkov, whose thoughts about different versions of this book were always right on target.

Last but not least, I can never sufficiently acknowledge the lifeline that was thrown to me by Maryann Wolfe as she put her needle-fine critical eye to many of the manuscript pages. I thank her for her patience and trials of endurance as I brought this manuscript to a close. Maryann and two of my favorite people, Joseph Manoleas and Lindsey Signorelli, give me sustenance, joy, and laughter, and above all, faith in the future.

THE SENSES OF DEMOCRACY

Introduction

In an Argentine newspaper of 1827, a writer conveys his hope to reach faraway readers and listeners. Toward this objective, he alerts us to a new kind of sound device still in an early stage of invention: a tool to transmit voice over distance, to close the gap between us, to capture the external stimuli that flicker many leagues away. This machine, which he calls an "acoustic telegraph," will enhance our sense of audition; it will satisfy our desire for contact and our need to be "in touch" ("Telégrafos acústicos" 1827). Reviewing inventions of voice technology that date from the early years of the nineteenth century, the author goes on to praise the advantages of telephonic transmission from the speaker's perspective: we can acquire enhanced sonority, a greater subtlety of tone; we can decidedly improve the attributes of the unassisted voice. More traditional acoustic devices also hold their appeal: our unnamed author reports the experience of a deaf man who heard a sonata through a pipe once used for tobacco; he points out the wood, water, and metal tubes that conduct timbre and tone of voice. The point is that with more modern devices, we will soon be able to hear and speak to each other over considerable distance; we will eliminate the gaps between us; and landscapes will shrink in size. No less important, telephony will carry clear religious and political advantage: acoustic aids will spread the Sunday sermons and also supply the news feed, keeping people abreast of spiritual and national events, as well as the rule of law.

This ambitious reflection gives support to a generally accepted nineteenth-century Latin American project: to elevate the capabilities of the human body in order to support the mission of nations, to disseminate the official word, and to train all citizens to perceive with a single ear and mind. But in other settings, perceptual devices might sustain less structured worlds, producing not a singular "common sense," but a diversified field of experience; an art of sensing that counters yesteryear's obsolescence or sustains increasing disruption, provoking fractious upsets in a disciplined public life. In this regard, telephony would function less to uphold church or state, but in fact to aid rebellion. It would also bring us fantasies of monsters with voices produced by machines. In 1827 and in Argentina, however, it was still too early to imagine a robotic technology that might test the authority of creole elites. In fact, it would take more than fifty years before a River Plate Frankenstein would surface; for the meanwhile, people awaited a monster of a different stripe, their tyrant Juan Manuel Rosas.

In *The Senses of Democracy*, I explore the role that the sensorium has played in defining democratic practice and rebellion, cultural crisis, and social change. Taking a wide arc of material that covers more than two centuries and focusing on the technologies and political events that interact with perceiving subjects, I look at the evolution of what I call "sense work" in Latin American culture—principally in Argentina and Chile—while also weaving events and experience from the United States and Europe. This study wends from the heights of romantic thought in both the North and South American contexts to the startling innovations of modernity that were embraced by the avant-garde of the 1920s and 1930s; it reaches the crisis of embodied knowledge that was provoked in the 1950s (here the voice of Merleau-Ponty sears through), and leads to the exacerbated "bare life" experience of prisoners under military rule. A final chapter follows sense work beyond the human by tracking art, literature, and cyber bodies that hurtle through globalized space. The idea is to trace the shifting representations of the sensing body over time as they respond to both new inventions and sociopolitical quandaries; in some cases, these representations collaborate with the nation's aims, while in others, they trouble models for citizenship and the norms of a well-regulated life. I am calling this book *The Senses of Democracy* to signal the linkage between the sensorium and political currents over an extended period of time. Far before democracy entered common parlance among Latin American thinkers (toward the close of the nineteenth century), we already experienced a political culture that was defined in terms of perceptions: most notably in Argentina, the "civilization versus barbarism" slogan that showed reason as separate from the senses gave an outline for the battles that would occur over cultural ideals and future direction. The sensorium captured dimensions of a larger political struggle.

Following the logic of Marx, who in the *Economic and Philosophic*

Manuscripts of 1844 wrote that "man is affirmed in the objective world not only in the act of thinking, but with *all* his senses" (1964, 140), I inquire about the ways in which the senses take form in culture. Shaped of course by biology and labor, but also by war and technology, and modernization and consumer desires, the senses are powerful agents to tell us about cultural progress. They illustrate how human perceptions protect us from danger; they announce the power of individual bodies against the authority of state; and they allow us to narrate stories of pleasure, pain, and resistance. Of course, the sentient body is the starting point for one's engagement with the world, but here I chance a further claim: when the discourse on democracy is altered—when public participation is engaged or foreclosed, when the concepts of the "people" are redefined, when we catch sight of nations in distress or hear repeated calls for war, when we feel the weight of modernity pressing upon the walls of tradition—then, indeed, we reframe the sensorium and the uses of human perceptions. The sentient body is a placeholder for a larger discussion of the effects of state practices on its people and, alternatively, it traces the ways in which the population resists or transforms social life. It also becomes a measure of aesthetic performance that captures the political drift. In some cases, we respond with shock or aversion (in the style described by Georg Simmel), but we also reconfigure the sensorial grid, giving privilege to one sense perception over others or rushing toward synesthetic response as a way to combine different strands of sensation with the illusion of wholeness. The representation of the senses, then, seizes upon different relationships between the individual in local or global conditions; it marks different eras of national culture and speaks to human authority and resistance. Finally, when the harsh realities of military rule leave us in a life system determined by captivity and torture, the representation of the senses registers injury and physical pain, in contrast to its postmodern antithesis that might indulge the intensities of pleasure or aim for pure sensation without any evidence of humans in sight. Sense work denotes a changing cultural landscape in ongoing transition just as it roots us in the "now."

A general claim here is that the senses are the way through which a culture finds its location; the senses stand as the basis of a particular experience in a particular time and place. They are relevant to how we see ourselves on the cusp of disorder or civil war, in the movement between tradition and modernity, in the tension between national and cosmopolitan yearnings, or even at the dawn of an age when technological innovation threatens the integrity of what we identify as human. Tracing sense work in culture makes abject experiences experientially available; it helps us organize cultural politics through a bodily, material presence. The senses, then, are part of the identikit materials that sustain the self or deliver it to chaos. At the same time, tracking the senses brings universalisms into question. To summarize: sense perceptions situate us in a time and place; they position individuals in a particular context. And although we all see and hear, touch and taste—universal activities that might define us as one—the specific example of culture or context alters the nature of these perceptions. Culture and context—famine or banquet; war or colonial impact; the conflicts of race, class, and gender; the shock of imprisonment and torture; even the hues of a particular mountain range, the scents of a special blossom, or the shouts of commercial vendors at a Saturday plaza bazaar—direct our attentions in a specific way and determine our range of perceptions. The idea is not to propose an unrestrained feast in the field of sensorial difference, but to maintain a local articulation of the senses in order to resist global sameness, to identify points of resistance from sense work, showing how its inflections deviate from any universal norm; to track history, politics, and culture through a representation of sensorial conflicts and breaks.

In the opening chapters of *Moby Dick*, Herman Melville begins with an encounter of characters from East and West. The different worlds that unite them in a shabby guesthouse onshore are linked by the narrator through a flow of uneven sensory perceptions: the narrator discerns the textures of quilted fabric and the crags of a lumpy mattress; he sees and smells an indescribable doormat, but cannot comprehend its purpose. Above all, his focus falls on the "strange guttural noises" (2000, 47) and tattooed body of the dark and foreign Queequeg, the character with whom the narrator shares a bed for the night. Everything in the perceptual field is regarded as "strange" or "queer," not to be understood by the reader until later on, when the characters board the whaler. The sea allows the men to smell and hear with freedom, to feel the graze of the wind, to expand the faculty of taste, to sharpen their acuity of vision as they let themselves embrace both internal peace and terrifying danger to come. Most interesting, the interracial contact that sustains them—the pressure of hand upon hand, the torsos within reach of each other—can be realized only in a context that is distant and free of US land and law. Though racial divisions on US soil cannot allow men to touch one another, the freedom of the traveling whaleboat permits all color bars to be broken. *Moby Dick* in 1851 responds to certain political situations of a country fissured by race, but parallel moments in Latin American history offer a representation of the senses for different motivations. Consider, for instance, the ascendant years of Esteban Echeverría, an Argentine poet who studied French sensualist theory and placed perceptions at the center of his work. Resisting the tyranny of the Rosas regime that had reduced all poetry to *materia prosa* (prosaic matter), Echeverría devoted his literary texts to the description of sensual assaults. Far from reaching for the heights of romantic love, he led his readers through mud, bog, pollution, and blood in order that they might experience the horror of Argentina at the height of its civil war. The good writer, inspired by dreams, would seek out poetic form by opening a course toward reason—or so Echeverría claimed—but for the moment, he called upon sensuality and shock to alert his readers to the political mire. Echeverría also made his point through food and degustation: showing his characters in pursuit of scraps of meat, discarded fat, and bone (in "El matadero"), he ponders the ills of digestion and shows bestial humans in pursuit of remaindered slop to relieve their persistent hunger. This is the world of bad food and bad taste, Echeverría tells us. Thus, if Melville is obsessed with modes of contact because of racial divides at home, Echeverría focuses on the construction of "taste" in a new Argentine nation still lacking in manners, etiquette, and refinement. Bad taste (literally and metaphorically) is a referent for a local political and social life gone terribly wrong.

The perceiving body is a particular obsession of American writers north and south to monitor the shortcomings and successes of democracy, to notice its grand omissions. Years later, John Dos Passos, traveling coast to coast and exploring modernity's triumphs as well as its sorry consequences for those who lived on its margins, continued to ask about the location and defining form of the American body. He acknowledged that we could not settle on one way of interacting with the American world as long as rich and poor debated the certitude of their respective perceptions. In those same years, Roberto Arlt could only describe the body in terms of extreme and violent abjection. The foul odors, the abusive contact between the sexes, the grating noises of urban movement, the humiliation of men's and women's bodies numbed to all sensation: these all conveyed the harsh oppression of Argentine working and middle classes as they moved into modern times. The question here is not just the location of bodies, but also the testing of senses under fierce duress. We travel between erasure and presence, between sensorial pleasure and violent assaults that affect our hearing and vision, and our perceptions as a whole. The senses record a political and cultural context that goes far beyond narrative scope. In this zone of detained attention, the senses do our cultural work and almost seem to stop time in the "now."

Critics who attend to the senses often defend the power of sight as the most valued of all perceptions. Marshall McLuhan (1962) wrote of the ways in which primitive communities were part of a synesthetic culture, blending tactility and olfaction, hearing and sight. He noted, however, that the printing press broke up this sensual mixture and instead imposed visual dominance over all cultural forms. Long after the Gutenberg break, Kant linked vision to authority and control, setting in place a discourse for nineteenth-century philosophers who regarded sight as the most important perception. In fact, their towering achievement was to link optics to the power of state. Jonathan Crary's (1990) lucid observations in *Techniques of the Observer* explain this nineteenth-century moment and the massive reorganization of social practices that altered the way people perceived. From the senses as an undifferentiated whole in earlier centuries to a state of pure visuality by 1850, Crary explores the ways in which sight became the dominant perception to signal rational power. Similarly, Martin Jay and Sumathi Ramaswamy (2014) understand the work of vision—the "imperial optic," they call it—as a systematic part of European overseas expansion. Foucault (1995) sustains the importance of social surveillance, the panoptic machine that looks over us and defines us from the vantage of state power, while Guy Debord (1990), referring to modern times, locates us in the "society of the spectacle."

However, a focus on the nonvisual senses lets other narratives of culture emerge. When touch and smell are featured, for example, we find ourselves in a perceptual track that fails to translate to logos. A more heterogeneous composition of experiences—less obedient, less hierarchical, less controlled—corresponds to what have been described as the "minor senses." This is perhaps a prerational experience, as many have noted; it appeals to an idea of an unschooled life, the antithesis of civilization. In this context, perception is intensely multiple and kinetic; it challenges fixed power. Walter Benjamin also attended to this diversity, reminding us of the importance of entwined perceptions as a guide toward embodied cognition and a profound understanding of self. Similarly, Walter Ong defended the inextricable mixture and bonding of all senses at once, while historian Mark Smith called on sensorial mixture to get beyond the privilege of vision and reach historical depth. Michel Serres called for a mingling of the senses beginning with receptors on the surface of skin and leading to synesthetic perception. And David Howes, editing multiple volumes on the anthropology of the senses (1991, 2005), deflected the stress on vision to examine a range of perceptions that emerge from the cultural and physical frame. Today many scholars—among them Constance Classen and Giuliana Bruno—celebrate hapticity, or the sense of touch, while Daniel Heller-Roazen traces the pressing importance of this sensation from classical antiquity to modern times. Our contemporary artists also take up the multisensorial challenge. We find experiences of tactility crossed by vision and sound in the work of the Argentine David Lamelas or the attraction of scent combined with rhythm in the "aromapoetry" of the US-Brazilian Eduardo Kac. Their art installations recall 1920s artists like the Argentine Xul Solar, who mixed color and music. They call forth the avant-garde's synesthetic attempts to register pressure and weight and tone in order to alter visual perception; they even connect us to today's banal market experiments to sell, for example, Napa Valley wines by immersing consumers in sensually altered environs (mixing taste with color, or bouquet with heat or cold), to introduce sensory substitution devices by which the tongue might learn to "see," to implant brain-computer interfaces that not only enhance existing senses but also carry the promise of developing new sensory receptors. All of these form part of a major undertaking to reorder the sensual grid. They endeavor to place experience under a wide range of accounts both in theory and practice.

It is not my intention to supply a ratio of experience, but to reevaluate events in Latin American cultural history as they cross with the work of the senses, and to explore a narrative—a way of reading—that has eluded our common purview. Beyond the naysayers who lament the loss of experience in our modern times, I attend to the ways in which the sensorium puts experience back within reach. The goal is to make accessible some stories whose meaning has been expunged from the atlas of historical achievement, to marshal events in culture that reassemble a territorial map. I am particularly interested in the local expression of what might appear to be a global commonality—how to see, touch, taste, and hear—and in tracking its representations. I am not attempting to defend the unmediated sense perception of an object as if there were no constructedness to the event and our responses; nor am I aiming to reproduce the debates about biopolitics and the state, a theme well-rehearsed by Foucault and later by Esposito and Agamben. Instead, my goal is to explore the articulations of sense work that consolidate a particular moment and place as they are plotted on the cultural field. Underlying this is a strong conviction that the ways in which we see or hear, touch or taste the world are driven by constructions of selfhood that are formed in local contexts; social norms cross with our daily experience of pleasure and pain.

When we speak of the sensorium, it is an easy leap to reach for a theory of affects. The considerable study on this topic, earning the rubric of the "affective turn," is in large part a focus on the agitation of the psyche in relationship to the passions. The scholars identified with this topic (here I think first of Deleuze, followed by Massumi; and more recently, the work of Berlant, Terada, and Sedgwick) insist upon the reciprocity between our power to be affected by the surrounding world and our power to act. But this form of affecting is not necessarily tied to a vivid description of visible, audible, or palpable events or objects of perception. Instead, it lingers on foreboding or joy, and often on the pressures of fear and terror, on the one hand, or pleasure and compassion, on the other. The mind's receptivity to external ideas—moods, forces, encumbrances, climates, or various unnamed powers—is the condition that constitutes important substrata of the social. This is a "felt vitality," as Patricia Ticineto Clough (2007, 2) has written, leaning upon Spinoza. Here we collect the unspoken effects of history—its ghosts, illusions, and nightmares—to see how they determine the subject. The opening scene of Sarmiento's *Facundo* (1845) brings us to this affective world of shadows and terror; Facundo's ghost appeals to unsettling residual effects that we can only capture by allusion or tone. This is the world of hazy fear and foreboding with which Sarmiento begins his famous book; only later will he turn to a physical encounter and clear, sensual data to organize his political world and give terror a name. It's strange that while thinkers like Sarmiento were reviewing the impact of indescribable emotion, a few decades later, Darwin was tracing this same expression in his book of 1872 on animals and humans, especially in later chapters devoted to the emotion of terror. A clear precursor to William James and Freud, Darwin undertook the study of mental dispositions to explain one's responses to movement. But the affective state also reminds us of a material connection to the real, and here the senses once again come in to claim a role. Sensation gives form to the affective state; it is both a precursor and a material follow-up to the work of emotion; it is the physiological entry point for a deployment of power. Here I am trying to assess the ways in which sensational encounters find meaning in a wider cultural span.

This book was not born in isolation and depends for its impetus upon some of my earlier intellectual obsessions with feminism, poetry, and voice. Work with my colleagues in the Seminar on Women in Latin America, a more than ten-year engagement that focused on gender and culture, resulted in my book *Between Civilization and Barbarism* (1992), which traced the placement of the female body in political debate and literary tradition. I continued writing about bodies in postdictatorship cultures (2001) but specifically addressed the materiality of literary texts and the physicality of the voice in a 2013 book examining contemporary poetry largely in the Southern Cone. The idea was that meaning in poetry is influenced by sets of perceptions that usually pass unnoticed: the rhythm of a phrase, the breaks in a line of verse, our dependence upon patterns of breathing, the tone and tempo that course through a given text from start to finish. I addressed the physical experiences that the poem places upon the reader in relation to the page. Julia Kristeva (1984) referred to the *chora semiotica* that brings the preoedipal experience to the surface of a poem through a basic contact of material and voice, sound and rhythm. In other words, the somatic experience of the poem sustains meaning beyond the word. Susan Stewart (2002) presented another version of this presemantic encounter when she observed that it is the experience of tactility that helps us learn how to discern and read. Poetry thus becomes a border experience, announcing a liminality that calls together presence and absence—placing, for instance, the sense of touch next to blankness or air—and lets us touch the materiality of words against a formless vacuum. The very palpability of the poem evokes a kind of friction between the different materialities of things or objects that cross our path in reading or listening to the literary work.

The somatic experience of reading is likened to a culture of effects, or so Roland Barthes (1989) once told us. It also announces, as many have shown, the importance of attention. Recent focus on "surface reading" (Best and Marcus 2009) or on the significance of descriptive passages over fictional narration (Jameson 2013) is part of this new direction that seeks out the materiality of detail, keeping things on the surface, and keeping the senses alert. We reach this through the unevenness found in a text, through descriptive distractions that stray from narrative just as in "real life" we are moved by the breaks in cultural flow, by the unexpected shocks and sensations that assault us in daily life. Bill Brown (2003) addressed this regarding the nineteenth century; the Argentine poets of the 1990s continue to sustain this theme. The idea is that meaning is formed from the solid encounter of the individual with the materiality of things. Thus, in the line of North American objectivists like Louis Zukofsky who began writing in the 1930s, some Latin American writers stressed in unfettered terms their slow encounter with the "thingness" of objects that stand on their own. Jorge Aulicino, national poet of Argentina today, reminded us regarding this meeting of poets with concrete objects: "the baroque is formed from plaster, not words" (2011, 26). The goal of literature and philosophy was to touch the materiality of ideas with "thingness" as the middle step in a chain of perceptions. But in modern Latin America, it is also a way to close in on the physical violence of the dictatorship years and beyond. It is a way to describe one's encounter with the torture machine triggering pain; it records the melancholia inspired by one's lack of knowledge regarding the fate of the "disappeared." Toggling between perception of pain and a state of waiting, one reconfigures sense work in terms of attention and absence or loss.

Sensible experience is conceived as a political act and also as an artful form of resistance. It cuts through the cultural landscape like a double-edged knife, piercing its fabric and texture. It registers perceptions of imprisonment just as it promises emancipation; it alternates between extremes of violence and pleasure. Jacques Rancière reminds us that the state distributes and controls the regimes of senses, but he also defends those aesthetic acts that open up new modes of perception that might elude the eye of the state (2004). Years earlier in Argentina, David Viñas insisted on the sentient self as the first line of access to political knowledge, while his colleague León Rozitchner, a student of Merleau-Ponty, wrote that it was centrally important to redefine political subjectivity in terms of experience and perceptual responses. Both sought a materialist reading of history, politics, and culture; and toward this, an insistence on the sentient self as a way to monitor social violence. Most recently, the Argentine essayist and chronicler María Moreno reiterates these lessons when she reminds us that democracy is all about governing the body, while literature, meanwhile, registers this experience through a strategy of *effects* (2016, loc. 597).

We are still left with a comparative question that haunts much of this book. As Latin Americanists working in the United States, we face the task of self-invention, the need to position ourselves and what we know so as to adjust to metropolitan desires. We wonder whether our account of the Americas can stand the test of the North, whether our regional sense of periodicity matches that of some distant center, whether the versions of literature that we produce and consume might compete with those of the mainstream, or whether *experience* as we define it can be the same across the hemispheric divide. Today's neoliberal market conditions, contrary to popular opinion, haven't leveled the field at all, and indeed, as literary and cultural critics, we are more often pressed into business by a certain retail allure: we used to think that we had to deliver the South as a feast for the marvelous real; today we dredge the rivers of sorrow in order to sell scenes of abjection. Latin Americanist scholars, along with writers and artists, continue to fuss with this question.

Ricardo Piglia, a consummate comparatist who spent his life writing about the travels of culture, addressed some aspects of these North/South conflicts in his novel *El camino de Ida* (Ida's path, 2013). A campus novel based loosely on Piglia's time at Princeton, *El camino de Ida* alludes to the *trials of comparison* that make North–South exchanges so vexing: the distorted readings that cross the continental divide or the inevitable violence done to peripheral texts that occurs as one tries to read them from metropolitan centers. In the novel, Piglia's narrator comes from Latin America to the United States to teach a seminar on William Henry Hudson, a nineteenth-century naturalist whose work has been largely forgotten by English departments here, though he continues to occupy a significant role in the Argentine literary tradition.[1] Writing in English from London, Hudson was able to recuperate a significant moment in the River Plate cultural history of nineteenth-century territorial expansion and is credited by some for having invented the landscape of the pampas. Even today, from the outside looking in, Hudson contributes to our thinking about exile, melancholia, and absence. From the perspective of Latin America, Hudson finds good company among the many who wrote far from home: the Cuban José Martí in New York, the Argentinean Julio Cortázar in Paris, the Brazilian João Gilberto Noll in Berkeley, and even Piglia himself, who wrote his classic novel about dictatorship while living in New Jersey. From these constellations, Latin Americanists come to understand cultural history as a series of displacements, mediations, and broken or interrupted flows. They allow us to lope through a field of murky transnational exchanges, often rendered opaque by the history of empire and by the empire of language. This canon in motion is marked by the discomfort of authors inhabiting more than one language as they try to come near to an original tongue that remains estranged and distant. Clawing through the sediments of language, grasping for a suppressed and perhaps magical word that might promise epiphany or redemption, living in more than one city at once and walking a double line, the exiled author bends the mirror of representation in order to announce her discomfort. In the process, the field of sense perceptions is reimagined as it pertains to a particular place; it also evokes the distortions of memory and distant political battles.

The sense work that I propose in this book brings up these local and comparative issues; it will foreground questions about how culture continues to take root in one single place and then moves beyond specific location. In times of civil strife or through the explosive growth of new immigrant populations, during the turn to 1920s modernization or in the moment of military rule, and now with the age of the global market so assuredly upon us, these crises test perceptions as well as embodied cognition. And, with this, sense work also accounts for our different experiences as they crop up on the North/South divide.

In these pages, I consider the scope of perception through literature and the visual arts, through history and political process. The examples give clues to the ways in which individualism and authority are asserted; they define class oppositions; they set terms for reading race and gender and let us focus on styles of attention. The first chapter starts with the early nineteenth century; a comparison of sense work in different lands is my point of departure. On separate visits to Paris, Thomas Jefferson from Virginia and Bernardino Rivadavia from Argentina met with the French Idéologue Antoine Destutt de Tracy, a philosopher who was known at the time for his sturdy defense of perceptions as a way to engage political life and the logic of economics. The statesmen from the Eastern Seaboard brought Destutt's books back to the Americas for eventual diffusion and study, but the resonance of his texts met dramatically different responses in the North and the South. At the University of Virginia, Jefferson's plan for a curriculum of French readings (from Condillac to Destutt de Tracy) was quickly abandoned; at the University of Buenos Aires, however, French philosophical thought signaled a resistance to the church and a step toward modernization. From this, we learn that neither direct perceptions nor their attending sense-based theory held universal reach and acclaim. Echeverría (a student of Destutt's material) and Sarmiento (an autodidact), both of the same generation, show us how perceptions are evoked for political and poetic purpose; they teach us to identify the weights and pressures defining political life. This stands in comparison, at the beginning and end of the chapter, to writers like William Henry Hudson, for whom the landscape evoked a sentient self in order to seek out a personal freedom, liberated from the burdens of industry, modernization, and war. Between these extremes, a politics of sensing gave shape to the nineteenth century and determined its canonical works.

While sensory responses among nineteenth-century Argentine thinkers were evoked to prove political acumen or to express the civilization-versus-barbarism trope in its full corporeal dimensions, women writers switched this model around and enunciated a particular sense work to show the weakness of authoritarian regimes. This is the focus of chapter 2. So while Sarmiento, for example, refers to his perceptual prowess to assert his right to power—"I heard, I saw, I acted," he boasts in *Campaña en el ejército grande*—women writers of his time break down this sensorial command to protest their ongoing exclusion. In an age of eavesdropping by the federal police of Rosas, for example, the Argentine Juana Manuela Gorriti describes an environment of listeners who learn to hear the wails of victims across a canvas of civil war. During extreme famine in the Andean highlands, the Peruvian Clorinda Matto de Turner describes banquets of gustatory delights as a political metaphor for class conflict, while the Cuban Gertrudis Gómez de Avellaneda studies the priority of vision endowed to the landed gentry, and Harriet Beecher Stowe insists on bodily contact—an encounter of black and white subjects—as a way to protest the national taboos that kept the races apart. Distinct sensory priorities also inform women's writings on travel; in fact, sights, sounds, and touch shape the voyager and define geographic location. The genre also celebrates technological innovation that enhances the living body; everything from the photograph to the transatlantic cable sustains or attracts the traveler's attentions and expands the breadth of perceptual experiences that could be described in the mid-nineteenth century. In effect, technology and politics were articulated as highly sensory affairs: we track this across the early chapters in stories of slave labor and military service or in the testimonies of those who narrated their in-the-field forays into desert terrains and conditions of war. In all of this, the senses point to the individual's encounters with forms of material culture, cutting through scenes of public disorder, good taste, and romances, and suffusing these moments with often dramatic arrangements of intensity and conflict.

The sensorial obsession of the early independence years through the midcentury romantics changes in later decades. Political events redirect sensory habits and expand the range of customs by which we feel and see. In the late nineteenth century and the beginning of the twentieth, when a liberal modernity captured the eyes and ears of individuals in the city, new inventions and products opened the appetites of the consumer. Technologies of sound and sight also held fascination for the urban public, among them early cinema and the wax cylinders that recorded voice. However, we should be quick to note, this adventurous spirit into sensual pleasure was not universally shared, and, here, the uses of science became the focus of discussion. What is the function of science? some Argentine journalists asked. And how could education modify raw sensual perceptions? A few were fearful about the new utilitarian approaches; others feared that the cultural sphere would be contaminated by excess. As an example, when Puccini's *Tosca* debuted at the Teatro Colón in Buenos Aires in 1900, critics complained that the excess of sensibility would lead spectators astray. Similarly, others reviled the public spectacles and carnivals and even the patriotic feast days insofar as they allowed unchecked sensory indulgence beyond all control and policing. Elite audiences felt the shock on the nerves that was triggered by popular masses. In 1903, Georg Simmel (1950) captured this well when he spoke of modernity's urban shock at the dawn of the new century, anticipating by several decades Walter Benjamin's well-known laments about urban stimulations; they both took to task modernity's sensational effects and with them, the decline of intellectual pursuits and the closure of a life of the mind. These preoccupations are a bridge connecting chapters 2 and 3.

The third chapter explores the sentient self under the quick modernization of the 1910s and 1920s, focusing on the ways through which writers in international debate sought to arrest the intensities of the new. Owing to the velocity and movement in cities, displacements, and the speed of machines, thinkers noted that a general intellectual fatigue was setting in, giving way to unfiltered perceptions. Poetry, cinema, and daily life absorbed this new disposition. Coining the phrase *un nouvel état d'intelligence* (a new state of intelligence), the French filmmaker Jean Epstein (1921) found an interlocutor in the Spanish poet Guillermo de Torre and secondarily in José Ortega y Gasset, while James Joyce—detailing an art of perception in his novel *Ulysses*—set the stage for a corporeal theory of writing that was based on sensations, a strategy that was quickly adapted by the Argentine Roberto Arlt. As a group, these intellectuals responded in different styles to the urgent shock of the new, recording the alienation of modern man in light of velocity and speed. Embodied thought thus became a guiding principle and banner: it marked the double time of the archaic and modern; it cut through distances over space and time; it overcame the gap between sense and judgment by appealing to the body as a precursor of thought. This was not without conflict. The ruckus of the urban masses, the strangeness of acousmatic sound, and the roar of airplanes and cars created at once an eerie discomfort and pleasure. They triggered an anxiety about unreachable distances and the loss of home; above all, the experience reminded individuals of their incapacities to resist the external stimuli engendered by the technologies of modern life. It is not surprising, in the midst of this frenzy, that many Latin American artists and writers grabbed hold of the reverse side of this much-flaunted sensational practice and looked toward a spiritual unity that would promise to affirm a collective whole. In other words, while for some, a highly sensational modernity was supposed to "do the thinking for us," for others, the body was experienced as a borderline register between material world and spirit; this incomprehensible "world beyond" was reached by tricks of perception. Roberto Arlt thought that this spiritualist turn was the con job of the decade, but he also considered with a jaundiced eye the much-vaunted "shock of the new." He was of course referring to a world defined by theosophists, magicians, and psychoanalysts—everyone from the heirs of Mme Blavatsky to students of Carl Jung who were driven to make use of sense technologies in an attempt to touch the psyche or soul. Nevertheless, in another avant-garde enclave, the synesthetic art of Xul Solar expressed his yearning for a collective spirit, the many fused into one. Through the inspiration of Aleister Crowley, from whom he learned theosophy and mystical thought, Xul indulged an art of blending senses and intense synesthetic crossings. The material thus became marvelous; it incited the imagination; it also provided the opportunity to cross the boundaries of reason and reach for a merger of spirit and sensation. Contrapuntal forces help us read the 1920s and 1930s: on the one hand, an obsession with the body and senses to register one's degree of alienation or pleasure; on the other, a turn toward the occult to prepare for intersubjective connections and stage a faith in the spirit. Both extremes respond to the wonders (and horrors) of modern technology; both need vibrations and electric jolt, and visual and sound combinations, achieving what one writer in *Martín Fierro* called the "collective synesthesia" of his times.

Following the age of high modernism, the approaches and uses of sense perceptions again take a different course. In chapter 4, I consider events of the second half of the twentieth century in which the sentient self, first, is used to express resistance to a populist program under the government of Perón, and, later, is evoked to register the pain and torture inflicted by military rule. This begins with a reconsideration of the influence of French phenomenology (especially Merleau-Ponty) upon dissident intellectuals of the Argentine *Contorno* group (1953–1959). I focus especially on its principal thinkers—David Viñas, León Rozitchner, Oscar Masotta—who claimed the value of embodied perceptions as a way to challenge the state. The *Contorno* writers thus set a measure for reading through the sensorial lens, for situating the body in history and the political present. Viñas installed a model for reading the physical history of Argentine culture starting from the early nineteenth century; Rozitchner tried to comprehend political subjectivity in terms of the perceptual field; and Masotta brought phenomenological thought to the doorstep of psychoanalysis in order to read the emergent visual avant-garde of the 1960s as it was tied to the Instituto di Tella (1958–1970), the prestigious Argentine art forum devoted to new technologies that captured human experience and perceptions. Nonetheless, the rapid intervention of military force in 1968 redirected this sensorial project in political philosophy and the arts; intellectuals from this point forward began to study the effects of torture. Accordingly, if the centers of state control were processed through the electric prod and the airdrop of bodies into the sea, avant-garde artistic communities would begin to describe the body as a marker of pain. The new biopolitical order is contested by artists and writers against the state. The works of the novelist Juan José Saer, the poet Raúl Zurita, and the visual artist Guillermo Núñez speak to the measure of this concern. Together, they establish a corporeal "ground zero" to give creative form to political protest and reveal the scope of victimization.

The close of the twentieth century and the start of the new millennium lead us to a crisis of experience of neoliberal rule and globalization, the focus of the fifth and final chapter of this book. Again, the discourse on sense perception shifts to different terrain. Replacing an interest in bare life conditions imposed by military regimes, the assaults by a volatile, global world and the pressures exercised by the free market now shape the field of representation in the twenty-first century. Perceptual violence often recalls an unfriendly past but is also a robustly physical response by individuals to market-run cultures. This is a bid for philosophical attention, directing the spectator toward minute details that guide us toward the terror of a vacant "now." Here we cannot ignore a late-twentieth-century longing to encounter and hold on to a reality that seems to be drifting away. This is seen in philosophical inquiry and also in the arts, inviting us to come in touch with the materiality of experience and objects. Bodies are the hub of this material landscape; their sensate condition, their perceptive capacities to take in what lies beyond the self—indeed, their accounts of pain or pleasure—become persistent modalities of art and literature in the late twentieth century, but in contemporary conditions these representations often announce a halting of time. In the extreme, bodily perceptions leash us to the *present*, a moment that suppresses the grand narrative of history as well as our longings for a future to come. Critics from Derrida to Gumbrecht have written of the power of this postmetaphysical epistemology of presentness that belongs to our current age, while thinkers like Jean-Luc Nancy, insisting on a posthumanist defense of the finitude of being, claim the body as the start for all philosophy and critical thought. Truth, writes the Mexican philosopher Luis Villoro, is found in direct experience (Ramírez 2011, 74). Taken to an extreme, the postmodern fascination with distance and semblance—with the measure of our experience with "things"—yields in its most exacerbated moment what Alain Badiou described as a "violent taste for surface and transparency" as we react "against depth" (2007, 64). Some have situated this as a crisis of belonging, part of a need to claim a place and location that we might actually own. It puts physical experience first; it situates the perceiving body as the first line toward the mind. Others see the transformation and contemporary aesthetics and ethics as ways to challenge the constitution of the individual self as the Anthropocene comes to an end. Hence, the interactions of human and machine, the rise of the cyborg, and the reworking of technology are triggers that incentivize paradoxical crossings: we now reach states of sensation without bodies, sensation produced by machines. Through these different critical lenses, a revival of what looks like phenomenology today extends over an arc of cultures and gives considerable attention to the place of perceptions sometimes unleashed from the human source that would anchor sensations in a physical place.

Some of Latin America's most compelling artists have interrogated this situation: from the Brazilian artist Nuno Ramos to the US-Brazilian sensory theorist Eduardo Kac and the Chilean artist-philosopher Demian Schopf. This last artist revives the neobaroque concern for permutations of form while also addressing the paranoia produced by machine-induced sensation. This problem also works its way out in a recent novel by Diamela Eltit, who helps me bring this study to a close. Here, in scenes that depict Chilean poverty in its fullest state of abjection, humans are dominated by machines and deliver themselves to global escapes via the World Wide Web; in a final effort to find a sense of self, they then meld with the cyborg world and therein find their creative potential. This is all promoted through the sensorial body that learns to perceive in the style of machines. Eltit supplies an allegory for reading the senses in the twenty-first century and speaks to what she calls the "larva state" to which the human has been reduced. The virtuality of new-age sense work, universal encounters without leaving home: in all of this, the local and global conflicts are resolved on the backs of Latin America's poor. Herein lies a final speculation: If materialism spells out a certain detachment from life (at least in the humanistic experience), and if humans merge with machines, will the anthropotechnics that have defined us until now find a different expression? Or will a return to the symbolic dimensions of art and writing save us from our demise? Perhaps this book is still about the portrait of the artist, longing for creative survival; or perhaps we're on the cusp of something new, a sense work without bodies.

CHAPTER 1

Sensing the Early Republic

Who am I and which places are these?

DOMINGO FAUSTINO SARMIENTO

In *Idle Days in Patagonia* (1893), the naturalist William Henry Hudson (1841–1921) surrenders to the sensual beauty of the Argentine outback. Freed from the shackles of English civilization, where he spent his final years, he delivers his body to the Patagonian South and recalls a direct contact with nature. Sandhills and shrubs come alive with the incessant humming of thornbirds; the hues of the sunset arouse him; the percussive tones of vizcachas and moles draw him close to the hillocks lacing the Río Negro. Sounds, sights, textures, and tastes wash over his sentient self. A receptive filter of the natural world, Hudson introduces his readers to the powers of vision and tone in the early chapters of his essay and concludes his book with an awakening to the countryside's enticing scents; from vision, the most intellectual of the senses, he delivers a final tribute to the most basic of all perceptions, evoking memory and emotion (2006, 104). The full sensorium is recovered in print.

Born on the outskirts of Buenos Aires to New England immigrant parents, Hudson supplies a pastoral that is clearly apart from the grand traditions of trailblazers and soldiers who purportedly conquered the land. Skirting the civil wars and the bloody battles enacted by Unitarians and Federals in the mid-nineteenth century, Hudson captures the southern landscape in its pristine, inviolate fullness. His version of the plains respects no partisan pull, nor does he take sides in the traditional versions of history that would separate political parties by the civilization-and-savagery dyad. Just as his grand biographer Martínez Estrada wrote, "What Hudson saw was always the truth. He had no commitment to political party or sect" (1951, 137).[1] From his later retreat in London, Hudson recalls a perceiving body, wounded and immobilized in the pampas and reconstituted in Argentine nature. He recruits the remarkable perceptions of taste, touch, and sight in order to share his experience with others. And almost funneling the lessons of Thoreau from the native New England of his family, Hudson through his solitude in the woods sought to see and apprehend without preconceived purpose and share his experience with others, always in pursuit of an ethical equivalent between the self and the land.

Perhaps his River Plate memoir is girded by a nostalgia for a life not lived. Written twenty years after he left Argentina, Hudson's book sustains a double course of past and present—not only guided by the trials of telling in a land he no longer inhabits, but also by the double experience of feeling himself a failed adventurer lost in England to perceptual darkness and without external enhancement of his fragile internal life. Hobbled by his inability to make deeper contact with nature and by a literary language—English—that doesn't match his Spanish language obsessions, he becomes a desiring subject in search of sensual form. And turning his voice against Darwin, who saw in Patagonia an "arid waste," Hudson reframes the South American landscape to supply a physical awareness that was simply unavailable in Europe; with it, he seeks the "recovery of the irrecoverable past" (2006, 110). It turns out that his approach to the senses was unique to Argentina, prompting later writers in the South to uphold this peculiar model as a way to cut through national malaise. For his direct engagement with the landscape unfettered from political life, Hudson gives us an anchor for a kind of innocent "sense work." From Ezequiel Martínez Estrada in the 1950s to Ricardo Piglia in a recent novel, Hudson stands for a kind of sensory engagement that fostered a peaceful exchange with landscape, a desideratum for many, though in truth it was rarely attained. By contrast, the full nineteenth century in Argentina begins with another project, a brutal awakening of the senses that rattled the early republic.

This chapter will focus on some notable foundational moments in the Latin American nineteenth century in which social, political, and literary life became tied to a regime of perception. I should say that I am not aiming to reproduce the current debates about biopolitics and the state, a theme well-rehearsed by thinkers such as Foucault, Esposito, and Agamben, and more recently in the Latin American field by scholars such as Andermann and Giorgi. Nor do I wish to reiterate the terms for a universal history of the senses, which has captured the recent imagination of scholars (among them, Howes, Jutte, and Jay). But here I explore the figuration of sense work as it emerges in specific conditions—during the postindependence years of new Latin American nations and, with Argentina as my anchor, beneath the shadow of the "civilization and barbarism" slogan that shaped nineteenth-century expansion and sustained the kind of sensationalist thinking that directed political and cultural debates. I will return to Hudson at the close of this chapter to see how this all makes sense.

Sensational Beginnings

This narrative begins with Enlightenment philosophy and its emphasis on the individual's perceptions insofar as this philosophy informs the early Latin American nineteenth century. With the call to arms against the Spanish crown and with the war apparatus well in place, the founding fathers in Spanish America turned to Enlightenment thought, and in particular to sensationalist theory, in order to challenge the colonial regime and the church doctrine that sustained it. In the midst of this new way of thinking, the human body claimed a central place. Here sense work was recruited in the larger project of bringing an end to Spanish hegemony in the Americas, just as it also sustained a narrative style that was vividly attentive to the audible, visible, and palpable qualities of objects perceived. On the one side, this was an endeavor of elites to mark a route toward independence. On the other side, sense work was often aligned with savage inclinations (a life of body over mind) and sustained those prerational feelings that would challenge a dominant logos. In the course of this chapter, we will toggle between these dramatic extremes in order to track their evolution over the nineteenth century from points both north and south.

What will become obvious is that the treatment of the senses is not always the same throughout history, but is modified according to national crisis, civil strife, and economic demand. Though empirical data of the senses supports a "regime of reason" (as Foucault would have called it), it was often, at the start of the nineteenth century and in the postindependence years, the materialist justification for asserting one's claims to power. Not only that, but as the century advanced, the discourse on the senses in Latin America was also coordinated by the "war machine" (I take the term from Deleuze), obliging us to look not simply at matters of life and death but also at the display of bodies as territory in the organization of provinces, states, and frontiers. Bodies observed and bodies observing shared a place in the political landscape. Civil war thus set in place an arsenal of sensual images imprinted on the national stage: it also guided writing and representation in the nineteenth century at large. So while we are coming to understand reliance on the senses as a way to affirm individual presence, we also see the sensually alert body (of the soldier, the military commander, or the backwoods outlaw) engaged in a conquest of land, subduing enemy subjects with the power of the eye and ear. From the underside of this portrait and as a private answer to public demands, the narrative of the senses—keep Hudson's example in mind—was certain proof that one was alive.

For the scope of this chapter, I consider three scenes from the Latin American nineteenth century in which the concern for sensory perception assumed unrivaled force. The first is based on a common connection that Americans (both North and South) sustained with French philosophy in the early years of the republics; the second is a scene enacted upon the conflict between civilization and savagery in the throes of civil war; and the third, a culmination of sorts, is the way in which sense work eventually takes us to a larger conversation about North and South, directly engaging questions of corruption and power, or eluding the state completely. Between a Baudelairean fantasy of "anywhere out of this world" (in the style of Hudson's nostalgic retreat to Patagonian nature) and a perceptual framework that cuts across poverty and war in order to theorize modernization, sense work organizes a perceptual experience that locates us in the "now."

Sensualist Philosophy as a Path to Revolt

The inaugural scene of this narrative is late eighteenth-century Argentina, when scholasticism, still the reigning discourse, began to lose its grasp.[2] The dismantling of this project occurred not only because the Jesuits had been expelled from their American holdings in 1767, but also because the scholastic vision belonging to the seventeenth-century theologian and Jesuit Francisco Suárez gave general evidence of resistance and wear. The prestigious centers of Spanish American learning captured the internal dissent regarding the course of theological doctrine: first, at the University of Córdoba (always considered the seat of Catholic learning in Argentina, and a former Jesuit stronghold), and second, in Buenos Aires at the Colegio de San Carlos, which by the 1780s was beginning to open to new lines of thought. Two figures spearheaded the reform: at the University of Córdoba new ideas came with Deán Gregorio Funes (1749–1829), and in Buenos Aires, with Luis José de Chorroarín (1757–1823), director of the Colegio de San Carlos. In Córdoba, Funes questioned Thomist doctrine and rejected scholasticism as a whole. By 1808, when Funes was charged with the task of mapping a new curriculum for university students, he included modern philosophy, for the time a radical proposal (Torchia Estrada 1961, 66–72). On this gesture, Sarmiento wrote that Funes "was accused, with absolute justification, of opening the way to Voltaire, D'Alembert, Diderot, and Rousseau, and the French Jacobins" (2005, 100).[3] Meanwhile, in Buenos Aires, Chorroarín was also putting cracks in the solid vessel of scholastic thought. Chorroarín understood that abstractions of theology could never guide the soon-to-be-independent nation, nor could the force of bloodline sustain the caste of elites. Instead, he expressed a new faith in ascendant notions of the individual and a defense of the biological qualities that defined a person in relation to his surroundings. And here comes the case for sensation.

Chorroarín was responsible for bringing new ideas into philosophy courses such that the Enlightenment's praise of reason began to occupy a place next to Catholic dogma (Chiaramonte 2007a, 59; Korn 1949, 103–104).[4] Moreover, he believed in the certainty of perceptions and in the human capacity, through the senses, to capture truths about the external world. "The sensations or sensory perceptions, when they are lived and are constant, steady and linked to reason, produce certainty about our bodies and they translate as a solid criterion of truth. In effect, no one who is reasonable, can doubt which impressions stimulate pleasure or pain in the soul or that these sensations are born for bodies that really exist.... Live sensation guided by reason and reflection ... can be considered a criterion for finding the truths of daily life" (Chorroarín 1911, 98–99). We're clearly in a materialist world that will carry weight in the sphere of ideas. These teachings continued in a second school, the Colegio de la Unión del Sud, founded in 1817 on the site of the Colegio de San Carlos (and in reality, an extension of the first), where the discipline of moral sciences was established to introduce new philosophies from France. At this institution, Enlightenment winds gained momentum especially through the sensualist philosophy taught by lay instructor Juan Crisóstomo Lafinur, who in 1819 taught Étienne Bonnot de Condillac and the Idéologue thinkers, not without considerable scandal.[5]

The philosopher and historian Charles Taylor remarks regarding this

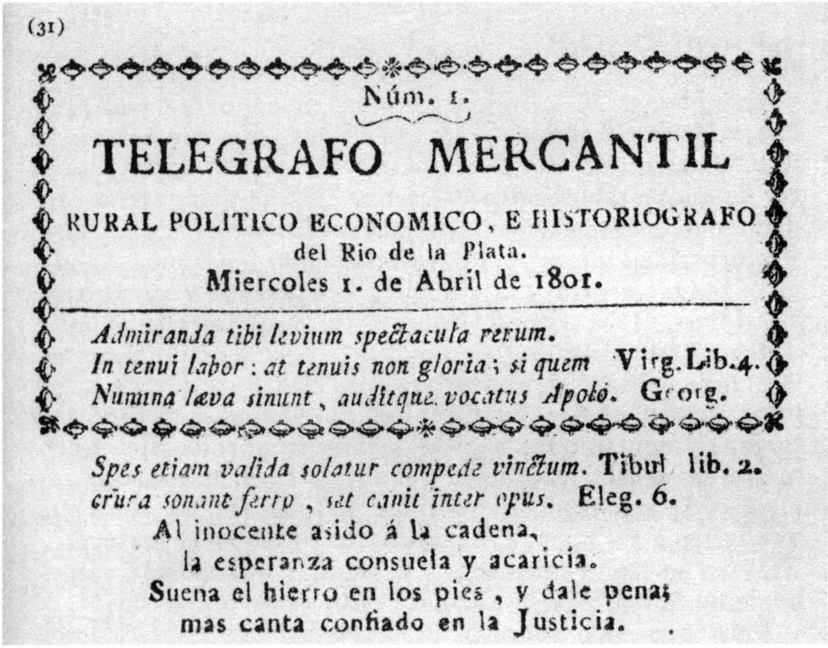

(31)

Núm. 1.

TELEGRAFO MERCANTIL

RURAL POLITICO ECONOMICO, E HISTORIOGRAFO del Rio de la Plata.

Miercoles 1. de Abril de 1801.

Admiranda tibi levium spectacula rerum.
In tenui labor : at tenuis non gloria ; si quem Virg. Lib. 4.
Numina læva sinunt , auditque vocatus Apolo. Georg.

Spes etiam valida solatur compede vinctum. Tibul lib. 2.
crura sonant ferro , sed canit inter opus. Eleg. 6.
Al inocente asido á la cadena,
la esperanza consuela y acaricia.
Suena el hierro en los pies , y dale pena;
mas canta confiado en la Justicia.

Figure 1.1. El telégrafo mercantil. *Biblioteca Digital Trapalanda, Mariano Moreno National Library of Argentina.*

nascent philosophy of sensations that "[i]t is easy to understand how the hope for wholeness and the rescue of the body has been used in the struggle between faith and unbelief" (2007, 616). In the Argentine case, however, the movement against scholastic thought was also linked to a repudiation of colonial control (an irony, of course, since the Bourbons, suspicious of scholastic thought, were responsible for expelling the Jesuits from colonial Spanish America). These points notwithstanding, the move against scholasticism became an important part of the American denunciation of Spain's retrograde ideas; it expressed the restlessness of philosophers and clerics in the preindependence movement.[6] See, in this respect, the editorial declaration of the first issue of *El telégrafo mercantil*, the earliest newspaper published in Buenos Aires: "Let new schools be founded here, so that once and for all, we can silence those barbaric voices of Scholasticism, which, while conceptually expressive, have obfuscated and have failed to transmit the ideas of the true Philosopher" (*El telégrafo mercantil* 1801). In another newspaper, the *Correo de comercio*, the editors referred sarcastically to the "scholasticist jargon" still in circulation, and sought to remand it to history's dustbin (Chiaramonte 2007a, 75). Overall, this negative reaction was fairly widespread, at least in the Southern Cone countries.[7]

The turn against scholasticism was accompanied by a rediscovery of the body in both philosophy and political texts, not to mention a turn in literary style that placed emphasis on experience and perceptions; it also linked in a single metaphor the physical and social body. Through the writings of the sensationalists and later Idéologues led by Antoine Destutt de Tracy, theories of perception guided the thinking of creole elites. In Argentina, this strand of philosophical thought gained prominence with the revolution of 1810 and in the university teachings that followed. Certainly Lafinur had introduced this material in the classroom, as noted above, but it wasn't until the young politicians took hold of these sensualist theories that the range of French influence expanded. Here, the *próceres*, or founding fathers, were active in bringing Condillac and Destutt de Tracy into the foreground of discussion—and with reason—since their theories of perception were seen as the preliminary basis for understanding an individual's participation in social and political life.[8]

How did this material reach Argentine shores? We know, for example, that Father Feijóo's reading of Condillac reached the River Plate from Spain, just as we know that the Spaniard Valentín de Foronda translated Condillac's *Logique*. We also have notices that Condillac's translation was introduced in Buenos Aires by Bernardo María de Calzada, while Destutt de Tracy reached Argentina through the work of Ramón Salas;[9] these texts circulated in bookstores and were advertised in the early years of *La gaceta mercantil*, the major newspaper of the postindependence years that began publication in 1823 (Parada 1998, 58).[10] The complete works of Condillac were held in the libraries of Liniers and San Martín. More important, the statesman and military leader Manuel Belgrano—a student of Chorroarín and Lafinur—began a campaign on behalf of the French sensualists in two articles he published in the *Correo de comercio* in 1810; here, he proposed that Condillac be taught in Argentine universities of the future.[11] From Condillac, Belgrano claims to have learned at least two guiding principles of metaphysics: "the more ambitious plan aspires to penetrate the mysteries, the nature, and the essence of being; the other, more moderate in scope, directs its investigations to the weakness of the human spirit" (qtd. in Chiaramonte 2007b, 6). If human weakness was apparent at all, it was because men hadn't been able to connect intuition with sensual experience and therefore were trapped in false reason. Worse still, they failed to engage with the spirit of progress; they failed to reach out for a shared commonality; and finally, they failed to acknowledge the missing link—found in perceptions—that gave the individual control over the environs and the political landscape. The sense work advanced by thinkers like Belgrano fell under the kind of scientific inquiry sustained by European thinkers, but Belgrano had in mind a plan for local modernity as well, setting the lessons of French sensualists and physiocrats in place in order to make labor productive;[12] as such, Belgrano demanded further education and training for Argentina.

Chorroarín's teaching was not lost upon his students, among them Bernardino Rivadavia, a man who became prime minister and then president of Argentina in a period that became known as "the happy experience" (*la feliz experiencia*) and was marked by relative calm.[13] It was during his term as prime minister (1821–1824) and under President Martín Rodríguez that Rivadavia publicly defended the mission of the French Idéologues, especially Destutt de Tracy, and pushed for the establishment of republicanism at home that would follow the French model in question (Gallo 2006, 2).[14] In this respect, Rivadavia also insisted that this French philosophical line occupy a central place at the University of Buenos Aires, newly established under his insistence in 1821. Rivadavia's familiarity with the Idéologues, stemming initially from his course with Chorroarín, was additionally nurtured by his six-year stay in Europe (mostly in Britain and France), where he was taken by republican thinkers such as Bentham and where he met Destutt de Tracy.[15] Though Rivadavia eventually turned away from the Idéologue project, accepting instead the philosophy of Bentham, he set in place a number of philosophy courses that would carry the Idéologues' lessons, especially seen in their models for a pragmatic individualism to guide the new republic.[16]

This, then, is Rivadavia's great contribution to the doctrines of the senses. Almost in the style of Thomas Jefferson, who did what was necessary to outline a similar plan for the University of Virginia, Rivadavia was responsible for setting the University of Buenos Aires on course. There, Rivadavia personally supervised the program in philosophy and appointed the teachers who would later communicate the lessons of the French sensationalists and the Idéologues who followed. Under the wing of Rivadavia's liberal influence, the major teachers of philosophy—Juan Crisóstomo Lafinur, Juan Manuel Fernández de Agüero, and Martín Diego de Alcorta—promoted the Idéologue project as a path that would guide the nation: here you could say that they crafted a version of the republic in need of a moral being that was never out of alignment with an instinctual, sentient body. The philosophy program where they taught bore the title of Ideología—an unmistakable tribute to Destutt de Tracy—and set the path for the kinds of learning that would circulate in the 1820s and 1830s. From the French philosophers, the Argentine professors had found the key to ordering human knowledge: from sense work—which was proposed as the originating point of their method—they could track the natural path of the spirit; more important, the Idéologues offered a universal plan to find a theory of experience that could undergird all public action and sustain the public good. The goal was to be up-to-date and follow the Enlightenment path.

But what can we make of these courses? From its earliest moments, the University of Buenos Aires placed Bentham and Adam Smith at the core of political economy courses, while Condillac and Destutt de Tracy became the pillars of the philosophy program (Cabanis's lessons in physiology were also represented in the lectures).[17] Here, in a university course that he offered uninterruptedly from 1822 until 1835, Martín Diego de Alcorta gave his most sturdy endorsement of these French thinkers.[18] In his course on ideology, for example, Alcorta defended the consciousness of the perceiving self as an epistemological anchor that would help one to understand the surrounding world and gain a moral bearing. Taking from Condillac a general idea about the sensate body, Alcorta was firm in these convictions as he introduced the first section of his course: "If we think of ourselves for a moment without hands, eyes, ears, etc., we would know nothing. These parts of our body . . . are like the doors to understanding" (Alcorta 2001, 34). Later on, in the second lecture, he described an arc of sensorial responses as a first step toward knowledge: "Certain organs are situated on the surface of the body; they make us learn about the existence of objects that surround us. They are our first access to knowledge" (36).

Alcorta's first unit, on metaphysics, reproduced almost verbatim sections of Condillac's famous essay on the statue and Destutt's *Éléments d'idéologie*, a text from 1801. A second unit of the course was devoted to logic (again, an acknowledgement of Condillac), and a third component was devoted to the interface of signs that help us think of the relationship between knowledge and representation (taken from Condillac's *L'art de penser* and Destutt de Tracy's *Éléments*). To a lesser degree, Alcorta referenced Locke, Bonnet and the encyclopedists, and Volney on natural law; he also showed a certain predilection for Adam Smith and made it a point to avoid Descartes. The goal of Alcorta and his colleagues was to argue for sense perceptions as a way to maneuver the body in the world, but also to prove that in our perceptual faculties we can find the basis of political will and eventual social duty.[19] Here, the sticking power wasn't Kant, as one might have expected, but that famous line repeated time and again by the sensualist philosophers and Idéologues: "I feel because I feel; I feel because I exist; and I do not exist but because I feel. Then my existence and my sensibility are one and the same thing" (Destutt de Tracy 1817, 42).

Alcorta drew upon several essays of Condillac, especially his *Essai sur l'origine des connaissances humaines* (1746), his most important contribution. In this book, Condillac argued for the necessity of signs and their connection to ideas, which in itself was not a new concept. However, the line of argumentation carried considerable appeal and was echoed by Alcorta and others in their various lectures. The exposition looks like this: First, the body is a source of language and speaks not only through words, but also through gesture, inflections, tone, and sound. With this understanding, we are then asked to read for both the materiality of the word and for what is expressed beyond language itself. Second, beneath the words and gestures, we can uncover human intention (this brings up questions of representation). Language serves to connect sensation and thought, to transform sense impressions into meanings and contribute to one's field of knowledge. In other words, Condillac—trying to surpass John Locke (whom Condillac had translated, though not without altering considerable sections of the original text in order to make Locke's logic conform to his own)—considers sensation as a "first thought" followed by a second in which the individual thinks about the effect of sensation. Critics dispute Condillac's understanding of sensation and reflection—whether the two are simultaneous experiences, sequential, or interdependent (O'Neal 1996, 18)—but for Alcorta, these are registered in the order of events, passing from sensorial impressions and, eventually, moving the soul.

By the time Alcorta came to teach Condillac's *Traité des sensations* (1754), perception clearly preceded and subordinated reflection. In this discussion, Condillac began by first imagining a statue that was blocked, because of its marble shell, from experiencing any sensation at all. However, its intellectual and moral life advanced as the various parts of this stone covering were removed; one by one, as the statue was exposed to different sensory stimulation, the statue came alive. The most important of these stimuli was found in the sense of touch. And similarly, all intellectual ideas—analysis, order, analogy, and language—are formed from memories of this sensation. In the end, the statue can remember, make comparisons, and find analogies between different experiences of things.[20] Alcorta continued with Condillac's lectures on logic (Logique, 1781), which served to harness sensation to the soul and ideas. Here, in this first turn toward the soul, we see the way in which Alcorta's lessons lead to an eventual plan for legislating morality, calling for the work of self-governance and reason as they derive from sensational experience.[21] We are observing here the emergence of both a discursive understanding of the body—its position within rational projects and the offshoots of meaning it carries—along with a literal body (the biopolitical body, Foucault might say) that suffers the experience of expansion and progress as it moves through uncharted terrain. And here, when Alcorta takes on a political position and enters the public sphere, he also brings in Destutt de Tracy.

Alcorta turned to Destutt de Tracy in order to define the science of examining ideas.[22] Here, Alcorta was concerned with human error and uncertainty; he resolved this by inevitably trusting to sensation and perception. In the complex reassembly of sense impressions, one could reach the clarity of ideas and moral choices and discover the road toward the common good.[23] This is clearly taken from the opening salvo of Destutt's *Éléments d'idéologie*:

> I have previously reduced the whole science of logic to observation of two facts. The first is that our perceptions being everything for us, we are perfectly, completely, and necessarily sure of whatever we actually feel. The second is that consequently none of our judgments, separately taken, can be erroneous: inasmuch as we see one idea in another, it is actually there. (Destutt de Tracy 1817, ix–x)

What follows is Destutt's long discussion of the ways in which the faculty of will emerges from the experience of perceptions. Wants, rights and duties, and concepts of liberty and constraint all derive from our ability to discern difference in a field of signs. Here, then, is the vehicle of representation that links perceptions to abstract ideas.

Foucault, in *The Order of Things*, was especially interested in Destutt's proposals insofar as they helped articulate the relationship between signs and representations (Foucault 1973, 105). In other words, Foucault was attracted to the investigations of eighteenth-century philosophy because here lay the classic quandary of how to represent thought as "thought represents itself" (80). But Foucault was also concerned with the ways in which Destutt identified bundles of experience such that perception, language, and representation were wrapped up as one. With reason, then, so much attention was given to the grammar of verbal order so that simultaneity and sequence could be better explained. This is a move from perception and the language of action, and from signs spoken by the body, to the field of discursivity and back to perceptions again; it takes us from the study of the relationship between vocal signs and gestures to the area of representation. Finally, Foucault observes with respect to the contributions of philosophers like Condillac and Destutt: "If language exists, it is because below the level of identities and differences there is a foundation provided by continuities, repetition, and natural crisscrossings" (122). The experience of perception marks the first step in an itinerary that eventually leads to freedom, happiness, and fostering the public good; most important, it confirms knowledge and leads one to matters of representation. There is an irony to this course of events if we admit that all knowledge is located in the space of representation and if, in the final analysis, the qualities of freedom and happiness cannot be represented; insofar as they depend upon unnamable feelings, they resist general definition. Hence, we return to Destutt's proposal in *Éléments d'idéologie* (and Foucault notes this as well): "I feel because I feel; . . . and I do not exist but because I feel. Then my existence and my sensibility are one and the same thing" (Destutt de Tracy 1817, 42). To feel (*sentire*) becomes the sole link between representation and knowledge. We are here in a sensory-affective world that appealed to Argentine thinkers.

There is a comparative reading that bears examination. Why is this sensual material so strongly enforced in learned circles of Spanish America while in the United States in the same period the matter is of secondary interest? Let's look at Rivadavia and Jefferson. We know that when Rivadavia traveled to France, he entered into a personal friendship with Destutt de Tracy; when Rivadavia returned to Argentina, he carried Destutt's writings as the basis for the new philosophy, and as we have seen, this model held considerable resonance at least through the early 1830s. In Virginia, meanwhile, Thomas Jefferson was publishing Destutt de Tracy in English. The two had met during Jefferson's stay in France in the 1780s, but it wasn't until his retirement years that Jefferson supervised a translation of Destutt's *Elements of Ideology* and his *Treatise on Political Economy*.[24] Destutt de Tracy, censored in France, circulated freely throughout the Americas, North and South. But there's a tremendous difference: if Destutt became the guiding force in philosophy at the University of Buenos Aires, in the United States, his entrance was far less auspicious. In fact, moral philosophy remained the unshakable matrix of US university courses, with Scottish common sense philosophy trumping the Idéologues tout court.[25] Moreover, if you look at the lecture notes of some early philosophy courses at the University of Virginia, the sensationalists are given short shrift. For example, George Tucker, a statesman and professor at the University of Virginia in those years, cited Thomas Brown and wrote in his inaugural lecture in 1828: "The subject which is to employ a large portion of your time is the Philosophy of the Human Mind—not that idle philosophy which enquires into the nature of the mind and its connection with the body, but that useful science which relates to the duties, the hopes and the destiny of man" (Hubbard 1828, n.p.).[26] In another course, from 1835, Tucker went on to observe that more than a claim on the present, we need to think of past and future:

> Sensations . . . always have a relation to the present. But thoughts have relations also to the past and future. We think of a past pleasure, a past suffering, etc., as readily as what is before us. Our wills have a qualified control over our sensation, from which our thoughts are exempt. This is by exertion of our wills over our locomotive faculties. We can touch or not touch a body; our eyes can exclude or admit lift; the mouth can refuse to taste . . . and . . . to smile, and the faculty of hearing can be diminished. But we have no such power over our thoughts. (Harris 1835, 31)

Mental philosophy is thus pushed aside for the moral underpinnings of thought.

This perspective effectively sets students at Virginia on a very different track from those in attendance at the University of Buenos Aires. Not only did the French Idéologues lack in the North the great reservoir of meaning that they held for elites in South America (after all, scholasticism had been repudiated by the late seventeenth century in the British colonies; hence, a turn toward sensation carried a different valence by the time of independence),[27] but there was no pervading acceptance of Jefferson's view (though he pressed for Destutt's circulation in English, in the end Jefferson himself came to reject Destutt's philosophical thought).[28] In fact, Destutt's teaching was never considered mighty enough to affect the United States academy as a whole. So why, then, is this sensual hold so strong in the South?

In a letter of 1816 addressed to Jefferson, John Adams wrote that philosophers from Catholic countries (and here he was thinking of France) appeared to produce atheists when orthodoxies failed them ("And what was their philosophy? Atheism; pure, unadulterated Atheism. Diderot, D'Alembert, Frederick, De la Lande and Grimm, were indubitable atheists. The universe was matter only, and eternal; spirit was a word without a meaning; liberty was a word without a meaning" [qtd. in Koch 1943, 95]). By contrast, he argued that in Protestant countries secessionists and critics eventually turn into deists. Perhaps Adams was right. By this late stage of his life, Jefferson's support of French doctrine had dwindled.

Sensationalist proposals upheld the initial thinking of a few of the US founding fathers—and Jefferson's case is the most compelling—although they never gained traction in university settings in the United States. Swayed by Scottish common sense philosophy in programs of "moral science," the sensationalists were seen to imperil sincerity and goals of common alliance. In South America, however, sensationalist thought offered the groundwork for a relentless reflection (at least until midcentury) about the role of the body in the training of Argentine citizen subjects. It also carried secondary consequences, allowing men in power to claim their authority within the new republic, underscoring an embodied knowledge that the later users of the "civilization and barbarism" trope would examine not without considerable conflict. In this respect, the body belonged both to savages and to men of intellect who evoked perceptions to repudiate the church's hold. By the 1830s, the tug-of-war over perceptions was far from neatly resolved.

From the University to Public Spaces: A Festival of the Senses

Alcorta's lectures in philosophy were addressed to a group of young men on their own paths to greatness; these would be the future liberal elite of Argentina, the writers and leaders who would oppose the dictatorial regime of Rosas in the 1830s and 1840s and who were about to map the future of their nation.[29] At the same time, this new investment in the study of the senses also enjoyed a life in the popular scientific journals and in public spaces. In the *Crónica política y literaria de Buenos Aires*, for example, Condorcet and Condillac were repeatedly praised as political economists of the highest order; Destutt appears as part of a discussion about the material pleasures to be found in science.[30] More important, in

La abeja argentina, a compendium of scientific material, new technologies, and inventions serving the fields of chemistry, agriculture, banking, and the law, a commentary on the senses brings us back to the lessons of Alcorta. In "Sofismas políticos: Culto de los antiguos, o argumentos a la chinesca" (1822), the anonymous author gives an extraordinary defense of direct experience.[31] The essay reviews advantages of sensory apprehension: how to capture the sublime beauty of nature, to reach into the cosmos, to understand the relation of man to the world and to the universe beyond him. After an almost lyrical defense of perceptions, the author poses a question: "In one word, wouldn't the universe perceived by the senses offer a vast field upon which we might develop physical and moral science?" ("Sofismas políticos" 1822, 245). This essay goes beyond the innocence of perception; it reaches thus for the connections between art and science, between moral philosophy and material inquiry; it urges a study of the senses in which objectives of equilibrium and beauty are present. Beyond the political framework, *La abeja argentina* was always attentive to the perceiving body in agricultural technologies, measures and weights, chemistry, and even mind-altering cures. In "Nuevas literarias: Inhalaciones" (1822, 147), for example, the anonymous author focuses on the use of sulfuric ether and laudanum. Can we alter the perceptual range of humans? Can we imagine experiments with corpses such that they will respond to electrical impulse? A commentary on galvanism forms part of a fascination with ways to make corpses move. Electrical forces, metallic charges, and a constant interest in physiological reactions to stimuli drive the interest of *La abeja argentina* in the bodies of medical experiments.[32] Nor is it of minor speculation for the authors of this cultural review to link discoveries in material science to public health correctives.[33]

While sensationalist thought occupied the university and the periodical press, another sector of the liberal government focused on the masses. The *fiestas mayas*, or May festivals, emerged as carnivals of sensorial display (see plate 1). Beginning in 1813, these civic festivals noisily celebrated the revolution of 1810 and promoted the nation's achievements.[34] Visual stimulation, loud performance, and decorated outdoor spaces were central to this promotion. "Theater is a tool of government," the Society for Good Taste proclaimed. Colorful and alive, the public fiestas were designed to entice the masses to join the liberal cause. Some might understand these demonstrations as a continuation of the Catholic holy festivals and processions, but the appeal of sensuality and color, dress, and movement (even phantasmagoria and visual tricks, according to Seibel [2002,

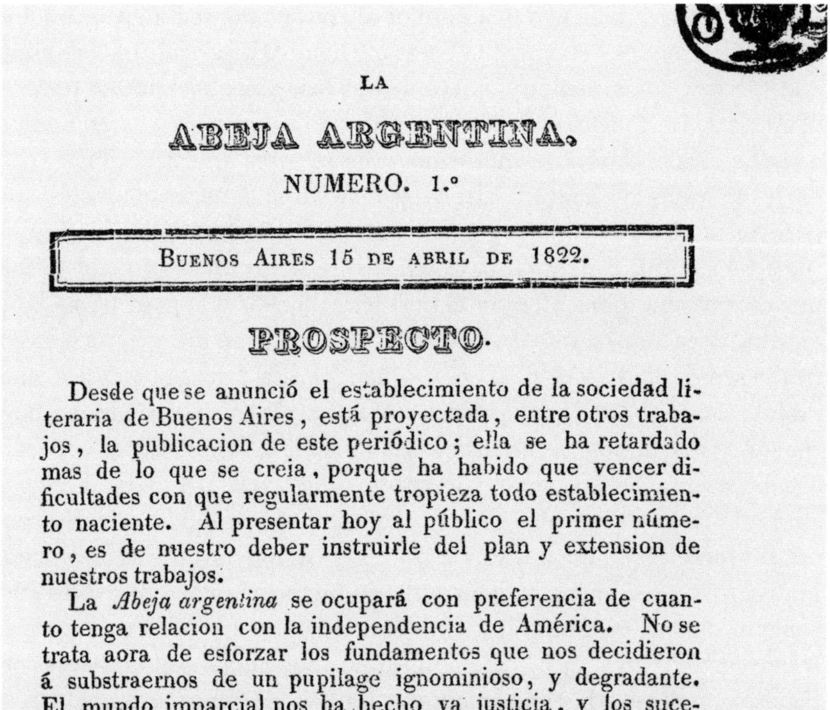

LA

ABEJA ARGENTINA.

NUMERO. 1.°

Buenos Aires 15 de abril de 1822.

PROSPECTO.

Desde que se anunció el establecimiento de la sociedad literaria de Buenos Aires, está proyectada, entre otros trabajos, la publicacion de este periódico; ella se ha retardado mas de lo que se creia, porque ha habido que vencer dificultades con que regularmente tropieza todo establecimiento naciente. Al presentar hoy al público el primer número, es de nuestro deber instruirle del plan y extension de nuestros trabajos.

La *Abeja argentina* se ocupará con preferencia de cuanto tenga relacion con la independencia de América. No se trata aora de esforzar los fundamentos que nos decidieron á substraernos de un pupilage ignominioso, y degradante. El mundo imparcial nos ha hecho ya justicia, y los sucesos han decidido la cuestion irrevocablemente. Sí: podemos lisonjearnos que es ya concluida la guerra de la independencia: este es el fruto de nuestros heroicos esfuerzos: con nadie hemos partido las glorias de este triuufo. Entretanto es importante que la América se convenza, que aun le resta que andar lo mas escabroso de la carrera, que tan gloriosamente ha emprendido. Nada habremos hecho con conquistar á tanta costa nuestra existencia, si no sabemos establecerla con solidéz. Este es el interesante objeto á que principalmente se contraheran nuestros trabajos. Convencidos que los gobiernos mejor intencionados caminan muy lentamente en este punto, cuando no estan los pueblos suficientemente ilustrados, nos proponemos generalizar por medio de este periódico aquellos conocimientos, que han acelerado en otros pueblos su organizacion social. Desenvolver los principios luminosos de esta ciencia; exâminar las bases, sobre que debe formarse un gobierno, para que pue-

Figure 1.2. La abeja argentina, *1822–1823. Biblioteca Digital Trapalanda, Mariano Moreno National Library of Argentina.*

64–65]), were especially designed to drum up support for new governing forces.

The early decades of the nineteenth century gave evidence of the construction of at least two kinds of subjects: elite leaders formed in universities who would take charge of the political destiny of the nation, and popular subjects whose identities were formed from mass events and carnival-like spectacles like the *fiestas mayas*. In both cases, the starting point was the body of a sentient self; and in both instances—for politics and for popular theater—a culture of effects seemed to matter.[35] Then, of course, there was the spectacle of horrors to be performed by the Rosas regime.

The Romantic Body

By the time romanticism took hold, with its intense pursuit of the collective soul and guiding moral compass, some among Alcorta's students had begun to rethink their lessons. Despite the fanfare expressed for Alcorta's university lectures, his disciples became embroiled in the significant political shifts in Argentina, moving away from the short-lived "happy experience" of the 1820s to confront the harsh rule of Rosas. Their philosophies also changed.

Here, we face a practical problem in the tension between theory and practice. If in the 1820s sensualist teachers in Buenos Aires were insisting on perception as the first step toward moral claims, a decade later the Rosas regime invented a new scenario, turning to sensation not only to attract the support of crowds but to discipline public dissent. This time, the Idéologues' slogan—"I feel, therefore I exist"—expressed the shock delivered to the Unitarian body by the tactics of Rosas's secret police (see plate 2). In other words, the sensual body that was so firmly installed in the consciousness of liberal intellectuals as a sign of liberation was now usurped by Rosas for the tactics of repression. Sense work under the Rosas regime served the rising technologies of torture; it gave a graphic reading of the savagery that liberals denounced in those years. Civilization became the equivalent of abstraction and reason, whereas savagery was understood as the presence of the literal body, a body that could be subjected to torture as much as it silenced the soul.

Understandably, and under the dangerous circumstances of the 1830s,

Argentine intellectuals began to fan out in different directions, abandoning the Unitarian course that had been set in place by Alcorta and also reevaluating the merits of his philosophical approach. In general terms, the theories of sense experience Alcorta taught to students were now subjected to a new evaluation due to not only rising political crisis but also a surging romantic will. In this context, the pursuit of a collective mentality would upend the belief that perceptions were a starting point to lead to enduring truth. In fact, by the 1830s in Argentina, romantics turned away from materialist science not only because it failed to account for internal conflicts but also because materialism was identified with Rosas. The spirit was elevated over coarseness: this became the *letrados*' cause. Juan Bautista Alberdi's pithy comments help make the divisions clear: "Intelligence differs from the senses, moral life from physical being, good from the merely pleasant, justice from utility, the soul from the body. This is not to deny the exchange of those principles, their identification of the one with the other. The soul obeys the body, but the soul is not the body" (1886, 240).[36] He then continues, "Sensualism denies man the consoling idea of a future" (240). Romanticism created a spirit with which to reevaluate these sense-based proposals; returning from Europe with new philosophies that made their political and aesthetic choices clearer, the intellectuals of Alberdi's cohort now sought a theory of action in order to restore moral obligation and seek out the absolute good (Alberdi 1886, 155–159).

Nonetheless, and despite Alberdi's admonitions to push sensuality aside, the romantics failed to abandon the sense-based theories completely. In fact, they relied on embodied perceptions to sustain their attacks against Rosas. Often this produced literary genres with grotesque sensorial effects that were draped around narratives of war and bloodshed; there was little space for nostalgia or for the literary sublime espoused by Victor Hugo.[37] We can occasionally see this in contrast to North American models of those same years. Compare, for instance, the expression of North American nostalgia as described by James Fenimore Cooper, with which he lamented the loss of a sensual world while he praised the march of progress, to the South American case that keeps the grotesque invariably alive. In this regard, the examples of Esteban Echeverría and Domingo Faustino Sarmiento are instructive. These authors celebrated the figure of the trailblazer as a way to come in touch with nature, and through it, to clear the groundswell of meaning that would sustain a future liberal republic. But with trailblazer stories, they also put the senses into play as central tropes for defining the individual in a land of savage indignity. The hunting trope of the 1840s in Argentina and elsewhere in Spanish America is not a site for nostalgic yearning (as we might see in the example of Cooper), but a course upon which writers might locate the various trials of perception.[38] It introduced a landscape ruled by terror, spouting carnal monsters and criminals, and exposing physical violence. In this respect, Hugo's sublime was out of Argentine reach.

Sensing Disaster: Echeverría and Sarmiento

Let's examine the case of Esteban Echeverría and Domingo Faustino Sarmiento, two pioneers of liberal thought in Rosas's Argentina. The nineteenth-century Latin American canon, both political and literary, stars these men in the opening act. Romantics who fought against tyrannical rule and who outlined a plan for government and law, these *letrados* found in the literary realm a way to awaken the sensibilities of the public. They put a theory of the senses to work for the cause of liberal freedom. Echeverría opted for poetry (although his short story "El matadero" became his most celebrated work); Sarmiento pursued autobiography and essay, always on the edge of genre and giving birth to new literary forms. Together they cultivated sensual violence to expose the Rosas regime.

Echeverría (1805–1851) was first a student in the courses of Martín Diego de Alcorta and then went on to study in France, returning home with fresh ideas from Leroux, Guizot, and Lermenier, not to mention the historical syntheses of Cousin that guided many Argentines of this generation (see Gutiérrez 1874, xvi). He later became the leader of the Argentine romantic generation and Rosas's strident opponent, finishing his life in exile in Uruguay. A sickly and reclusive man,[39] Echeverría wrote about intense corporeal violence delivered by the adversarial agents. Exposing physical torture is thus central to his work; his poetry and prose insists upon sensation and perception, and also *sensibilité*. An essay of 1827, written in French during his years in Paris, sums up this position: "The existence of ideas is subordinate to sensibility. Man cannot think without feeling, such that the source of his thought is sensibility.... Sensibility is to the realm of ideas what friction is to electricity" (1870–1874, 5:421). Although Echeverría in later years reneged on this youthful interest, his prose and poetry never lost the affective-sensational draw; material horror pursues him. Consider, in this regard, these few verses from his long poem *El ángel caído* (The fallen angel, 1846):

Dreaming, perfection from mundane ideas

Add to that war and filth

Hearing cries and curses
Seeing vast injustice
And more than any other deplorable thing.
Seeking poetry in nations
Where you touch prosaic matter
With your eyes, ears, and nostrils. (1870–1874, 2:353)

A poet and philosopher who railed against authoritarian abuses, Echeverría constructed a literary discourse full of "prosaic matter" (*materia prosa*); palpable horrors invade the space of dream and verse. Incapable of evading these vile attacks, he writes a poetry of effects, with lightning bolts, darts and arrows, and rivers of blood described with such intensity that they appear to gush on the page. In the final verses cited above, touch, sight, audition, and smell sustain prosaic matter. The good writer, inspired by dreams, will seek out poetic form to open a course toward reason, but for the moment, sensuality and shock immerse us in the mire.

But how is this logic shaped? A conduit for recent ideas in philosophy, Echeverría returned to Argentina in 1830, after five years in Europe, and was dismayed by the material culture that awaited him in Buenos Aires. His turn against Alcorta is sharp, as if the fault for Argentina's failures depends upon his teacher alone. Thus in a late-life poem, "Avellaneda" (1849), Echeverría directs his anger toward the philosopher mentor whom he followed so eagerly in his youth:

I was a believer recently converted.
There in the capital of Buenos Aires
The doctors taught me to doubt
God, virtue, valor,
Good, justice, and my own ideas.
They taught me how talented conquests
Of the human spirit were prepared over the years
How false and ego-filled dogma
Stuck like a rotten plague
To social body and nation
And paved the way to enslavement and death.

Sophists or unwise sectarians
Of philosophy . . .
They failed to calculate the moral weight
Of the very doctrine they taught.
Quickly, abolishing
Social virtue, smiling
They rendered tribute to the brutish despot.
Corruption invades and like gangrene,
Poisons
The guts of a nation (1870–1874, 1:340–341)

Echeverría reminds his readers that the climate of sensualist ideas requires a second look. By 1849, Alcorta's teachings were seen as far too inadequate to assess and comprehend the range of present-day ruin. Because the throat slittings and spectacles of beheadings continued under Rosas, we have proof sufficient—or so Echeverría tells us—that sensualist philosophy had clearly gone astray.[40]

In his five-volume edition of Echeverría's works (1870–1874), Juan María Gutiérrez tried to right the misperceptions of his friend, correcting (in his annotations) the passionate excess of the poem:

> The philosophical teachings to which the illustrious poet refers, more systematic than emancipatory in both form and content, opened the eyes of youth to the frank study of philosophical problems in general, breaking with old scholastic methods and the yoke of dogmatic doctrine.
>
> The consequence of this direction is placed in evidence . . . by the apostles and martyrs who reacted against the politics of Rosas. Indeed, they were disciples of the University of Buenos Aires, beginning with Mr. Echeverría himself. (in Echeverría 1870–1874, 1:438)[41]

Perhaps because Echeverría begged for more attention to the soul and to a Catholic spirit (albeit with modern inflections that were designed, as Halperin Donghi explains, more to reach the ignorant masses than for any deep spirituality that Echeverría might have possessed as his own),[42] Gutiérrez rewrote the late narrative of his poet friend and saved the value of Alcorta's lessons.

Here we might consider that Echeverría had learned the lessons of the French sensualists only too well, since in many sections of *El ángel caído* he seems to acknowledge—and, indeed, affirm—that material perceptions formed the basis of all his work. Invaded as he was by visual images (and sanctioned by the romantic creed that exalted local color), his poetry is full of violent details—of "bloody torsos, vampires / hands covered in blood / always knives and skulls" (1870–1874, 2:18). In this context, Echeverría laments, our brains are only fleshy matter deprived of reason (2:14). But just as materialism describes the carnal ferocity of a terrible world, another unexpected force describes the soul's attractions. In the second section of *El ángel caído*, the poet represents figures at a dance:

> Living passions began to cross.
> With latent rays,
> A magnetic force
> Let love flow through the soul. (2:82)

A strange science enters here; again, Echeverría's editor Juan María Gutiérrez is quick to set us straight. In a long note appended to this stanza, Gutiérrez observes that electromagnetism in the 1840s was beginning to capture the imagination of Argentine writers: "Magnetism. Magnetic action exists beyond doubt. Like electricity and galvanism, it allows surprising and inexplicable phenomena. Its magic agent is magnetic fluid. Some confuse it with electrical fluid, others with galvanic; but magnetic fluid alone seems to live and work on the human body" (in Echeverría 1870–1874, 2:546). We are in the presence of a technology that not only alters perceptions but also awakens the spirit. Echeverría, hoping to turn to the heart, places the drift of love in the arms of pseudoscience, just as Edgar Allen Poe—in the same decade—found fascination in those inventions that opened hidden worlds.

Echeverría wavers between materialist science and the callings of the soul; he pulls away from violence only to be drawn back in its thrall. I have already shown with *El ángel caído*, cited above, that Echeverría needed to struggle against the "prosaic matter" in order to find the poem. In his short story "El matadero" (The slaughterhouse), the inaugural text of the national canon, Echeverría again addresses the materialism guiding the Rosas regime. A fiction written from 1839 to 1840, though not published until decades later, this text reminds us that literature carries an ethical challenge: to expunge the contagion of barbarism and put all readers on alert. The slaughterhouse at a distance from the city is thus described as a scene of mud and pollution, judicial violence and disorder (see plate 3): it is part of Echeverría's pervasive show of uncontrollable instincts and sensory indulgence that will lead Argentina to ruin. To top it off, Echeverría makes his point through food: showing his characters in pursuit of scraps of meat, or suffering the ills of digestion, he gives a vulgar (and ironic) slant to the eighteenth-century idea of good "taste" as an attribute that defines a nation.[43] A vision of a slaughterhouse of discarded fat and bone, blood mixing with the mud of the streets, with images of the rabble crying out for morsels to quell their hunger, "El matadero" is a fitful scene of a nation that cannot be born. The text, for this reason, is bespattered with mire, leaving us stuck in a weighty morass that is the stuff of an aborted future. Is this the birth of genre as Noé Jitrik proposed? Perhaps another story might intervene. Years ago, Sandra Gilbert and Susan Gubar, in a now classic feminist study, sought to portray romanticism as a moment when male writers, needing to give birth to a literary work, took up the pen not as a sword but as a phallus. The blank page was its corresponding vessel, a womb that might give birth. But Echeverría in this instance uses the pen to produce chaos and error; his text is a mass of undefined flesh refusing to take human form. What is left, in the mode of Dr. Frankenstein's creature, are perceptual subjects alert to sensation; receiving or delivering pain, and always deprived of reason. This failure is then translated through the inadequacy of genre. Is "El matadero" a fiction, an allegory, a chronicle of daily life, a *costumbrista* sketch of mores? Similarly, is *El ángel caído*, nearly 550 pages in length, a poem or an epic monster resisting its containing cage? Both are pulsating masses, triggering the reader's perceptions; and in spite of himself, Echeverría extends sensual imagery in order to awaken the soul.

I referred earlier to the proposals of Victor Hugo, who defended the sublime. But Hugo also realized the value of the literary grotesque. In the encounter of these two modes, grotesque and sublime entangled, the earthquake of poetry explodes, Hugo once told his readers.[44] Echeverría, familiar with Hugo's text, picked up on the message. In fact, in *El ángel caído*, he praises the winning combination—"And pretend to see grotesque / And sublime together / A huge work represented" (1870–1874, 2:25)—though in Argentina, he reminds us, this combination cannot work as long as tyranny reigns. By 1841, there is no space for tranquil beauty. Rather, human bodies are locked in vulgar pleasures or they stand as victims of torture imposed by savage mobs. Despite his frequent protests against this sensorial route,[45] Echeverría shows terror's imprint though material form.

This is where the lettered class is redirected; now they are like butchers exposing blood and bone. A few verses from *El ángel caído* illustrate this point:

And the poets will be the butchers
The gauchos and landowners men of letters,
And others will steal the diploma from Doctors
Whose wit is only alleged. (1870–1874, 2:257)

This is a radical departure from the confidence that French philosophers had placed in the capacity of men. Now *sentire est percipi* (to feel is to be perceived) finds living proof in the effects of authoritarian regimes; the human is a set of sensory receptors, experiencing pain and distress, and the poets—uncouth butchers—now lead the savage charge. The only objects of poetry are forged from knife and gun. How, then, can the poet stretch the limits of literary form? Where is the poem behind the *materia prosa*, or prosaic matter? And how can genre expand the capacities of poet and reader? There's more to these questions than meets the eye.

In the prologue to *El ángel caído*, Echeverría observes what he calls the "two sides of our being"—the spirit and the flesh (1870–1874, 2:6). Absent liberal thought, we only have sensation. This angry binarism structured all of Echeverría's work and set in place a break, a strategy of rupture, to explain this double life. Let's look at *La cautiva* (The captive, 1837), Echeverría's classic work, where the device of the caesura determines the entire poem. *La cautiva* begins with an ode to nature, but already in the first stanza, we witness a defining break:

It was evening, and the hour
In which the sun shines over the
Andean crest.—The incommensurable
Desert, open and
Mysterious, extends
At its feet—sad was its sorry face (1870–1874, 1:35–36)

From the height of the Andes, a dash cuts the text, dropping us from the mountains to the open desert below. From the sun-filled peaks, we descend to sadness. This initiates a pattern of breaks and uneven pictures that elicit sensual perceptions appealing to image and sound, and secondarily to affects. This double experience is sustained through the strategy of alternating cantos. The vast beauty of nature, recounted in the first section, is cut suddenly by an unpleasant sound ("in the calm plain a deaf clamor was heard" [1:40]). This prepares us for the second canto, "El festín," where the poet writes: "The field was covered with corpses, with trunks, limbs, blood and bones, mixed among the living. / Covered was the field" (1:56). In this poem, where death always lurks near life, Echeverría's second canto is anything but sublime. It is filled with sounds of hissing, shrieks, and screams, deliberate acoustic breaks in what might have been a harmonic poetic horizon:

> He rises and stumbles,
> falls like lead and, growling,
> turns over like a beast;
> This one screams, the other cries
> And others begin to drink. (1:49–50)

Here, the natives howl, they snort, they crave the blood of humans and horses; they lick their chops after devouring the remains of the slaughter; they stage a general uproar expressed in unrepresentable speech. As readers, we are asked to bear witness to these ravenous sounds as cannibals "suck, drink, and savor the blood of the dead" (1:48). If "perception is being" as the sensualists proposed, here Echeverría displays the grand performance of savagery to excite the senses of the viewer. We are asked to link word and representation and to be shocked by what we read. But the rhythms broken by the caesurae of the text introduce another dimension, such that the break, the incapacity to find resolution, is what most steadily forms the poem. This is where the poem turns from an affective mode to a poetry of effect. In the rhythm, we hear the constant gallop of horses, the dust that the rabble whips up, the continuous, uninterrupted flow of vulgar, unrestrained habits identified with the mob. But the caesurae offer a dissonant jolt, and perhaps a moment for reflection. In the crevasse, thought is born. Conflicting sentiments travel through the cantos, emerging at points of rupture where different sensibilities or ideas collide. Thus, if the first section of the poem was structured by a décima of rhyming couplets, the second section ("El festín") holds on to the octosyllabic verse yet dispenses with the conventional final rhymes. The horror of the tribe is recounted, but the many caesurae invite us to pause along the way to take stock of what is lost. Between these extremes, *La cautiva* takes form while Echeverría gives us literary figures working out their perceptions. The third canto thus signals surrounding noises and introduces María: "She moves—she's all ears, walking over the sleeping savages,—she listens,—she sees— / she stops,—she breathes" (1:59). Note again how the caesurae and breaks in rhythm are made visible through the dashes in the text. At the same time, María is described as a subject with senses on alert. Here and there, through movement and stops, Echeverría pushes Maria from one point to another while all the senses move her. She is a living, sentient form.

The need to see and hear is central to this canto; Argentina's wilderness disallows any time for slumber. The fourth canto synthesizes in two pages the contrast between cantos 1 and 2; quickly we pass from the silent beauty of the night to the clamor of the mob. With this, the flight of María and Brián begins in earnest though their path of escape becomes foul and infected: far from sublime, nature becomes grotesque. Reminiscent of a scene from his earlier epistolary narrative, "Cartas a un amigo,"[46] Echeverría paints stagnation and death:

> The sun burned like a forge
> On the mired swamp
> Of stagnant water, the filthy fish
> Swam among the dead, below stench-infested air.
> Or among the impure waste,
> At times they chewed on corpses (1:79)

Nature is more than the pretext for pathetic fallacy; it determines how we come to live on the underside of beauty. As the poem advances, the human bodies lie front and center. Echeverría asks his readers to see Brián's wounds, to feel Maria's Amazonic strength, lifting up her lover's weight in her female arms. Is this gender shift provoked by the savage regime, where nature turns against itself, defying all the rules (surely when the Unitarian is sodomized in "El matadero," we sully a similar question)? Or are these the preconditions for love in unbearably horrid times? In the long run (as the poem concludes), Echeverría tells us that neither love nor heroism will be remembered; we can only score effects upon the reader's mind. The fire of canto 7 attests to this spectacle of destruction; it razes land and love, leaving only "Mud, straw, vile remains" (1:95). A poem formed by cuts and breaks and alternating rhythms, radically thrusting between beauty and horror, between different scenes exposed on each side of the caesurae, between the easy rhyme of ballad form and the asperity of broken meter, *La cautiva* pleads in the end for "the harmony / of invisible creation" (1:136) that is only found in death.

Deleuze and Guattari, in *A Thousand Plateaus*, signal the value of rhythm as a moment of continuation against potential disorder (1987, 311–350). In this context, rhythm keeps the forces of chaos outside and protects interior space; it pushes back utter confusion; and owing to the repetition, it reminds us of the comforts of home. "One ventures from home on the thread of a tune," they write (311). Rhythm is the environment's answer to the formless abyss. Others, from Kristeva to Agamben, have found in poetic rhythm the space of maternal protection, where preverbal signs wash over the infant's body as a touch of love. Similarly, in Echeverría's verse, gentle vibrations appeal to the ear, encircling a safe space that protects the reader from the perceptions of horror that permeate the poem. Moreover, the octosyllabic verse, despite its breaks and frequent ruptures, keeps the rhythm of Spanish poetry from the time of the *romancero* alive for modern readers. The Argentine poet writes to this effect in his essay "Fondo y forma en las obras de la imaginación":

> Rhythm is the music through which poetry captures the senses and speaks with great efficiency to the soul. Vague and measured, it corrects melancholia and guarantees repose; in full sound, precipitous and quick, it is the torment of the affects. . . . It wounds with dissonance; it bewitches with harmony, and through consonant endings and onomatopoeia, it gives voice to inanimate nature, and lets the soul fluctuate between memory and hope. (Echeverría 1870–1874, 5:119)

Rhythm appeals to the constancy of recall and to hope for the future. It places memories of sheltered space apart from the lines of fire; it overrides the shrieks and screams that savages convey. Rhythm works against the rupture that dominates the form of the poem.

What, in effect, is found in the caesurae? When we hear that a poetic measure is missing, we know from the phantom absence that a prosthesis is needed. We need to cure the body of verse, to fill in for the cuts and absence. Equally important, we need to remind ourselves that poetry from the time of antiquity keeps the body alive. It allows severed heads to sing, it permits the corpse to breathe new life. This is the condition of possibility for the survival of literature, but also for reaching out to give birth to a new republic. This is the hope invested in poetic genre that sustains Echeverría's dreams.

Cultural tradition here supplies another order that stands against savage effects; history enters through remembered rhythm, sustaining a national song upon the bloody expanse of the plains. And although we see the broken body of the poem, we retain in our hearts and ears a clear recursive order. In turning to the *romancero* inherited from early Spain, Echeverría gives us a rhythmic memory that remands us to historical time, evoking the murderous violence belonging to the Rosas regime; like the medieval battles between warriors from the time of the *romancero*, this too will come to pass. Echeverría thus writes in unexpected combinations: in *sextinas*, *décimas*, and heptasyllabic verse, all of which give vent to the full adventure that Spanish versification might offer. It is memory of history through recursive rhythm; it is home that haunts the ear. The text leaves us doubly awakened to savagery in the present moment—and to the grotesque image that it inspires; it also announces the palliative of versification to build a continuum in history.

Echeverría considers literary form in order to rattle the reader; the broken verses lead to a crescendo, and violence infects the word. This appears in the blocked flow of verse, it shows up in the darkened visions, it is felt in the sluggish impediments to movement and political progress. Violence and writing thus combined place our *experience* in the center of the text, making us, as readers, one and bound to events from Argentine history. From the morass and ruins, we as readers are urged to start anew, to grow reason from the body's wounds, and to awaken from cultural slumber.

In a prefatory note to a recently edited volume on Echeverría, Alejandra Laera and Martín Kohan remind us that Echeverría, who died in Montevideo, is a *prócer* without a tomb (Laera and Kohan 2006, 9–10). Perhaps this is the writer's revenge against the deep materialism that informed his poetry and prose—to disappear without a trace, to escape the captivity scene that defined Argentina (as well as the title of his famous poem), to achieve over the *materia prosa* the invisible ideal beyond reach.

Sarmiento's Sense of Power

Echeverría's response to the material cultures of *Rosismo* takes on the thrust of grotesque encounter. And though his romantic spirit lifts him up over what he calls the "corruption ... error and ... material" of the Rosas years, he nonetheless turns to sense perceptions to describe the world that he finds (Echeverría 1870–1874, 2:540). The goal is to denounce the tyranny of matter over reason, to reject crass sensuality in order to sing the poet's spirit, and to seek the communal idealist ties that promise modern freedoms. But above all, Echeverría's path, as many critics have argued, was to establish himself as a writer, to shape his legacy as a man of letters, albeit with an anguished heart (Laera and Kohan 2006). In the eyes of some, however, this plan was a simple failure (Halperin Donghi 1951).

Against this, Sarmiento's reach is far less modest. From his early writings, Sarmiento (1811–1888) writes against the regime in question, but positions himself as a man destined to lead the state. Sensual triggers dart out to reach his perceptual grasp; he captures them, explains their power, and on the side, he proves his mettle for leadership and future control. To see how this is deployed, let us consider his two major works, *Facundo: Civilization and Barbarism* (1845) and *Campaña en el ejército grande* (The grand army campaign, 1852). These composite texts—part fiction, part history, part personal account and political pamphlet—daringly unmask the arrogance of despots and set a blueprint for government and law. We could pause once again to reflect on the ways in which literary genres are born, the ways in which the confusion of untamed fragments of prose ignites a particular literary flame or provokes a national problem. Josefina Ludmer linked the emergence of genre to an emergency of state (1988, 11–14). In his writings, Sarmiento anticipates Ludmer's claims. He evokes a state of national emergency so grand that we need to convoke all our perceptions: to see and hear the enemy, to register its terror, to taste the blood of victims. The unformed combination of essay/fiction/theory is Sarmiento's choice of writing form to embrace these sensorial prompts. No single genre has sufficient thrust to capture the blatant violence. Secondarily (and not least of all), Sarmiento prompts us to question how the body is created and sustained in words, how an author lets us taste and touch, how we come to feel the wounds of the other's suffering limbs. This strategy of representation is deployed over multiple bodies: the body of the text, the body of the republic, and of course the body of abject persons exposed to a villainous regime. These emergent bodies respond to the emergency of state that defines Argentina under *Rosismo*; they are the substance of the unformed text.

To intertwine this cluster, Sarmiento begins *Facundo* with the body of land; the introductory chapter is the "physiognomy of the republic." Second, he addresses human bodies born of contradiction: insofar as corporeality is the very basis of barbarism (by contrast to the abstract reasoning that should belong to civilization), he shows how the wounds delivered by savages are felt on the bodies of liberal men. Finally, Sarmiento gives a dense corporeality to the text itself; he makes a word shriek out on the page and lets us feel the flesh of narration. From the tropes of the body that course through *Facundo*, Sarmiento begins to construct a model for experience and sensation despite the fact that he defends a life of the mind and spirit.

In short form, we could say that experience became a central theme of his work, but indeed it's much more than that. Sarmiento observes a world in which reason, bound to a savage, carnal culture, has fallen on its back and needs once again to be lifted. In this service, he rescues the trope of civilization against barbarism, a phrase he borrowed from Europe, and makes of it the lasting stamp that continues to pervade Latin American culture up to the present day. Sense and mind become joined together.

But how can we speak of the dyad? Sarmiento's writing is of course seeded by Rousseau's idea of a social contract and by the pages of his *Confessions*, texts that were amply cited in midcentury Argentina and which situated a sentient being at the dynamic center of thought. To be sure, Rousseau's organic images of the political and sensual bodies formed part of the *sensus communis*; they defended the human body as the first step to political engagement. But if Rousseau had hopes for political unity by letting the body speak, Sarmiento was after something else: the sensual self as a conduit for his own political dreams.

Let me show how this is played out within the two books I mentioned. In *Facundo*, Sarmiento goes in small steps to reach his agenda, first working through the affects—feelings, fear, and foreboding—and then, further on, getting to the uses of sensory perception of objects and things within his reach. In both cases, the description of the affective and physical apperception is not a course to contemplative thought, but serves instrumental reason. In his first mention of Facundo Quiroga, for example, Sarmiento ponders the outlaw's ghost and brings him back to life: "Terrible specter of Facundo, I will evoke you so that you may rise, shaking off the bloody dust covering your ashes, and explain the hidden life and the inner convulsions that tear at the bowels of a noble people!" (Sarmiento 2003, 31).[47] On the surface, this oft-cited opening sentence promises to unveil the pressing secrets of barbarism that have wreaked havoc upon Argentina; savage terror externalizes a complex moral drama. But there's another point. The body named in the initial text is a ghost; we need to bring it back to life so that readers may perceive it and feel its terror. Sarmiento needs to teach us *to feel* this disturbance, and, of course, he cannot perform this operation only upon a corpse. From the nonbody, the phantom, Sarmiento then appeals to the affects; he invites readers to acknowledge the prodigious weight that puts pressure upon our bodies. He brings this ghost to life when Facundo makes an entrance in the text, represented as a living being with palpable, breathing form. You could say that we need the figurability of fear—its performance, its theater, its staging—first to shape our affective response and then to lead to a physical sensing, and finally as a way to wait for something to change.

Samuel Monder (2010) has called attention to the sweep of Sarmiento's gaze as a way to fill the Cartesian blind spot, so named in the *Dioptrique*, a way to have the affects close in on the empty center of unnamed meaning that we cannot yet behold through reason. In this regard, the "terrible specter of Facundo" comes to occupy that empty center: we approach it by seeing through the dense layers of fog and mist; we approach it through different landscapes; we animate our senses through the legendary fear that Facundo poses. We thus move in on the outlaw, piece by piece, to get near to his commanding terror. Our feelings fill in for the incomprehensible missing center, a way to locate experience, and eventually lead us to understand the perversions not just of Facundo but of the Rosas regime as a whole. In the world of phantoms and repetitions, we feel the effects of gothic terror; at the same time, we are asked to claw around and try to encounter the real. This double operation fascinates me, for it exposes contradiction: Sarmiento leaves us in the presence of ghosts as much as he outlines a desperate need to get to the hard rock of reality, to put it onstage and display it. From this, a new national literature is born, whose configuration will last to the present day.

Sarmiento understood that all bodies—those of cultured elites and bandits, members of opposing political factions—were implicated in a larger narrative that might one day lead to modernization. But they had to be drawn out for his readers; he needed to show readers the pressures that were placed on the literal and discursive body. It follows then that Sarmiento would need to tell a tale that not only derived from the affects, but then moved on to the senses with vivid descriptions of palpable, audible, and visible stimuli that crossed his path. In that way, more than a *feeling* of terror, sight, sound, and touch would rattle men from their slumber, urging them to rise up and rebel against the powers that held them captive. Experience of the sensual kind was, in Sarmiento's case, used to disrupt inertia and break the complacency of passive readers. But there's more. Perhaps in combination with his readings of Pierre Leroux and Herder regarding experience and understanding,[48] Sarmiento was striving for an image of man as a sentient being in search of community and striving for a secure base of knowledge. It is *civilization combined with barbarism*, as the title tells us; there is neither an antithetical frame nor a choice of options. Both extremes are looked at under a single lens. In other words, we have to combine the work of reason with the exercise of sentient bodies. And though Sarmiento is recognizing community, his is a community guided by a vibrant, new leader; in this case, by Sarmiento himself.

Let us stay with *Facundo* for a while, trying to keep track of the world of perceptions that emerges in this classic work. Sarmiento begins with a sense of foreboding, a vague unnamable unrest, and then proceeds to use sense data in order to shape an argument; in this second instance, despite his autodidactic training in the province of San Juan, Sarmiento nonetheless comes quite close to the lessons of those first professors of philosophy in Buenos Aires whose reputations reached him through his intellectual confreres. And by 1845, when Sarmiento was in exile, he also had access to theories of sensation and perception spread by his Chilean colleagues. There are of course significant shifts. In *Facundo* we see the physiological treatment of the terrain, but we also read about the natural stimuli that appear in the text as the bases of a creative wisdom and political knowledge. From the first chapter, then, we learn of the "physical aspect" of the land, described as an infirm body; its clogged arteries and sluggish blood are in need of stimulation. Beyond that, we get what seems to be an inspiration from Rousseau, in which one's interactions with physical or sensuous forms affirm the priority of consciousness; from here, we find a route toward cognition that allows Sarmiento to reach for a theory of state.

To get there, Sarmiento toggles between the mediations of image—through language, consciousness, and feeling—and the lure of pure immediacy that will give proof of what we need to know. In some cases, he acknowledges the mediations of language and consciousness that are necessary to rewrite the chaos of barbarism; in others, he stresses the performance of the enemy body and the ways in which this staging will excite the reading public's senses. The opening epigraph on the title page of the 1845 edition lays bare these major conflicts: "On ne tue point les idées" (One can't kill ideas), Sarmiento writes in French, stealing a line from Diderot yet attributing it to Hippolyte Fortoul. His ensuing Spanish translation represents another challenge: "You can sever the heads of men, but never their ideas" (my translation). Much has been made of this faulty citation. Some see it as Sarmiento's way of challenging the hegemony of European thought, a gesture against authority. Others call attention to the inaugural quote in French as a way to introduce a double language system that anticipates the binomial of civilization and savagery itself, with French occupying the site of civilization (a language that few in Argentina would have understood in 1845!) while the Spanish language must be regarded as an instrument of the barbaric other.[49] Beyond this, Sarmiento installs the body in his Spanish translation: he tells us that even if we attempt to decapitate a body (*degollar* is the verb he uses), the free flow of ideas will be available for those who wish to pursue them. Body versus thought. Throughout *Facundo*, Sarmiento mounts a series of contradictions about the property of word and body. There is a first uneasy opposition contained in the inaugural phrase: in order to reach the ideas of men, we first have to acknowledge the severed heads that litter our national path. Even if we remove the body, the ideas of men will remain. Is the body irrelevant to the world of ideas? Can Sarmiento override bloodshed in order to let philosophy rise alone, defending an unfettered contemplative life that lacks material basis? Here, the resources of print culture enter: in order to let ideas survive, we must trust to the *materiality* of words. The real body is swapped for the body of narrative; against the severed heads, the free press will survive. We find ourselves ensconced in the mirrored halls of representation as Sarmiento presses further. He acknowledges that through the power of narrative, and of literature in particular, he can awaken the bodies of readers. Although the inaugural epigraph does not directly allude to this struggle, Sarmiento will use the exercise of writing to speak both to the world of ideas and to the world of *effects*. There is a second feature of Sarmiento's prose that draws from the famous initial citation. The realm of ideas, the work of the intellect that overrides the immediacy of the body, is born in Argentina from a lawless land of material bodies in conflict; in other words, within the framework of a culture for elites, even the world of abstract reasoning comes from the same kind of sensory alertness that is required of backwoods bandits. Again, it's not civilization *against* barbarism, but a pairing: civilization *and* barbarism, coexisting, mutually dependent, each sliding into the other's arms so that we can't tell one from the other.

Several details from the early pages deserve our notice: First, the land as a place of sense stimulation requires vigilance and attention. Attuned to its range of impressions, we need to control nature both as part of a national project and as a personal resource for survival. Recall, in this regard, the opening pages of *Facundo*, where Sarmiento tells us of the caravans of settlers who cross the plains. They need to be on the alert in order to stay alive: "If their ears hear no sound, if their eyes cannot pierce the dark veil that covers this quiet solitude, to calm themselves down, they turn their gaze to the ears of some horse next to the fire, observing if they are at rest and easily inclining back" (2003, 46).

There's a fundamental problem announced in *Facundo*: How can we survive and control this land if we have limited sensual acumen? And how do we compete with the men of the outback? Sarmiento makes this clear in the oft-cited chapter 1, where he praises the popular figures who roam the Argentine plains—the pathfinder, the tracker, the outlaw, and the wilderness bard. In his descriptions, Sarmiento shows immense admiration for these men yet refuses to veil his envy. And when he comes to understand that sensual experience is the basis of poetry, he really gets himself stuck: If barbarism is the equivalent of living by the senses, then only the barbarians will be poets; and if the savages are the true poets, then how can civilized men ever compete? How can they be expected to write?[50] Here, on the side, a comparison is helpful. Recall, along with Sarmiento's proposal, the ambitions of James Fenimore Cooper, who at the close of *The Last of the Mohicans* praised the natives of yesteryear for the authenticity of their poetry and voice. Unlike Sarmiento, Cooper reached back to an age before the republic, struggling to find a moment previous to the turmoil of his present time. Accordingly, Cooper gave dignity to the vanquished in a move that we might liken to the idea of "imperial nostalgia" to which Renato Rosaldo (1989) once alluded; first you kill the natives, then you stamp their images on a national coin. Cooper glorifies the natives in *The Last of the Mohicans* precisely because he knew that history had already left them behind.[51] But in the Argentine case, the backwoods poets of the 1840s were still very much alive, threatening Sarmiento's potential; a wistful competition emerges between them over matters of voice. Here there is no instantiation of friendship or brotherhood, as in the case of Cooper; nor is melancholia expressed for any brave lost race. Rather, in the absence of social institutions, the intellectual must somehow figure out how to sing *better* than the natives whose voices haunt him still. After all, Sarmiento needed to leave an enduring effect on the ears and eyes of his readers, to be a better poet than the woodsman, to surpass the woodsman's skills. And here Sarmiento takes these lessons to the scene of language itself.

Sarmiento's prose is deliriously palpable. The rhythms of the sentences rock us back and forth; at times they seem to graze our skin. His prose shrieks out its utter materiality and makes us feel the weight of print on the page. Exclamation points pepper the text and are there to awaken our feeling. Moreover, he understands that these features form the power of narrative, swaying an audience of listeners to see the correct course for political change. Here voice is not an agent of absolute truth, but a device to shake readers up, a means of finding through tone and timbre an alternative to conventional reason; Argentines are thus called upon to react, asked to experience the terror in the flesh, to feel the rhythm of the prose and to be carried away by its power. Sarmiento strikes for the world of instincts in the hope of expanding perception, but he also uses the rhythm of prose to remind us of a time of waiting,[52] that empty time that eventually leads to the doorstep of action where men will challenge the enduring horror of the Rosas regime.

The sensorial aspects of Sarmiento's language, his drive toward the poetry of prose, are ways to remind us that poetry from the time of antiquity keeps the body alive; it allows the return of the dead; it permits tattered bodies, victims of tyranny and oppression, to inhale new life through words. And indeed Sarmiento knows of the power of voice, of its impact on the body of others. Note, then, how Sarmiento records the voice of a man he encounters: "The voice of that honest and innocent man made every fiber in me tremble and reached my very bone" (2003, 56).[53] Here, it is not the communicative value of words but the phatic function of voice that vibrates on the listener's body. For its palpable effect on the body, it is akin to the orality belonging to bandits and gauchos. It is the voice that shapes the "democratic personality" that Nancy Ruttenberg (1998) once identified in the founding gestures of the preachers in the United States during the colonial period.

The ideal and the palpable are paradoxically joined to impact body and mind; it is as if to say, through the material features of voice and land, and through the intensity that they stir within us, that eventually we might be able to fashion ourselves as republican men. In other words, if we learn to forge links between the sounds, scents, and material effects of the land and the rhythms of the language we hear, we might also learn to configure an ideal, to allow thought to guide us to freedom.[54] So *Facundo* begins as a manual for learning to feel the pressure of enemy voices; it continues as a lesson on learning to see and hear.

Sarmiento's book projects a steady awakening to poetry that is stoked by the flames of rural adventure; but it also lumbers through the disorder of civil society, registering the din of unruly crowds, the obscenities of catcalls and unpleasant slogans. In this vein, Sarmiento asks us to identify cacophonous sounds and hear how they form the basis of meaning: he structures binomials in his text (civilization and barbarism, Argentines and Arabs, the Middle Ages and the nineteenth century) in order to break them down; he builds up the idea of narrative coherence only to destroy it, and he winds up with a textual form that defies adherence to any single genre. Neither novel nor essay, neither autobiography nor romance, neither political treatise nor melodrama, the ambitious prose of *Facundo* begs for an awareness of proximate and distant effects (of sound, voice, and matter) insofar as they startle the senses. It goes along with Sarmiento's appeal that we learn to listen and see. Not only does he make a point of teaching us to hear the sounds of nature, but he also teaches us to use our senses in order to perceive the tyrant's threats. So Sarmiento encourages his readers to distinguish between the colors of flags, to reject the crimson ribbon of Rosas, to identify the phrases and slogans that separate the despot's bluff from expressions of authentic freedom. "The apple of discord has to do with naming," Sarmiento tells us (2003, 127). And he goes on to explain: "I lie, the fun is not over yet: for Rosas has taken to calling his present and future enemies, 'savage, vile unitarists,' and twenty years from now, just as today all those who wear the label he has put on them are federalists, one will be born a *savage*, according to these stereotypes" (127). Naming, like the sound bites that will appear on media screens more than one hundred years later, centers a political debate. But Sarmiento gives a final lesson when he offers to the best observer and listener the grand rewards of freedom (and, for some, the power of state).

"¡¡¡Barranca Yaco!!!," chapter 9 of *Facundo*, offers a remarkable final episode in Facundo's life; it is the story of his murder. In this chapter, Facundo finds himself in Buenos Aires, where, despite his base inclinations, he acquires a certain sophisticated view that belongs to men of the city: he wears a jacket along with his poncho; he places his children in private school and obliges them to don the tailcoat; he takes on the airs of a gentleman and gains the respect of urban elites. But with this, he also loses his instinctive ways, a flaw that will cost him his life. The narrative has interesting twists leading to this denouement. From Buenos Aires, Facundo precipitously decides to travel west to Córdoba, although his lieutenants advise against it. Bullheaded and resistant to the counsel of others, Facundo refuses to hear. He thus departs on his journey. En route, his carriage is assaulted and Facundo is shot in the eye and killed by the bandit Santos Pérez. So what is the possible lesson in this conclusive example? Sarmiento reminds us of the importance of perceptual skills in order to survive in the nation. In the city, Facundo lost the intuitive alertness that had endowed his person in the outback. He forgot to listen to his perceptions that would have helped him survive. To be a successful leader, then, one must not let down one's guard. Absent the sensual alertness, no individuals in Argentina of the 1830s and 1840s have the chance to prevail.

In order to keep up with the demands of both civil society and life in the savage wild, one needs to awaken the affects and senses: on the one hand, to be attentive to signs of oncoming disaster, and on the other, *to see* the bodies and blood, *to feel* the weight of the corpses. "The words tyranny and despotism," Sarmiento writes, "awaken in the mind a painful memory; when pronounced, they make all the wounds bleed once again, reminding us of fifteen years of ongoing fright and fear" (2003, 242). This experience produces a language incarnate. From the assault on the body, a clamor eventually comes forth, rebelling against brutality and demanding political reform. "The voice will escape from the wound," Sarmiento observes in the final pages of *Facundo* (241).

A last observation about Sarmiento and his trials of perception: If Sarmiento wrote *Facundo* while in exile in Chile, distant from the action of civil war and from tyrants whom he had never encountered, he also understood that this gap had to be filled. Perforce, he needed to enter in direct contact with his opponent, to feel the breath of the enemy, to stare him in the eye. This need was realized in his later travels and is captured most notably in *Campaña en el ejército grande* (The grand army campaign), a book written while Sarmiento was on the trail with Urquiza fighting against the Rosas regime. This text is a composite book: it consists of letters, excerpts from earlier publications, travel reflections, chronicle, and memoir; it is diatribe, denunciation, and debate about military tactics in time of war. It is unevenly written, repetitive, dogmatic, and anecdotal, but it also exposes incomparable lyric moments as Sarmiento ventures through rural terrain. For the sensuality it captures, *Campaña en el ejército grande* evokes the travel genre; for the military planning, it tracks the mind of a man as he stakes out a claim on greatness; for the marvel the author expresses before landscapes of incomparable beauty, the text stands as an intimate diary of a key moment of personal transition. This is also a book that communicates the urgency of perceptions in mid-nineteenth-century culture. Sarmiento thus refers to optical games: he introduces the *gabinete óptico* in order to understand what he has seen; he evokes the name of Houdini to make a case for his sleight-of-hand talents. He reveals his interest in galvanism, electricity, and ether; and he obsesses about the telegraph and its ability to make words fly through space and time. These are all part of the nineteenth-century attempts to supplement the senses, to use technology and a host of prosthetic devices as tools to test for the body's weakness, and to register the shock of these sensual attractions upon our perceptual skills. But in Sarmiento's case, this exercise is not gratuitous. Rather, the sensual awareness lets him enter political life, as if mastery of the tricks of representation assured him control of political detail.

Travel literature allows us to take this material to a heightened mode of perception, to explore the engagement of the individual with an environment that is strikingly new, possibly dangerous, and always fit for adventure. A literature of attractions, perhaps more pertinent as a framework than the oft-cited "contact zone" that Mary Pratt (1992) used so efficiently to describe the colonial encounter, travel discourse allows the individual to speak from direct experience, to feel the pressure of new encounters and the challenge of the unexpected. From the prologue of his *Viajes por Europa, Africa i América* (Voyages through Europe, Africa, and America, 1849–1851), Sarmiento begins with the following words: "In the following pages, I offer my friends a miscellany of observations, reminiscences, impressions and incidents of travel.... They know that toward the end of 1845 I left Chile, with the goal of seeing with my very eyes and touching—to say it somehow—the state of primary instruction in nations that have made it a unit of public administration" (1993, 3). "To see and touch" (a phrase that Vicente Huidobro would later use for his own poems about the senses): that is, to come close to new experience, to capture materiality in its fullest dimensions (even if Sarmiento often invented scenes that never occurred or directly copied them from other written sources!).

The advantage of *Viajes* at this point in our chapter is to check on Sarmiento's aesthetic reflections on the senses, to show how he constructs an intermediary zone between the barbarism of *Facundo* and the wartime events of *Campaña en el ejército grande*. Written as a diary of his sea journey on both sides of the Atlantic, an adventure that, as the title indicates, took Sarmiento through Europe, Africa, and the Americas, *Viajes* gives remarkable evidence of Sarmiento's theory of perception. Of his travels through North Africa, he writes:

> The delicate tissue with which nature covers itself during nocturnal repose ... brought to the senses that sweet sleep that, ceasing to look outside, lets the imagination engage with memories and impressions, like a child who finds new objects within reach. Thought also has its spontaneous acts, and all the sensations transmitted by the brain, without use of our will, come forth in moments of rest, and are ordered by their affinities until they become part of our spirit and logic. . . . That way, the most practiced intelligence, when it faces a basic idea that it has digested for a very long time, takes paper, and effortlessly, a whole book is sculpted from a single piece the way a silkworm weaves golden threads. (1993, 199)

Sensation, first; absorption, second; finished book, third. Sarmiento maps out a plan not only for observation and writing, but also for locating a strategy to put his perceptions toward gain and profit. From the raw material of sensation, he writes a complex book. In this respect, Sarmiento insists on a temporal interval to allow for the work of the spirit to mature and engender, from the basic perceptual stock, a field of new ideas. Direct sensual encounter ("palpable and immediate" [199]) even allows the subject of these charges to invent a fantasy of the future. Introducing temporality and representation into the debate on perception, Sarmiento here exceeds the parameters of sense theory for his time. His is akin to a double vision, insofar as an isolated sensual experience extends itself and occupies multiple time schemes; it serves present, past, and future. We saw this in *Facundo* insofar as Sarmiento laid claim to an experience that he had never directly enjoyed (he described Argentina from the vantage of his exile in Chile), setting him on course to later events and later direct encounters. Travel literature, even more than *Facundo* in its hybrid state, sustains a coordinate between present and past; and we see this in *Viajes*. Here, Sarmiento observes a new event and likens it to the literature of previous eras. See, for example, Sarmiento standing at the edge of the Mount Vesuvius crater: "Two more steps and we were at the crater's edge, from which I could see—Oh horror!—What Titus saw in the Sanctum Sanctorum—nothing!"(1993, 246). The ruins produce a double focus: Sarmiento's immediate observations trigger a remembrance of the experiences of others that have been recorded in print. An event of retrospection, to be sure, but also a doubling of time. Analogies allow him to grapple with history and events, as Sarmiento displays affective memory as an effect of representation. Like the dioramas and optical cabinets,[55] the loose references to photographic images, or the abundant allusions to telegraphy—all present in Sarmiento's writings—sense stimulation is useful not only because it leads us to the soul or a rich interior life, but also because it situates the reader in the mirrored halls of repetitions and echoes that belong to the art of representation. Finally, in order for an experience to survive, it needs to be shared with a friend: "All the travelers to Italy try to find a friend. Since the object is to be moved by the spectacles of monuments and nature, the person who can't share with another the ideas and emotions he feels will have to die a martyr" (254–255). If you can't represent an event and convey the experience to another, the impact of the experience dissolves.

Among the textual strategies that travel literature puts in play, Sarmiento's *Viajes* allows him to tell his own experience and put his feelings onstage for readers. Here you can be honest and tell the truth or poach upon the described sensations of others and claim them as your own. More important, in the style of autobiography, the travel genre allows you to test the relationship between inner life and external sensation, and, ultimately, because it's written from afar—usually after the voyage—it allows you to test the limits of the copy, to expose the free play of representation. The travel journal thus helps Sarmiento to speak his perceptions, to differentiate among them, and to make a case for his view of difference; to register the shock of the new and bring it into line with known phenomena and events. Of course, the travel journal may be a simple excuse to compensate for the *horror vacui* of the moment, but it also shows the agency of the author as he exercises it on objects and landscapes. The travel journal is thus the perfect instrument to record perceptions and to project and measure personal experience within a broader horizon. It is also the perfect venue to launch a distant critique of home.

Charles Olson, writing on *Moby Dick*, observed, "I take space to be the central fact born to man in America" (1947, 1). His claim could be applied to any number of nineteenth-century texts that explored American frontiers, seeking out limits of civilization on the border with savage others. This literature of liminality, a defining moment in the Americas North and South, also depends on sensory perceptions that became entangled with rational forces. In this respect, Sarmiento's texts enjoy the fertile company of writers such as Poe and Melville. Poe, for example, in *The Narrative of A. Gordon Pym* (1838) describes an exploration of the New World South that is adrift in perceptual excitement. Full of cannibalism and a mutinous plot, the sea adventure is a sensual affair, testing the effects of shock. “We had seen and felt; but we could neither think nor act” (1914, 9:108), Poe’s narrator tells us toward the end of the novel, putting the materiality of sensual prompts on a par with the materiality of writing. The blood and gore of the explorer’s travel plot is recuperated by the letter in blood. A novel that in 1838 competed with the travel accounts of Darwin, whose famous voyage took him around the coast of Tierra del Fuego, and that anticipated *Moby Dick* by more than a decade, *Gordon Pym* organizes a pastiche of sensations, leaving us with an intense awareness of not only the experience of the new and palpable but also the materiality of writing.

In the various texts that make up *Campaña en el ejército grande*, Sarmiento also gives his readers a literature of intensities and effects. On the surface, it would appear that Sarmiento has no intention of engaging in travel accounts (his *Viajes*, after all, more than covers this genre), but takes on instead the role of lowly “reporter,” a man with a political axe to grind against both Urquiza and Rosas. Sarmiento’s memoirs become a sturdy testament to the experience of war and power, and to the dreadful personalities that form part of the political opposition. Like *Facundo*, *Campaña* is a hybrid text in search of order. In both, Sarmiento tries to shape experience and assign a name to power. But *Campaña* is less about the historical past than about actual experience, relocating perceptions in both the warring body and the competing body of texts that describe it. Toward that end, we are made sensitive to the unevenness of the trials of military conflict; we come to hear the sounds of destruction, we learn to hear the rabble, we are taught to smell the body of the filthy Urquiza as he advances in the campaign, we read of the perceptions of a man who listens for the cry of macaws (Sarmiento 1998, 234). We even hear the fussy voice of Sarmiento as his adversaries would hear it: he is, according to Urquiza, a “squealing reporter” (283); he is, of his own admission, “a buzz in the ear of Rosas” (107). These allusions to preverbal sounds are triggers of meaning; they alert the audience to a need for change, they signal a call for rebellion. They emphasize the power of voice and ways to make oneself heard. Sounds are also accompanied by the nonrepresentational experience of the horror we feel when we perceive that death surrounds us. Sarmiento thus alerts us to the pestilence of rotting corpses (234); he shows us scenes of mass execution (told from the perspective of the women who avert their eyes before the theater of blood); he also describes the noise of the parades that welcome soldiers to Buenos Aires. “Shots, furious shouts and threats of decapitation, with accompanying drums and bugles, were enough to warn the ‘savages’ of the dangers of their critical voice and to put the entire population in a state of consternation," he writes (91). Moreover, we see the red ribbon as a sign of Rosas's control, and in these cases, we are asked without fail to abhor it (226). The red tag, or *cinta colorada*, so important in *Facundo*, is also a leitmotif in *Campaña*; it is a color that Sarmiento refuses to wear insofar as he links the color red to the Rosas regime. There's logic behind this choice, he explains; the color red holds sensual danger. In this regard, he writes: "God made the leaves of the trees green; if he had wanted them to be red, he would have given us different eyes; because with the eyes we have, red tires us and all the more makes us suffer" (237).[56] By showing how the color red fatigues the senses, he also proves that the tyrant Rosas dishonors the norms of nature.

The tirade against Rosas continues throughout the pages of *Campaña* as Sarmiento signals the cast of misperceptions that always leads Rosas astray. In one case, he gives the example of Rosas trying to fill the swamps on his land by altering the flow of water (222). Unless you attune your senses to nature, Sarmiento points out to his readers, you can never change the landscape, nor will you triumph in history. Less philosophically, Sarmiento also shows Rosas as a man bereft of common sense insofar as he ignores measures of weight and balance. Sarmiento thus tells the story of Rosas, who has ordered his soldiers to lighten their loads. No, Sarmiento claims, Rosas has no idea of the necessary dynamics of transport: "To take the backpack away from the soldier is to remove a mechanical counterweight that he balances against his gun" (188–189). In order to render politics visible, you have to touch its physical expression. And from the mismatched weights and improper exercises that Rosas demands of his soldiers, Sarmiento accumulates sufficient proof to signal his opponent's faulty perceptions; Rosas is deficient not only in sensual detail but also in tactics of war.[57]

Worse still, on the battlefront, Rosas deprives his soldiers of normal affections. Sarmiento reports that the *rosista* troops fail to respond to the rain and cold, or to stimuli on the flesh; they execute orders like corpses on guard, while their lofty commander refuses to show any sign of respect for the bodily needs of recruits: "To kill and to die. This was the only faculty awakened among this immense family of bayonets and regiments. What was Rosas for these men? Or better, what kind of beings had he made of the men who joined his ranks? He turned them into statues, into passive machines to endure the sun, rain, brutal weather, temptations of the flesh, with instincts only to kill and to receive the blow of death" (138). Rosas suppresses the positive aspects of a sensual world that Sarmiento, by contrast, upholds. Only with the end of the Rosas regime will men be able to mount a horse and travel; only with Rosas's end can men return to sensual awakenings that correspond to peace and freedom; only with Rosas's retreat will the soldiers return to a full set of physical responses. You could say that state oppression shuts down the range of senses, whereas liberty promises to rouse them.

The military mission allows Sarmiento to report on his direct experience in war, to overcome his bookish character. His travel thus becomes an affair of the senses as he delivers himself to nature. But he's of two minds about this adventure. After all, in the countryside, sense perceptions are separate from the intellect. In the country, we are animallike and unthinking, only receptive to sensory prompts. In this regard, Sarmiento writes: "So the impressions pass through the senses without leaving a trace on the spirit: one vegetates, changes place, without realizing what really matters. . . . Where am I? I asked myself, without being able to shake off the lethargy in which I was immersed" (101–102). Sarmiento thus needs a supplement to sense work in order to feel less estranged and, ultimately, to discover his purpose. Finally, after describing a long list of places he's seen ("observing what my eyes could see, and what my ears could hear" [103]), he comprehends his mission: "I'm again traveling through the lands in search of a teaching tool for the *pueblo*" (103). It would appear that direct experience is most expedient if it leads us to a political truth. Listen, in this respect, to his reflections in the concluding pages of his notebook:

> I touched all things up close, I witnessed all the events, I treated all the actors in the drama and, owing to a rare combination of circumstances, I was able to put myself in all the vantage points from which the events could be seen; from the East, when I lived in Montevideo; from Entrerríos, where I took the side of the General Urquiza; from the military position, in Buenos Aires, where I could see the troops as they traveled to Rio de Janeiro; and from Chile, whence I could see the negative effects upon the provinces. From all these points of view, I found one thing alone, and that is that the General was obstinately causing trouble, raising obstacles when there were none; he was devoted to destroying everything he could, and forcing everything—events, men and matter—to become hostile to him. (292)

From life on the front lines, Sarmiento saw the war up close and was able to reach an insight; it allowed him to denounce the villainous generals and expose their wayward actions. In this respect, his memoir is used to keep our eyes trained on the dangerous other in order to attack and defeat him; but Sarmiento also focuses on the need to alert Argentina to the extent of the damage done. We have to construct the body of the other (the body of the human enemy and the body of the landscape), as well as the liberal body of the person who uses the capacity of sensory perception. Here, the goal is to show Sarmiento as a perceptive and quick-fire machine.

For his commanding perceptual acumen, he issues a powerful phrase, reminding us of Caesar: "I saw, I heard, I acted" ("Yo vi, yo oí, yo hice" [119]). Similarly, he often writes, "I've seen it with my own eyes" (118), a sign of authenticity and presumable control. The map is a satisfactory device for representation, but real, close-up experience gives him a deeper sense of the land: the sounds, the dew, the shrieking macaws, the scent of dying embers all serve to prove the author's presence on the march. The experience fills the time of waiting, waiting for tyrants to fall:

> We camped a bit further on, the night was powerful, and until very late, I savored the nocturnal spectacle of the Pampas, silent despite its 15,000 guests, my surroundings illuminated by the bivouac fires, which at a distance resembled a flame that intermittently scarred the horizon. The scent of wild vegetation, moistened by dew, the shout of a few aquatic birds, an uncertain harmony within the silence; that infinite extension gives the Pampa a certain solemn majesty, which seduces, attracts, imposes fear, and awakens our melancholia. The spectacle was new for me, and I continued to enjoy it without ever feeling sated. (190)

Sarmiento also turns this into a lesson about the value of seeing and hearing, which allows him to dig deep into nature where his perceptions most certainly guide him, but where he also takes the sensual prompts to find his way through the war campaign.

Jonathan Crary (1990) tells us that the early nineteenth century produces a new kind of observer, overturning classical space. No longer does the observer respond to prescribed sets of possibilities; rather, modernization attacks our sense of experience with novelty and speed, and with various motion devices that test the power of vision. "Modernization is a process by which capitalism uproots and makes mobile that which is grounded, clears away or obliterates that which impedes circulation, and makes exchangeable what is singular," Crary writes (1990, 10). Viewed in

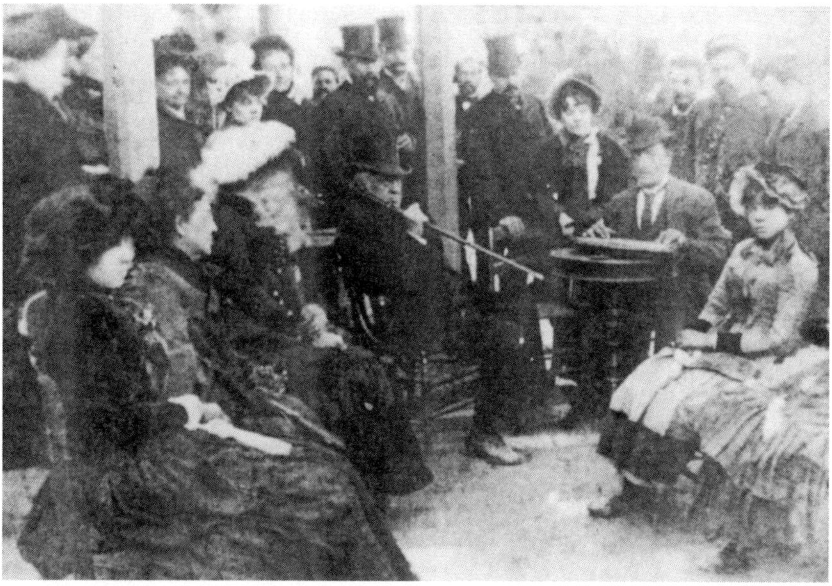

Figure 1.3. Sarmiento with his hearing trumpet, undated. Archive of La gaceta.

this way, modernization forces us to reimagine alternative landscapes of the real; it lifts all anchors and leaves us floating in the present. It also leads us to rethink the effects of war and military advances in sustaining one's quest for control.

The war apparatus makes the sensate field palpable and present and proves, through Sarmiento's interventions and descriptions of what he perceives, that *his authority will prevail* in politics and cultural life. From the floating present, he begins to imagine a future. But there's another point worth noting. The silent body of the nation also needs awakening; it needs men to come to their senses. It is a wake-up call for freedom. And here Tulio Halperin Donghi is insightful when he writes in his introduction to *Campaña* that Sarmiento's turn to polemical words is designed to move against "the immobile and obstinately mute body of the nation" (in Sarmiento 1998, 53). The *pueblo* needs to learn to listen, to see the present disasters of the Rosas regime; they need to break the range of expression that keeps them between noise and silence (Sarmiento 1998, 286). Dissatisfied with what he hears, however, Sarmiento seeks out new voices.

In this respect, and writing seven years after *Facundo*, Sarmiento is the new *baqueano* of the nation, the backwoods scout who informs his readers about how to walk through hostile terrain. His task in this fragmented memoir is to make sense of *broken* letters, teaching us to feel the *broken* body of men, and to experience the *broken* nation that needs one day to be whole. Another way of saying this is to remark that the body that belonged to barbarism is now possessed by civilization.[58] And as readers, we join in community with the *bolitinero*; we experience violence together through his disordered textual form, and learn to find a voice to spread the news. But the irony of Sarmiento's lifelong tale about perceptions lies elsewhere, appearing at the close of his presidency (1868–1874) when he is left in deafening silence (Nelle 1993, 66). With a nearly complete hearing impairment, deprived of the voices of others, Sarmiento loses his ability to understand the national community that he tried to build throughout his career. He misses the sound of the assassin's bullets that nearly take his life; but, more important, at this crucial stage, he fails as *baqueano*. As he loses his sense of hearing, he misses the call of the *pueblo* that he so intently attempted to rally.

Comparing Senses

This brings me to a final reflection on the role of the perceptual enterprise in shaping the political arena of the nineteenth century. Here I take loosely from Davide Panagia, who tells us that in the first act of nation building, the work of the perceiving body is both political and aesthetic; in the second act, however, perceptions come to stimulate reason and move the individual forward into contact with others (2009, 9). As we have seen in the span between the early philosophy teachers and the midcentury writings of Sarmiento, sensual alertness was evoked time and again to build community and contact, to set the nation on course. But this model fails to suffice in all historical settings. And here we need to acknowledge that the reflections on sensation were never consistent over geographic divides; rather, they responded to different social crises and the necessities of political encounters. In this regard, we are not dealing with a universal body, but bodies that are particular and present, tied to specific moments of political change and history. That said, let me return to the comparative measures that I promised at the start of this chapter.

Keeping aware of the articulation of the perceptual field as it was shaped around political challenge, I want to note briefly a few scenes from the United States, covering the period from independence through to the mid-nineteenth century insofar as they correspond to the Argentine discursive alignments covered in these pages. Consider, for example, the sensual experience that guides Jefferson as he outlines a plan for the state of Virginia, or the detail for architectural design that corresponds to his gaze upon Monticello;[59] think of the sense work that directs Cooper's trailblazers, those who need to hear and see their surroundings in order to clear space for the nation; or recall the work of Thoreau and Emerson, who sought to open their senses to nature, while at the same time, the abolitionist writers (most notably Frederick Douglass) sought to put visceral images of degradation and torture within grasp of their mass-market readers. The gothic excess of nineteenth-century fiction, as Leslie Fiedler once wrote, displaces onto the somatic realm all the conflicts of interiority far before psychoanalysis would eventually name them; it emerges along with the shock-and-awe thrills driving circuses, carnivals, and medicine shows, along with spectacles of popular ritual, in all cases shaking the public to its core with hope, illusion, and promise, or providing sufficient distraction to relieve them of their despair. On the surface, it would seem that the US writers followed a sensationalist course similar to their Spanish American confreres insofar as both linked the world of perceptions with their hopes for democracy and communal experience. But this fails to explain the differences between them.

In pursuit of this distinction, let me briefly allude to Melville. A tortured and solitary man, aggrieved by the deplorable state of a nation enslaved, Melville explored the range of perceptual skills that life on the sea demanded; but in a more quiet way, and distinct from his Latin American colleagues, he also used perceptions to explore the depths of the soul. And in *Moby Dick*, as he delved into the human reach of the sea-bound crew, Melville linked the sailors in a communal tie through the perceptions and instincts they shared, while he also created a literary text based on the sensate body. An embodied cognition is central to *Moby Dick*, and its effects have been noted by many. D. H. Lawrence, for example, writing of *Moby Dick*, shows that Melville depends on "a bodily knowledge [that] moves naked" with a "sheer physical vibrational sensitiveness, like a marvelous wireless station" in order to register the "effects of the outer world" (qtd. in Otter and Sanborn 2011, 3). Though hyperbole may dictate Lawrence's phrasing, what is certain is the sensual power that affects both the bodies represented in the book as well as the body of its textual form. *Moby Dick* is a novel that demands attention to the pulsations of rhythm and form along with the bodily pulsations of the characters who take the novel to its final explosion.[60] It may be that Melville, like Sarmiento, crafted an art from the thunder of the sentence as well as from the liquid flow that courses through human and animal bodies.[61] We might say that just as he dissects the monster's body, with its layers of bone and flesh, he also dissects the corpus of literary history in hopes of reaching its soul and meaning.

On the *Pequod*, the men are introduced as bodies: they are the eyes and ears and hands and legs that make the sailing enterprise go forward. Their sensibility—their anxiety before the threat of the whale, their perception of the shifting winds and currents that signal present danger, and their longing for home and family—puts them on alert; it is their check against the absolute power that belongs to Captain Ahab. Their sensory awareness and regard for each other stand in contrast to the destructive force of their captain; what's more, these scenes allow Melville to build a critique of power. Unlike Sarmiento, who claimed in good regard that sense work was the necessary step for seizing power from tyrants, Melville shows us the abuses of sense work in a figure like Ahab, who uses his thrashing authority in order to argue his right to be right.

But there is a second consideration that agitated both Melville and Sarmiento. Both make much of the signs of identity that are found on the body: Sarmiento studies the wounds on the flesh that will eventually produce a voice; Melville studies the tattoos on Queequeg or the scars on the body of the whale, constructing a history of violence along with signs of self-affirmation. But for both writers, it's not entirely certain that the markers have transcendent meaning. "Signs taken for wonders," that celebrated phrase of Melville, also calls for reader perplexity: Perhaps the signs lack the symbolic force that we hope for? Through our use of signs, will we fail at representation? Or is the valance of perception beyond the scheme of signs? And can the single sign explain the complexity of an interior life full of conflicts? And finally, is there a grade of physical human cruelty that exceeds symbolic form?

Here, recall the famous doubloon scene in which Ahab dissuades his crew of sailors of the certainty of their own perceptions. In the hope of buying his sailors' allegiance through the promise of gold, Ahab disabuses them of their sensual alertness and their finely tuned perceptions. Only the captain can lay claim to authentic perceptions of nature; he is the only one (or so he claims) who reads the winds, who understands the seascape. The others must follow in the path of their indefatigable leader. This scene may be an allegory for Melville's preoccupation with slavery in the United States in 1851, a commentary on the ways in which bodies are moved around like bulk without attention to the mind or soul. As if to tell a counternarrative that runs against the tales of Sarmiento, Melville offers another fable when he tells us that the despot who halts the perceptual alacrity of the masses severs the popular connection stretched through each individual's internal world. This action will only lead to disaster and announce collective doom.

The relationship between the body and the collective was the topic of philosophical inquiry especially from the time of the Enlightenment through the nineteenth century. David Bates, writing on the political body, observes:

> The body was now understood as an effort to defend and preserve the association of free individuals who made it up. The political was therefore inherently legal; it required a certain institutional embodiment so that it could act in the world. This embodiment was defined *not* as a capacity to represent or articulate a preexisting will or set of interests but instead as a genuine process of integration and decision. . . . There is no general will of the political community until a series of institutions make possible that synthetic operation and then deploy it through the body. (2012, 212)

Melville's doubloon scene in *Moby Dick* brings this together as much as Sarmiento's commentary in *Campaña en el ejército grande*, where Sarmiento insists on a unified body in order to heal the nation. Both would seem to acknowledge the corporeal basis of knowing and the value of the collective voice. And when they show that adversarial relations among men are represented as disputes about sensual perceptions, they dismount the abstract basis of power and forge a path beyond universal abstraction. Nevertheless, the paths of these two great canonical figures separate at this point in the story, for while Melville exposes the abuses of perception instantiated by Captain Ahab, Sarmiento evokes perceptual skills to *bring himself to power*; the community of men who are joined through sensation can only serve to advance his mission. Melville establishes his critique of power by revealing Ahab's relentless drive and by acknowledging that the strength of democracy lies among an assembly of workers. Perhaps we can say by contrast and in regard to Sarmiento's case that it all goes back to himself; his narcissus guides his motley ship, whereas Melville plumbs the communal soul. The success of Sarmiento's discourse leads him to become president in 1868, while Melville, the son of a revolutionary officer in the war for independence, will later sink into near oblivion.

Or perhaps we can say that the conditions of war in midcentury Latin America were not yet focused on an interior life, or that intellectuals failed to uncover the conduits that could in fact lead to the spirit. In the long run, the sense work of Latin American literature translates the foundational violence of a political reality out of sync with social need. It captures the litter of undead corpses or of ghosts inhabiting social spaces that should have belonged to the living. From its fractured textual form and unrelieved attention to bodies in pain, Latin American literature maintains its open wounds, which—as Sarmiento said—were the signals to awaken a voice for the nation.

The Argentine philosopher and statesman Juan Bautista Alberdi, lamenting the effects of the civil wars and the slow modernization of Argentina, expressed his dismay about the impoverished reality of Latin American life: "Isn't it time that South American history has more than accounts of its war and its soldiers, as we know up to this point?" (1876, 4). But he also launched an invidious comparison with the United States, and in particular with New England: Argentines should imitate New England men for their intelligence and perseverance ("To study men of that cut; copy them, repeat their acts; be like them, advance like them, worry like them: this is the way to introduce and acclimate South America to the society of the North" [297–298]).

Alberdi's New England pastoral was never realized in his lifetime, but he carried with him a number of important texts that guided him toward an appreciation of nature and its ruins. As he told in his autobiography, "Mi vida privada," first Rousseau and then Volney were available in his personal library in order to take him, when solace was sought, beyond the lessons of Condillac and Locke; they carried him to a natural space not yet devastated by cities or war. They pressed him toward a sensual appreciation of nature that was far from the maddening crowd (Alberdi 1900, 294–295). Second, his nostalgic reflections on his native Tucumán (dating from 1834) were dedicated to the quiet refuge that nature supplies, to the simple appeal to perceptions of light, sound, and color: "For the son of a warring nation, whose history is full of sad and glorious memories, this music has incomparable force!" (1900, 329). In the final appeal of this essay, he confessed a desire for the memories of his childhood landscape;

he also hoped that Argentine men might partake of life in the outback and the sensual relief it provides.

Truth be told, Alberdi's hopes were frustrated time and again, and indeed we find few Argentine writers in the nineteenth century who followed the pastoral path free of political mission. For this reason, William Henry Hudson, the Anglo–Latin American writer whom I mentioned at the start of this chapter, the man who found in the preindustrial world of Argentina a grand melancholic enchantment, occupies a special role for Argentine intellectuals even today. Hudson found in recovered sensation a way to return to the past, a way to touch the wilderness of the mind as his last frontier. It allowed him to assume the identity of the woodsman without ulterior goal.

Hudson learned from the English romantics that the imagination grows in nature, and that nostalgia is the pathway leading to the full differentiation of the senses in order to capture the past. *Nostos* plus *algos*: to return, but with burning pain. To feel through remembrance and to experience loss in the flesh. Sensual perception, as Nadia Seremetakis observes, becomes a way to link the body to the experience of history (1994, 3–4). And Hudson, in this respect, gives a legend of sense material in order to grasp from London the distant Argentine past. His books skirt the civil conflicts that surrounded his days in the River Plate, and instead they turn to the countryside for sustenance and prolonged reflection. Patagonia, Río Negro, and rural Uruguay are all part of his autobiographical accounts. Above all, these are provincial areas that bring time to a halt, detaining a common sensual memory that overrides division and war. In order to think in this way, Hudson necessarily fled from the military actions for which he was deliberately recruited; he also forgot the colonial legend of Britain's stake in the distant South (this is the gist of Hudson's novel *The Purple Land*). With these disavowals, announced loud and clear, Hudson could then move back to barbarism and find his place in nature.

I asked at the beginning of this chapter why Hudson offered such great appeal to Argentines in the late twentieth and early twenty-first centuries. Perhaps it is due to a flight from violence of the kind that Sarmiento knew, a violence that pervaded national life from the time of the conquest and lasted well into the dictatorships of the 1970s and 1980s. Perhaps Hudson's Patagonian world allowed a retreat from the unending political struggle that the body must endure; for Hudson, the *locus amoenus* of sensual pleasures was both a respite and a promised cure, a place where, after so many failed encounters that a return to action promised, Hudson finally could surrender to the tranquility of a bookish imagination and incorporate innocent details of nature to awaken his sentient self. It's no surprise, in all of this, that Hudson's most devoted Argentine reader was Borges, a man who renounced the truculence of political debate and the intrigues of national power, a man who turned the tale of the trailblazer into a reader of signs and who in the end sought to sustain the body through incessant puzzles of mind.

CHAPTER 2

Troubled by Gender

Technology and Perception in the Women's Nineteenth Century

It's as if there were an electric wire between us.

MARIQUITA SÁNCHEZ DE THOMPSON

How can you shut your eyes and ears?

HARRIET BEECHER STOWE

In *Extravagancias de 1834* (Extravagances of 1834), César Hipólito Bacle, a Swiss-born lithographer residing in Buenos Aires during the years of the Rosas regime, played enticingly with the details of local custom that defined Argentina. In effect, during the early years of the Argentine civil wars, while Echeverría was writing about filth and disorder, Bacle turned his attentions to daily folk and urban life and the cult of women's fashion. Among the prints and engravings included in this last collection, the series on the woman's *peinetón*, or hair comb, continues to provoke critical interest.[1] In this sequence, Bacle poked fun at the excesses of feminine fashion, ridiculing the disproportionate head ornaments that attracted female fancy in the 1830s. The images pointed to women's persistent devotion to style, signaling their desire to be up-to-date regardless of the rules of decorum; in particular, the artist toyed with the female desire to see and conversely to be seen by others. But the lithographs also guide us toward a new sensibility with which women challenged the limitations of physical space; the images invite us to behold an emerging realm of the sensible that invaded nineteenth-century life.

Take the image in which a worker must break open the wall of a home so that the señora with her *peinetón* might gain access to the street (see plate 4). For a start, the print shows domestic space as little more than a jail (the window rails on the left side of the frame, in addition to the building's exposed-brick walls, loudly bespeak enclosure); but it also invites the viewer to *feel* the prison of fashion to which women have devoted themselves. Hence, the dark colors of the home break open to brightness and light; one needs to parade in public in order to capture the zest of the times. Here Bacle isn't shy about his opinions: as if to announce that the trend is rampant, he draws a second head comb, equally as expansive as the first, that takes over the full space of the scene. The volume and extension of the *peinetón* compete with the weight of bricks; the accessory invades the city streets and fills the airspace and ground. But there's more to this discussion. As if the first lithograph were not sufficient to expose this trendy accoutrement, in a second print (see plate 5), Bacle takes the joke in another direction, pointing not so much to the weight of the hair comb, with its prodigious extension on earth, but to its winged resemblance; the *peinetón* lifts the female subject above land, free from gravity's shackles. As the woman is rendered weightless, an instrument of flight, the *peinetón* now carries a force that eludes the gentlemen below. There's a wistful commentary here; the women in these images lack the very agency that would allow them to regain their physical bearings. Sailing through the sky, they become the objects of general laughter in Buenos Aires life.

In short form, and despite the laughter that these images provoke, Bacle's prints point to a new Argentine style in formation. They also signal the constant mobility and change that new sensorial effects engender. Indeed, as Argentine women pursue the ends of fashion, everything is set into movement. As an archeological document, then, or a clip of peripheral history, the *peinetón* invites a reflection on the engagement of women with their environs while also revising the boundaries of public and private spheres. In this regard, we see bodies pressing on obstacles: against walls, on doorways, on the stones separating home and street; we see bodies working against the laws of gravity that contain women and keep them close to earth. While these pressures mark the physical space where flesh encounters the resistance of matter, they offer new scenes for staging somatic experience in the nineteenth century. They show the feminine presence as a challenge to the regime of the senses that had been set in place by men.

In general terms, the nineteenth century brings Americans North and South into a world of technological invention: machines and scientific devices affect the work of the senses. This is seen grosso modo in the major transformations of industrial production, but also in the small-scale gadgets that enhanced the body's capacities to perceive and feel. With a dazzling set of tools—cameras, stereoscopes, lithographic reproductions, and a variety of telephonic devices—image and sound were reproduced in unusual ways, yielding a new kind of observer who understood that signs might be infinitely copied as they traveled through time and space. This replaced the "old" way of looking in which the auratic singularity of an image or sound enjoyed prestige and value. Now, even the mechanics of image or sound reproduction tended to excite the senses. Photography, as an example, became the great "democratic leveler" (Crary 1990, 13), allowing the multitude access to images and sights of experiences far out of their reach; it exceeded the direct and singular contact that the "live" image demanded.[2] Bacle's prints, as prime examples of the new lithographic techniques of the first half of the nineteenth century,[3] served to capture the multiple experiences of cultural life, reproducing them in extended series for a wider public. Of course, this carried consequences for politics and everyday existence.

The war machine, as we saw in chapter 1, set the tone and direction for a kind of technological base dominated by a need for the rapid communication of events (notably through telegraphy), a means for efficient transport (vehicles to move provisions and people), and lenses of amplification to sight the distant enemy in the battle camps beyond.[4] But there's another field to consider. If it is true, as Jonathan Crary and others have told us, that new contrivances resulted in an epistemic shift, or as Crary calls it, "a new set of relations" between the body and the observing subject (1990, 3), then it is also true that the nineteenth century gave wide attention to the ways in which gendered bodies interacted with new technologies of the times. Of course, domestic appliances were never far from the imagination. It is reported, for example, that the Rumford stove and chimney (invented in Massachusetts in 1790) was quickly brought into Buenos Aires by the soap makers Cerviño and Vieytes, and placed in homes of the city by the empresarial family of Manuel Belgrano under the colonial regime (Halperin Donghi 2014, 80). This was followed by the introduction of the sewing machine and the gas lamp, which women considered as required necessities for the home. That said, later innovations of the century—appealing to sight and sound, to communications and reading, to movement and temporal shifting—more notably captured attention, exciting the imaginations of women on both sides of the hemispheric divide. With reason, then, the Peruvian Clorinda Matto de Turner, in her important cultural journal *Búcaro americano*, celebrated the technological age of the *fin de siglo* as a moment dominated by new invention and by none other than the man she identified as "Edison, the Marvelous" (Matto de Turner 1906, 639).[5] Many events intervened from the time of Bacle's prints until the age of Edison, but one thing is certain: women stood by as observers, consumers, and critics of the novelties set before them, and eventually they took on a role for themselves as creative voices for change. Far from conforming to Bacle's images of ridiculous women in flight, female journalists like Matto de Turner carved a clear role for themselves as protagonists in modern life. They considered science and female education, philosophical materialism and fashion. As a whole, they assembled a chorus of laments about a world of inventions over which they held scant power. But they also sustained the perceptual advances that new technological networks enhanced.

Throughout the nineteenth century, trains, telegraphs, and telephones captured female attention. In the *Album de señoritas* from 1854, the Argentine editor Juana Manso de Noronha celebrated these innovations: "The creation of the electric telegraph would closely follow the inauguration of the train and the other marvels of civilization.... Onward!" (Manso de Noronha 1854b, 59). Though the first telegraphic link (between Buenos Aires and Montevideo) would not commence until 1866, Manso waited with eager anticipation. A world traveler who spent many years in Brazil, she cast an envious eye on progress abroad and hoped for modernization in Argentina. But she also had a political agenda. A longtime friend of Sarmiento and in tune with his plans for progress, Manso praised the achievements of the liberal post-Rosas years, and especially anticipated the arrival of foreign inventions on Argentine shores that would credit Sarmiento's authority: "With a little activity, within two months, we will have gaslight; in two years, with a bit of goodwill, the trains will begin to extend their routes into our open and uninhabited country" (1854a, 21). The railroad entered Argentina belatedly in 1857, but because it had been working elsewhere (in England since 1825, in France since 1832), its imminent arrival excited the imagination of Manso; and because of Sarmiento's many references to the need for rail services in Argentina, her interest in the train was all the more persistent. In another column, she also showed enthusiasm for the first steamships to sail South American rivers: "On January 1, 1853, the steamship was inaugurated on the inland rivers of America that connect Brazil, Peru and Bolivia.... In South America, the first signs of the *Silent Revolution* were given: to defeat the tyrants forever and kill the seeds of fratricidal wars" (1854d, 24).

Along with the train and the steamship, the new contraptions that harvested image and light also attracted compelling interest. The daguerreotype, the magic lantern, the photograph, and the stereoscope extended their appeal to women readers. Widely considered the foundational female voice of liberal Argentina, Mariquita Sánchez de Thompson, who pitied women for their lack of strength and turned to masculine valor as a sustaining model, wrote consistently about new discoveries in the technological landscape.[6] In 1840, she observed the advantages of the daguerreotype, of recent invention the year before:

> Yesterday we saw a marvel. The execution of the daguerreotype is admirable. Try to imagine a camera obscura in which you place a plate already loaded with the proper additives. The plate is like brilliant silver. Once in place, you set in the direction you want and in six minutes you remove it and add another substance, using a thermometer to check the temperature you need . . . and then, after all these precautions, you see on the plate the landscape you had focused upon: it is as if you had sketched it with a black pen with a perfection and likeness that would be impossible to obtain through other means. You can see the smallest objects with great detail; you even see the mortar between the bricks and the luster on the limestone walls as if you had looked through a magnifying glass. What an object of meditation! How ignorant we are! (Sánchez de Thompson 2003, 168–169)

The quoted passage shows a fascination with technology as well as a desire to be à la page. Sánchez de Thompson is arrested by the novel properties of the photograph and also by the depth of detail that the new invention affords. Here, the mechanical device surpasses the strength of the human eye.

Several decades later, and also in praise of scientific advances, Juana Manuela Gorriti, the main female creative writer and journalist of the Argentine nineteenth century, invited a colleague to share with her the thrill of scientific progress. In *La alborada del Plata*, Gorriti's famous cultural review for women, we read the following unsigned article:

> The expectation of success fuels the spirit of research. Man gained confidence in himself and took a valiant chance on the most daring endeavors: he took up a detailed study of nature and he multiplied and perfected his means of observation: the *microscope* put him in possession of infinitely small beings; the *telescope* shrank large distances;

> the *chronometer* measured time; the *barometer* and *thermometer* measured moment by moment the variations of atmospheric pressure and temperature. Man studied matter with a powerful will of experimentation, and matter revealed another world of unknown phenomena. ("La ciencia" 1877, 9–10)

Like Mariquita Sánchez, Gorriti also found personal pleasure in the new technological advances. In one of her many letters to Ricardo Palma, she wrote on September 7, 1885: "The telegraph keeps us up-to-date with political news from around the world" (2004, 16). And in a second missive to her Peruvian friend, on December 28, 1885, she explained that telegraphy kept her abreast of news specifically from across the Andes: "The telegrams kept me up-to-date with the news on [an] hour-by-hour basis. In that way, we know everything—perhaps without all the details—but we find out what we want to know" (18).

Just as the daguerreotype drew the attention of Mariquita Sánchez in the 1840s, Gorriti was also taken with photography and its power to shock the observer. Although the technology wasn't new in Argentina—aerostats and the first daguerreotypes were in use by 1845, and journalistic photography was utilized in the war in Paraguay (Alexander 2005)—it continued to attract the attentions of those who were interested in modern devices to capture image and action. In a letter of the 1880s, Gorriti wrote: "I will send you some photographs with my letter. Meanwhile, get ready to fill your curiosity with these new villages of the pampa; they are no longer raw and empty, but now populated by colonies and cities" (2004, 42). Photography facilitated the exchange of strange and arcane knowledge; it sent local information across transnational borders; it let individuals catch a glimpse of conditions of life as they were experienced in distant lands. It awakened the appetites of the senses and kept people up-to-date.

Finally, there was sound technology, which was a source of fascination from the time of independence. Just as the telegraph was largely employed by diplomats and men at the war front—it was first introduced by the Paraguayan army in the War of the Triple Alliance (Buch and Solivérez 2011, 190)—photography later came to the service of women, as Gorriti's letter shows. At the same time, other sound technologies were deployed in the interest of community, used by both men and women. Take an article from Sarmiento regarding the transatlantic cable. In an oft-cited passage from 1874, he conveys his awe for the new transatlantic connection between Europe and the Americas: "We behold an event so important that if earth and land had sensible feeling, they would tremble with pleasure as they felt their molecules traversed by the grains of human thought coursing through electrical currents" (Sarmiento 1899, 374).[7] When in proximity of the near-erotic vibrations sustained by the teletyped message, all of nature quivers; human thought, acquiring sound and movement, cuts through earth and sea. But Sarmiento's proposal also hints at a reversal, an inverse personification: as land and water pulse ahead and acquire feeling, human thought is streamed through wire. In this transposition that occurs in the sensual world owing to invention, Sarmiento finds a source of joy. What is absent here is a sense of rebellion that these new technologies might stir in the hearts of listeners; also lacking is an obvious use of sense stimulation to test the rule of state. This would change as the century advanced.

By the *fin de siglo*, the first telephone cables were set between Buenos Aires and Montevideo. This dramatic step toward modernization occurred in 1889, fully two years before one could communicate by phone between London and Paris (Buch and Solivérez 2011, 325). Indeed, telephony was everywhere in the popular imagination, and women journalists were no exception in writing about the new invention in their weekly columns. Caught between expressions of wonder and a cynical laughter about the confusion that voice transmissions might trigger, they wrote repeatedly about this intriguing new cable for voice. Clorinda Matto de Turner, for example, insistently gave playful attention to this modern invention. In a column entitled "Teléfono" (Telephone) appearing in *Búcaro americano* from its inaugural year and then continuing as a feature throughout the magazine's nine-year run, Matto de Turner tested the power of telephony not only to capture the banalities shared over long-distance wire, but also to shift the identities of speakers and confuse those who listened in. Lost voices, mismatched names, and missteps in social graces all emerged from the novel experience of voice as heard through a machine. But in another vein, and beyond the playfulness that the telephone inspired, Matto de Turner also offered a considerable evaluation of the public-health benefits and hazards presented by technology in her time.[8] On the third anniversary of *Búcaro americano*, Matto de Turner grandly praised the successful inventions that changed daily life not without a critical eye:

> The sewing machine saved the lungs of women from consumption while mechanical progress . . . created new jobs that were not necessarily healthy.

> The electric current of civilization . . . reveals a new redemptive power: it saves the horse that had been tied to the wheels of a streetcar, a bit like the image of avaricious throngs who inhabited Dante's hell.
>
> And it's the power of light that descends from ether to the earth, cutting the chains of the oppressed living being. . . .
>
> We're referring to electricity and electric streetcars, whose development should contribute to the well-being of noble and humanitarian hearts, and above all the lives of women. . . . [T]housands of draft horses will be saved from the cruel work that tortures the human mind with memories of chain gangs and forced labor. . . . [H]appily, this era is coming to an end as civilization now condemns these habits.
>
> The presence of electric trains in the United States supplies convincing proof of their important . . . superiority compared to our streetcars of blood. (Matto de Turner 1898b, 342–343)

Technology is framed in a humanitarian light: it speaks to a gesture of liberty and progress, freeing not only humans but also animals from the burdens of labor. Matto de Turner, moreover, uses technology as a temporal marker, separating an earlier period of enslavement and forced labor from the modern age with its new inventions.

While technology was equated with comfort, easing the burdens of workers, it also offered a sideline chance for distraction with new forms of entertainment. Not coincidentally, it served the minor industry of supernatural conversations with the dead. Mesmerists, hypnotists, and spiritualists took advantage of new devices. In that way, the famous "knock on the door" that made spiritualism an overwhelming source of interest for North Americans at midcentury also drew upon experiments with electromagnetic forces and electrical currents. These scientific tricks allowed the faithful to open communication with the world beyond; they promised to sustain a route of access to the dead through electric charges. It might be difficult to explain why writers of the *fin de siglo* continued to cultivate the phantasmagoria that Poe made famous in his stories of the 1840s, but even Juana Manuela Gorriti, who began in the same decade as Poe to covet a style of gothic writing before she went on to historical fiction, returned—in the final years of her life—to seek out extrarational cues to give depth to her literary world. Some regarded the attention to fantastic literature—with its ghost stories and uncanny reversals—with gnawing suspicion. Elites saw this as bad food for social actors who barely knew how to read, and signaled the immigrants and rural crowds who began to

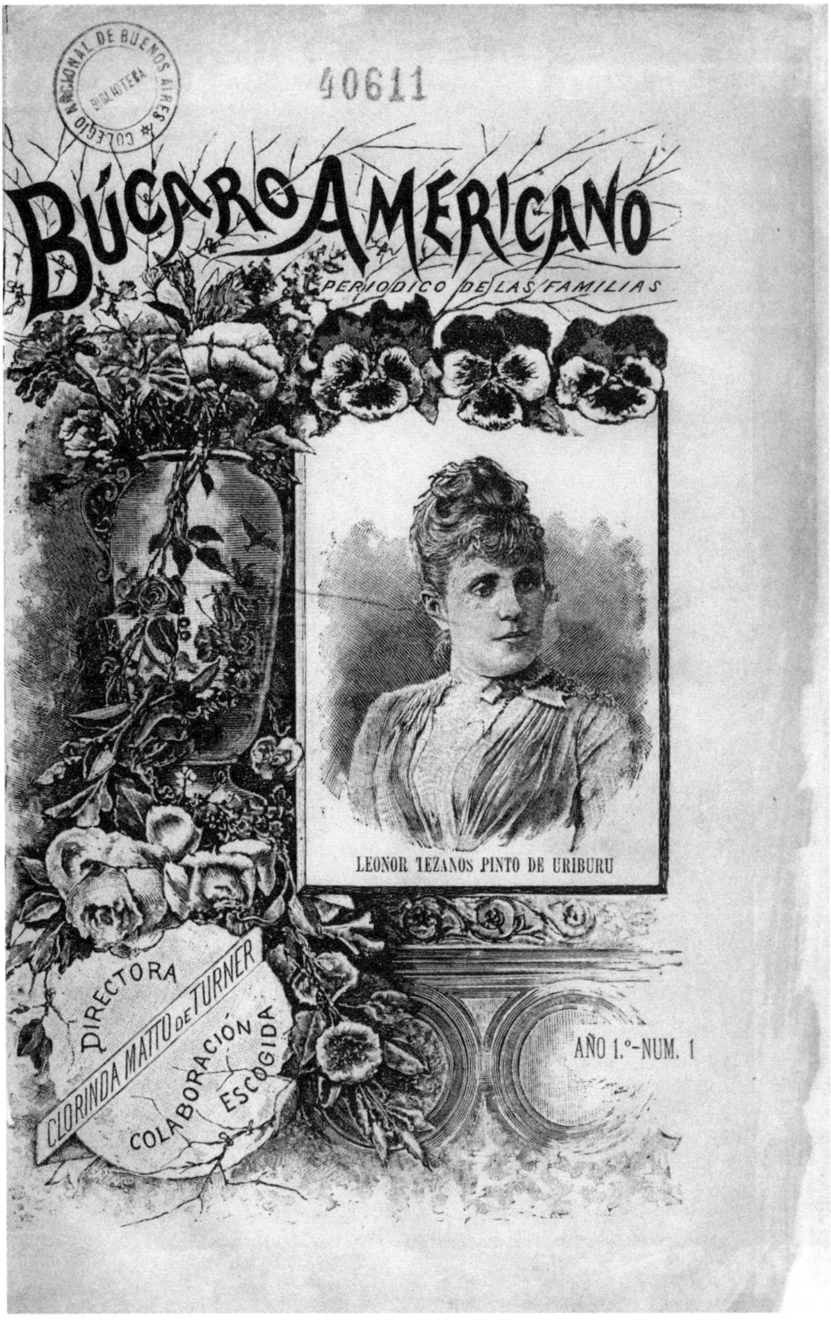

Figure 2.1. Búcaro americano, *Buenos Aires. Courtesy of Colegio Nacional de Buenos Aires.*

move to the city and were too easily captivated by fictions of otherworldly encounters. Others knew that the fantastic and gothic genres allowed an outlet for repressed psychic desires; long before psychoanalysis held sway, such writing performed the work of unearthing our deepest fears and then bringing them within fictional order. A third speculation is that fierce resistance to materialism led many writers—among them Raimunda Torres y Quiroga (a.k.a. Matilde Elena Wili) and Eduarda Mansilla de García (author of *El ramito de romero*, 1874), and especially Eduardo Holmberg (the major writer of the fantastic genre of the Argentine generation of 1880)—to seek in the supernatural experience a linkage to the soul.[9]

But an interest in the illusionist's art and its attendant electromagnetic devices also corresponds to the strange experience of time-space travel that new technology affords. The moving tables, the Ouija board, the "fantascope" or magic lantern, and the pseudoscientific investigations that manipulated the human body under the spell of electrical charges were, as early as midcentury, the material of newspapers and cultural reviews, literary texts and essays. See, in this respect, the interest in electromagnetic trances that populated the pages of the *Album de señoritas*, Juana Manso de Noronha's magazine for women. Therein she gives vivid accounts of the broad appeal of new technologies used for "magic":

> The dancing tables, the speaking boards, the divining rings, the coins that stick to doors without nails, the jumping keys, etc., etc. All these things are born in the sphere of the marvelous and extraordinary and, now for several months, have had delirious effects on European society. In Paris, in London, it's the only topic of conversation.... We in the New World who never want to fall behind Europe, have also bitten the bait, and a short while ago, we heard in Rio de Janeiro phrases like this: "Today I asked my table if there would be any important event for me, and the table answered in the affirmative!"
>
> It's an error to think that magnetism would produce these apparent miracles; the vital fluids, magnetic fluids, electrical currents, and ether do not have any effect on inanimate things; rather, they only affect humans. A magnetized object can provoke an artificial or magnetic dream in a subject as long as the person who controls the magnetic effect has also been magnetized himself. The effect of the turning tables can be explained through the simple phenomenon of electricity, which unfolds from the contact with different fluids that form in the

> atmosphere whose gases, so remarkably unique, produce an electrical stimulus that exercises its power on wood or some other object....
>
> The phenomena of magnetism are very extraordinary, but they should not be confused with electricity, which is not any less interesting, after all we believe, and of all the arcane metaphysical sciences, animal magnetism is the most powerful. We have seen experiences so supernatural, so beyond everything that the human mind can explain, that we wouldn't know how to reproduce the character of *events* so that they would not be labeled as apocryphal. We would like to see our doctors dedicate themselves to a study of magnetism as the most powerful agent of medicine, of that enormous chaos where one walks in the dark, and which they fear illuminating by saying: "*Non plus ultra.*" (Manso de Noronha 1854c, 11–12)

As in the case of Edison's inventions that were first refused by science and industry only to be sought out by spiritualists in the vein of Mme Blavatsky, magnetism here becomes a force of attraction for women writers like Juana Manso, providing an alternative entrance into the worldwide conversation and sometimes surpassing the draw of formal research and study that was largely prohibited to women.

But scientific inquiry of the scholarly stripe was never forgotten by women writers who sought to avail themselves of educational training that was reserved largely for men.[10] Two items deserve our attention: first, the ways in which women writers evoked the need for a scientific education in order to train the senses; and second, the moral lens through which women assessed the advantages of science. From the start, the earliest feminist journals of the Argentine nineteenth century insisted on educational rights for women. Whether in *La aljaba* of 1830, in which the anonymous editors demanded education for their daughters ("For how long will we have to see the female sex suppressed in the obscurity of an oppressive system?" ["A los que se oponen a la instrucción de las mujeres" 1830, 1]), or more than twenty years later in *La camelia*, a publication of Petrona Rosenda de Serra, where an unsigned editorial demanded training for women ("Oh! Opened wide, our eyes see the harmony of nature, the immense mountain chains, the dense sky above, and the immensity of the seas: we anxiously seek within ourselves the necessary intellectual tools to examine these grand works, and we find nothing to rely on except our own admiration" ["Moda" 1852, 3]), pleas for female education are the red threads of women's periodical culture. The petition culminates in the editorials of the *Album de señoritas* in 1854, where a training of the senses is demanded as part of a rigorous philosophy for women. The objective here is to understand sensibility and soul, as the anonymous author writes:

> Let's worry about sensibility and let's study the ways in which it's reproduced.
>
> First: Physical sensibility
> Second: Moral Sensibility
> Third: Intellectual Sensibility
>
> The soul suffers or enjoys, not only because of its contact with the physical causes of the organism, but also because of the impression that it receives of the sight of just and unjust behaviors, of beauty or ugliness, of the knowledge of error or truth. Etc., etc.
>
> This explains the subdivisions of sensibility in physical pleasure, moral and intellectual pursuits, and in the expression of pain. ("Ilustración de la mujer" 1854, 42–43)

The training of women also carried a moral dimension. Clorinda Matto de Turner, for example, insisted that women take advantage of scientific instruction that had first been reserved for their brothers. In an editorial of 1898 in *Búcaro americano*, Matto de Turner defended the right of women to enter scientific fields but warned that in a materialist society, with its emphasis on the acquisition of wealth, women should not lower the threshold of reason to which they have aspired (1898a, 318).

This is not to say that women writers were always liberal in their visions. Conservative interpretations also attacked materialist science. Elia M. Martínez, for example, was frank in her assessment of the utilitarian project: "[T]he materialist school . . . plants seeds of corruption. Out of this, shaped by a poorly interpreted science, the utilitarian school was born along with fraud, corruption, hate, and ingratitude disguising with refinement: envy with its court of calumnies and intrigues, limitless theft, and murder with impunity" (1898, 329). In another essay in the same review, Martínez became more vitriolic and even disputed the merits and power of the "colossal inventions" of the nineteenth century. Even the steamship and electricity come under her critical lens: "[B]etween harmony and real progress, we hear an unexpected protest by those who diffuse good doctrines. They complain of those who rebel against order, delivering themselves to chance, or those who cultivate leisure and vice and take disciples who believe they can disturb the social peace, provoking the unhappy masses who think they can change the world" (1897, 288). Here, materialist science is located in the sphere of rebellion; it promises to upset the social order with its focus on material things. This reproduces the trepidations expressed by Esteban Echeverría (see chapter 1), who separated himself from early materialist theory of the French sensualist school in order to move toward harmonic ideals of spirit and social order. Embodied cognition as philosophy and pursuit threatened the social whole.

By the late nineteenth century, conservative women became impatient not only with what they perceived as social uprising, but also with the ways in which scientific inquiry neglected the inner self. We are listening to an emerging narrative in which the spirit is protected against the sensual being. Consider, in this regard, the following essay in which Teresa Mañé observes the excessive rationalism of scientific thought. In "Las enfermedades morales" (The moral illnesses), she writes: "There's no pain that cannot find relief; there's no wound that cannot be healed; there's no illness that can't be cured; but science crashes in on itself when it loses sight of the heart. This organ cannot be cured with animal substances or with vegetables. The heart cannot be reached with anything that comes from pharmaceuticals; it is only healed by the word, by pain, consolation, or death" (1896, 32). These critiques, however, are always crossed with protests against gender exclusion. Reacting against Lombroso, for example, Mercedes Cabello de Carbonera observes that science should not be used to reinforce the inferiority of women: "How is it that the moral and social code is so severe and strict with women when it is liberal and generous with men?" (1896, 54–56). An even more aggressive attack on technology was placed in evidence by Clorinda Matto de Turner. When reviewing the kaleidoscopic events of the nineteenth century as she crossed into the twentieth, she wondered if technology had improved the human condition: "Next to the steamship and electricity, countless bodies that man has enslaved in his service are screaming through wars of conquest, the intransigencies of religious creed; they announce a thirst that can only be satisfied by a materialism that sacrifices ideals and lets the powerful exercise injustices on the weak" (1901, 590). Science must lead to faith if we are to be sustained in the modern world.

A Literature of the Senses

The literary fictions of nineteenth-century America, both North and South, reveal a textured landscape of sensory material captured by the bodies of women, while, of course, they also incorporate the debates about technology and learning as they emerge in the age of invention. From the River Plate to Caribbean cities to the rural and urban United States, feminine cultural production takes up these issues in nation-building narratives (melodramas and romances) and in pamphlets, newspapers, and manuals that register female experience. They put women's sensory reach at the center of wide discussion. It's not surprising, in this regard, that Mary Shelley's *Frankenstein* (1818) inaugurates the literature of a century, placing the monster as the amalgam of unsorted senses. But we never should forget the political dimension of this exploration. The goal is to make legible the connection between body and soul, to show the soul leading the way out of the body to knowledge and feeling, as when Hawthorne through his character Hester Prynne in *The Scarlet Letter* (1850) seeks to find the "tooth of remorse"; or when Poe in "Ligeia" (1838) studies the decomposing body of his beloved; or when John Brown focuses on the body parts of the black man in order to locate the essence of blackness. We are witness to a fascination for grotesque and gothic experience combined with an insatiable desire to know and control perceptions, linking bodily sensation to affect and then leading to reasonable truths. Baudelaire made this apparent in "The Painter of Modern Life" when he spoke to us of the double composition of all works of art, joining beauty through historical theory and then through the contemporary moment with its fashion, its peculiar moral life, and through modernity's emotions. "The duality of art," he concludes, "is a fatal consequence of the duality of man" (1995, 3). In not a dissimilar way, the attention to the senses is caught in a web of interlaced threads: on the one hand, it locks us in the present moment of experience that keeps us aware of the circumstantial sweep at the moment of perception; on the other, it leads us to a historical dimension rooted in the link between sensory effect and thought. Behind the instances of perception, we reach for an intelligibility of history, the path of Hegel and Marx.

What concerns me here is the response of women, who show how emergent sense theory and technological networks serve a larger goal to modify politics and shape historical critique. Toward this end, this chapter focuses on midcentury women—Argentina's Juana Manuela Gorriti,

Cuba's Gertrudis Gómez de Avellaneda, the Peruvian Clorinda Matto de Turner, and Catherine and Harriet Beecher from the United States. As a group, they are indicative of nineteenth-century writers who take *experience* to be central to their texts, aiming to position sense and sensibility as necessary for literary form and then, beyond the text itself, for community engagement. In this vein, they unsheathe the blade of documentary knowledge surrounding new technology about the senses and use it to question the heady partisan politics of American life at midcentury. In the process, they thus reroute the maps of battle, considering another version of history anchored not so much in abstract debate, but in the very bodies of slaves and natives who have been excluded from history and in the lives of women who try to intervene in political direction. We might say, then, that this is the war machine as seen from the distaff perspective, but there's also something else: women offer a plan for a material reading of culture that draws directly upon female experience. They rely upon the senses to engineer a kind of political work that speaks to gender and freedom.

Let me start with small steps. The insistence on sensual experience (how we hear, see, and touch; how we interact with the world around us and feel the weight of those exchanges) is more than a path to explore women's interiority (often developed and expressed in the private sphere, removed from the realm of public debate, and separate from the perceptions of men). In effect, what will surface in this chapter is a claim that individual perceptions, and a trust in the sentient being, work as part of a larger project both to define the bases of governmentability (whether colonial or newly independent) and to expose its shortcomings and flaws. In this regard, work with the senses offers a resistance to despots and unsettles our faith in a universal divinity; in the end, it admits that perceptions are necessary to give testimony in the shadow of silence. Women's writing, developed from the sensual aspect that I am outlining here, attests to the participatory role of individuals in shaping democracy; but rather than discussing the *exclusions* of women from the literary canon, or arguing alone for the ways in which women insist on their *difference* from men, I am making a case for "sense work" as a way to question the limits of writing and the limits of the law; sense work, then, for all its constructedness, is a prerequisite for reading politics and history, a way to capture a social milieu in the process of major transition.

A caveat is in order here. I want to move beyond the erotic sensibilities of women, a topic that has enjoyed the attention of many scholars over the years; this tie has led us to read, among other things, for the relation between erotics and reading, an obvious link that finds a place in the vast canvas of nineteenth-century literature, from Flaubert's *Madame Bovary*, the urtext that gives full heft to this bond in fiction, to the defining realist novels of the Hispanic world: among them, Leopoldo Alas's *La regenta* (1884), in which the protagonist is erotically aroused by the fictions she reads, or Soledad Acosta de Samper's novel *Teresa la limeña* (1868), in which the female figures shape their ideas of love by literary works and music. The pairing of eros and reading continues among the authors considered in this chapter: Juana Manuela Gorriti gives us "The Dead Man's Fiancée," a story in which Vital is accused by her aunt of reading novels that inflame the senses; or Gertrudis Gómez de Avellaneda's *Sab*, where the slave and Carlota read novels together as children, a near-primal scene that inspires Sab's later passion; and Clorinda Matto de Turner, whose character in *Aves sin nido* teaches his beloved to spell through a board game resembling Scrabble (Matto de Turner 1998, 84), such that love is borne through the letter. Similarly, in *Uncle Tom's Cabin* Harriet Beecher Stowe has Tom learn the forbidden act of reading through the aid of his white female tutor; pedagogy here is crossed with the generosity of love. Beyond this, the chapter will flow in a different direction, showing sense work as a prerequisite for reading the dramas of politics and history.

The sensual responses developed in the female version of nineteenth-century debate are situated within the reigning philosophies of the time. Riding upon the work of the sensationalists (Locke and Newton, for starters), and more important for the Latin American case, the philosophers associated with French Enlightenment thought (most notable among them, Condillac and Rousseau), the intellectuals of the new republics were deeply concerned with experience, with the ways to explain the material world through sensory apperception, a problem established in chapter 1. In this line, the body was the starting point for all access to knowledge, and, more than the Cartesian cogito, in its Americanist version it extended a preference for the immediacy of contact and for the sensuous path that underlies comprehension and fortifies our judgments. Listening, seeing, and touching the "real" were a preamble to American freedoms. We also remember that the American experience, north and south, was marked inevitably by blood and war: not only expressed through the "civilization and savagery" tropes that defined the Americas during civil conflicts, but also through the discourses on race that marked human worth by terms of the color of one's flesh. Whitman famously sums up the corporeality of this racial encounter in "I Sing the Body Electric":

> A man's body at auction . . .
> Gentlemen look on this wonder . . .
> Examine these limbs, red, black, or white, they are cunning in tendon
> and nerve,
> They shall be stript that you may see them.

They are visible bodies, bodies put on display, but also bodies that we perceive through our senses; bodies that we inevitably see, touch, and hear. From this, we learn a path of reading for the politics of matter, corporeality, and place. Literature offers this map of sensual exploration; it also shows that literary bodies engage distinct perceptual resources at different moments in history; as such, the interpolated sensual knowledge provides, in each instance, varied technologies that allow us to read by extension for the complexities of social life.

Terry Eagleton was right when he observed that "[a]esthetics is born as a discourse of the body" (1990, 13). But I am more immediately interested in the ways in which the senses, registered in the cultural text, somaticize our understanding of gender, politics, and the state. The latent pulsations of sense work are clues to ways of comprehending political and historical becoming. In this regard, and as evidenced thus far by the two lithographs by Bacle or the inquiries of journalists such as Matto de Turner, women can be seen as disarticulating the basis of a national project. By focusing on becoming—encounters of opposing forces, collisions between sound and matter, or chrysalidic breakthroughs to meaning that begin with a sentient self—they allow us to reach an understanding of social and cultural life not yet registered by history or law. Bacle's prints also tell us that one cannot achieve this "becoming" unaided. Rather, the use of technology—anything ranging from a hair comb to an electrical impulse—will come to the rescue of those who are pursuing a wider experience in the modern, trans-American world.

But we also encounter differences: Gorriti steeps us in an *auditory* world, while Gómez de Avellaneda proposes an *ocularcentric* dimension; Clorinda Matto de Turner takes us to the scene of culinary offerings that elites enjoyed in Peru to stress the importance of *taste*; and a writer such as Harriet Beecher Stowe emphasizes the moment of flesh-on-flesh *contact* as central to the antislavery awareness that needs to capture her readers. Each corresponds to a different phase of government and capital, and with it, a different use of bodies in the national landscape. In other words, particular economic systems produce special categories for sense work and different rules for reading not necessarily tied to erotics alone. Indeed, the American world of the nineteenth century featured a special attention to perceptions as a way to define social and cultural differences and modernity on the rise.

To this effect, Peter Gay (1984) reminds us of the emerging French nineteenth century as a space of social pyramids, of social distinctions and boundaries, of neurotic distortions of privilege. The American world also contained its fair share of stories about poverty and abjection, resulting in the fall-from-glory narratives that depicted once-wealthy landowners now deprived of their fortunes. Matto de Turner represents the corruption by money exercised upon the privileged classes in Kíllac; Gorriti and Gómez de Avellaneda tell of fallen wealth and status; and Stowe in much broader strokes paints the moral vices of a social class whose economic gain depends on the trade of flesh. In the process, these writers make us keenly aware of social exclusions and the ways in which different social groups rely on their perceptions in order to redefine the barriers that would separate class and race; through this, they draw complex portraits of national disorder. We come, then, to a dual experience: while subaltern bodies teach us to define the experience of abjection (hunger, torture, coldness and wet, the lash upon the flesh), elites are also shown in their own codes of sensual privilege (consumer excess of items of luxury, sumptuous foods to entice the palate, even musical choices).

The disharmony of this experience sustains an ongoing "battle of perceptions" that defines in its fullest range what it means to be modern (Gay 1984, 35). Zola observed the nineteenth century as a time of transition, a world in which nothing was still. Due not only to the disruption caused by civil war or migrations from farm to city or from European to American shores, the movement recorded in nineteenth-century texts was amassed as a compendium of detail showing people in constant transit. It was the work of the eye and the ear that created a picture of this world; it was the representation of palpable matter drawn close within the spectator's reach that awakened nineteenth-century reader perception to a new world on the brink of change. The women writers of the mid-nineteenth century brought this sensual matter to life, and with it, they called attention to their potential of becoming human in ways that had not yet been catalogued in the archives of liberal men.

Hearing Argentina

In these terms, let's think of the stories of Juana Manuela Gorriti (1818–1892), an Argentine from the Salta elite whose life was in constant movement due to the urgencies of political exile set in place by the Rosas regime. Her early fictions, written largely in Peru but with scenes traversing the Americas and Europe, describe characters on the run: bandits, patriots, and kidnapped women; a sabre-bearing cast that spans the treasure-hunting adventurers of the colonial period and the later civil wars, and reaches a pioneering moment of modernity in the urbane *fin de siglo* replete with its technological innovations and consumer delights. In the process, crossed identities lie at the center of Gorriti's fictions such that no one seems to know who's who. Women are disguised as men; Incas are crossed with Spaniards; and most of all, in her early fiction, written during the regime of Juan Manuel Rosas, Federals are blurred with Unitarians, forcing a collapse of partisan reason. It is the regime of the sensible that allows Gorriti to wend her way through the shock of an unsettled world, to use the power of experience to explain injustice and civil war.

As she maps the Andean corridor running from Salta to Cuzco and Lima (and in one case, California), Gorriti also pays particular attention to the material aspects of bodies. It is from "mi ser material" (my material being) (2003, 46), for example, that she tells the narrative "La quena," a gothic fiction in which the protagonist's bones are used, in the end, as an Andean flute, a source and inspiration for song. Her stories are also about wounded bodies in need of healing; tourniquets, bandages, and strips of cloth placing pressure on injured flesh. In many cases, characters carry emblematic physical signs—scabs, incisions, birthmarks—that give proof of identity and political allegiance. The scar carries the name, but it represents internal turmoil, a gateway to the soul. It also reveals a political economy in which women register norms of justice and disorder.

"The Mashorquero's Daughter," one of Gorriti's better-known stories about the conflicts between Federals and Unitarians, is a tale that sustains the "civilization and savagery" trope made famous in Argentina by Sarmiento in his *Facundo* (1845).[11] Here, the evil Roque Alma-negra, or

Roque Black-Soul, a henchman for the notorious *mazorca*—the secret police force of Rosas—stands in contrast to Clemencia, his pious and loving daughter, who protects her father's victims and tries to deter his feckless abuse of power. For its structure, the fiction depends upon the use of the senses and, from "that terrible vocabulary of cruelty and irreverence" (Gorriti 2003, 86), the ineluctable power of the name. Roque Alma-negra thus lives out the foul predictions of his name, just as Clemencia, through her own name, prophesizes unfailing kindness. But these essentialisms are crossed by active perceptions that reveal a different access to truth. In this regard, Clemencia and Roque Alma-negra are opposed not just for their moral purpose, but for the ways in which they register reality and act upon their perceptions. Agency and affect become important to the fiction; they expose the folly of ill-guided men and often lead to wisdom.

Roque, of course, is attentive to his daughter's voice ("So sweet and melodious that it sounded like it came from a choir of angels" [2003, 86]). Likewise, he treasures the eyes and blonde curls that belong to his only daughter. But nature will not allow Roque to act on his perceptions: instead, he splits his affective world from his political mission, continuing in the odious job of murderer for the Federalist service. The only sensuality that counts for Roque is thus tied to blood and revenge, and it is inspired by rumor. The secret listening of the *mazorca*—with its attention to eavesdropping and snitching—defines the sonorous age in which Rosas comes to power. By contrast, the sensual world in which Clemencia lives is intelligent and moral. The senses teach her principles of fairness and give individuals an idea of value. As a teacher of music and drawing, moreover, Clemencia turns to the feminine arts to nurture her finely tuned ear and her perceptive eye. These talents are not wasted in the ethical assessments she later deploys. First, she sees the arms of her father appallingly stained with blood; she also hears the vile language of the crowds who rebuke her father's actions. The plot thickens as Clemencia eavesdrops on her father's domain, hearing the words of henchmen who join with Roque to menace the Unitarian crowds. Forewarned through this act of espionage, Clemencia hopes to save the targeted victims by disguising her identity with a veil; eventually, she will switch places with a woman who has been imprisoned in Roque's jails, and only then will she guarantee the other woman's freedom at the expense of her own.

Here it is revealed that women have the capacity to use their senses to fully comprehend their surroundings, whereas men, stunted in their perceptual experience, fail to learn to interpret the signs they see or hear. In other words, men can't link sensuality with ethics or political justice. This understanding comes to the reader in steps. First, Clemencia, wearing the traditional veil of nineteenth-century women of Argentina and Peru, receives the gaze of a stranger who mistakes Clemencia for his betrothed. Even as he embraces her, he cannot discern that the woman is not his beloved Emilia. Other scenes of misrecognition follow in which Clemencia's acute vision and hearing allow her to track the path of the hated *mazorca*, but the police in return are helpless to read innocent faces or listen to cries for freedom. The final scene of misrecognition is all the more astounding. Having traded places with an imprisoned woman in order to set her free, Clemencia enters a dark cell where, disguised, she encounters her father. He, bent on revenge, reaches out for her throat and stabs his daughter to death: "He stormed toward her, reached out with his bloodstained hand and, feeling a woman's throat, plunged in his dagger" (2003, 102). Full of melodramatic collisions and reversals, Gorriti's story makes it clear that Federalist men cannot take care of business, nor can they use their senses to protect the women they love. Indeed, in the romantic world in which the civil wars took place, only the women seem to set things right due to their gifts of audition and sight. Awakened to the sensible encounter (Clemencia hears the wails of the widows, she sees the bloodstained hands, she listens to her father's plots to murder Unitarian families), women then act on their gained experience. Female agency is conditioned by direct encounters with the world. The rest, as the moral of Gorriti's story alludes, is left enshrouded in darkness upon which only divine redemption and judgment can eventually work their effects.

One might claim that the American nineteenth century always sustains a literature thick with sensual perceptions. Whether we focus on the work of the trailblazers in forests or the military incursions into enemy territory, or even on the sensationalist press, we march through a world that requires heightened attention to the senses. Danger lurks in the woods and cities for those lacking alertness; the threat of defeat or death stands for those who can't get their perceptions in line. In chapter 1, I considered the spectacular presence of the Rosas regime—the enforced codes of dress, the red ribbon, the public parades and banners—and touched upon the ways in which Sarmiento responded to these displays. But Gorriti, also a Unitarian, takes her sense work in another direction, underscoring her ability first to perceive the horror and then to discern through the ear. The female abode retains a memory of both of these perceptual responses. While visual arousals were evident from public celebrations, they also entered the home through the anti-Rosas clandestine journals: newspapers such as *El grito argentino* and *Muera Rosas*, for example, provided ample visual evidence of bodies that were subjected to state violence. The home harbored these horrific images of diabolic celebration, with blood pouring from the throats of victims to quench the thirst of Rosas; as such, even the texts most notoriously critical of the Rosas regime carried a theatrical, almost camp spectacle of the horrors of Federalist crimes.[12] Creative women writers like Gorriti certainly acknowledge these visuals, but also bring the role of the female intermediary to teach us to experience terror through the alerted ear. While it may be claimed that Gorriti's obsession with masquerade and disguise are running tropes in her stories, she also sought out antidotes to the visual loyalties demanded by the tyrant Rosas. The work of hearing became more important for her early stories written during years of civil war.

It is of small surprise that audition became an obsession among the liberals opposed to Rosas. For example, in her correspondence of the 1840s with Esteban Echeverría (then in exile), Mariquita Sánchez de Thompson from Buenos Aires alerted her reader to the power of the ear, centering it as the major trope with which to report the news. In each letter to Echeverría, she focuses on the noise and rumors of the city, and gives him to understand that murmurs and whispers constantly tickle the ear: "All we have is this noise that each person records according to his ideas, desires, and interests," she writes (Sánchez de Thompson 2003, 54). Her letters begin time and again with verbs that designate rumor and alert us to sound: "it is announced," "it is said," "it is heard," "it is rumored." But Buenos Aires is also a city of "silent noises" (67), the soft whisper of rebellion that the anti-Rosas cohort sustains against the regime's mistruths. Gorriti's work with the ear follows in this direction, using the human body to reveal a sensibility not controlled by the Rosas police.

Feminine sensorial responses perpetually remind us that the body lies at the center of political struggles. For the nineteenth-century women who are the later focus of this chapter, eyes and ears and, later, structures of taste and touch become the organs of knowledge to catch a world in constant movement, a world in which sense perception is key not only to undoing the knowledge of men in power, but also to discovering new routes of expression, detaining the fleeting sensations that are bypassed in appraisals of history. In this state of affairs, sense perceptions offer a medium with which to capture a feminine stake in material culture, trapping the markings of race and gender on the body for other kinds of experience and

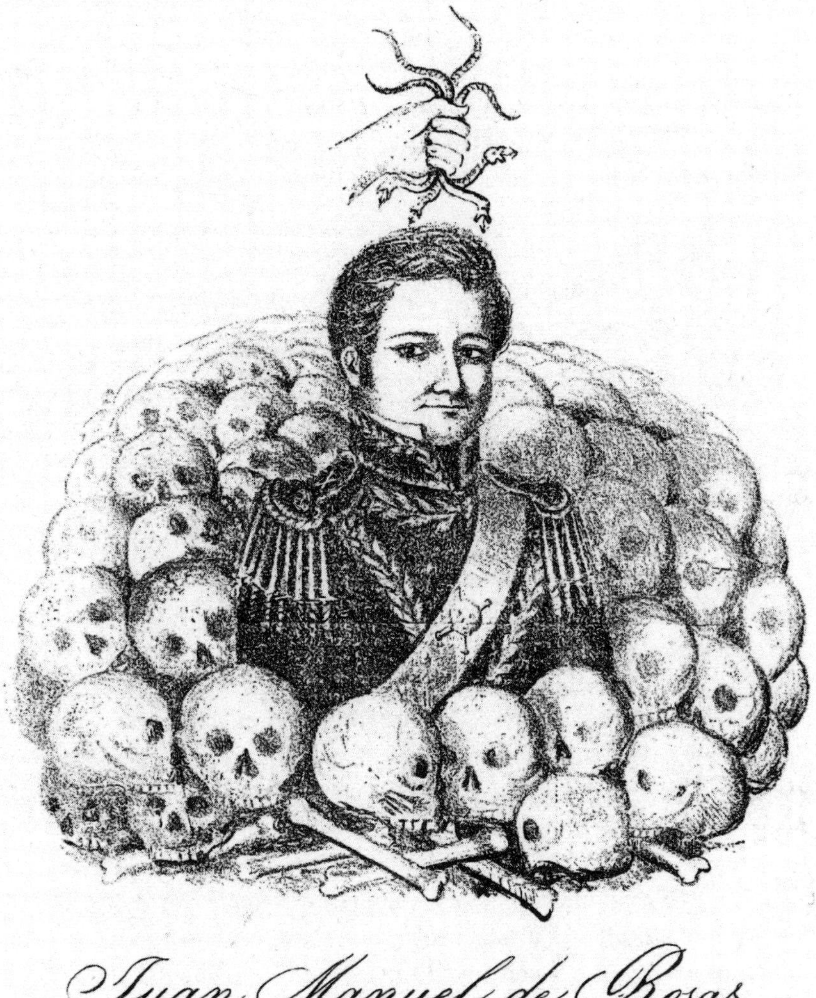

Figure 2.2. Antonio Somellera, "Juan Manuel de Rosas." ¡Muera Rosas!, *no. 10, March 5, 1842, Montevideo. Courtesy of Mariano Moreno National Library of Argentina.*

gain; and it is sense perception that marks the world of appearances as a first step for women to reach and comprehend the political choices set before them. "People are the slaves of their eye and ear" (Stowe 1981, 433), writes Harriet Beecher Stowe in *Uncle Tom's Cabin*, as she begs us to step beyond the material to link experience to the spirit. Her goal is to rethink the use of the senses in order to propose *another* version of politics that puts an end to enslavement.

Sensibilité

We can situate the affective drive of women writers of the nineteenth century within the age of sensibility that preceded in France and England and was carried into the Americas through popular literary texts along with the philosophies of sensualism that I mentioned in chapter 1. *Sensibilité*, in the European eighteenth century, was tied to benevolence and kindness; it also promoted tear shedding as a way to awaken our compassion for others. But *sensibilité* also carried latent meanings that escaped the force of language. It taught one, for example, to identify the meaning of a blush, the feeling behind a rise or drop in voice, the flirtations signaled by a woman's lowered lashes. Sensibility referred to one's power to make meaning beyond words themselves. We saw this in Crèvecoeur, who in the North American landscape was considered a "farmer of feelings" (see his *Letters from an American Farmer*, 1782); we perceived this also with Jorge Isaacs as he evoked sympathy in his novel *María* (1867) through scenes of agonic confessions that brought his audience to tears. Moreover, for the men of the founding republics, sensibility was considered a kind of discipline: any man who wished to evidence public spirit had of necessity to show force of feeling.[13] We also saw this with Thomas Jefferson in *Notes on the State of Virginia* (1787), praising the humanity of the Mingo chief Logan who mourned his murdered family with deep and unrelieved compassion. We later saw this in Tocqueville, who in *Democracy in America* observed that the increase of sensibility in Europe and America was linked to emergent democracy (1945, 2:172–177).

Sentiment as moral superiority, as part of Enlightenment discourse, was later cultivated by those of lofty ambition who could justify westward expansion (in the United States) or the conquest of the outback (as we observed in countries of South America in moments of territorial expansion). In both cases, the conquest of the desert and plains was tied to residual concepts of the "noble savage" and a collision of races that was explained by the perceptual depths of each group. Both natives and foreign invaders in the fictions of James Fenimore Cooper (in the United States) or José de Alencar (in Brazil) remind us of the power invested in sensible, feeling men. Then there's the question of gender. Do women have something to add?

Sentimentality in the hands of women takes a different direction. One might recall Mary Wollstonecraft's *A Vindication of the Rights of Woman* (1792) or, closer to home, the Seneca Falls Convention of 1848 for its "Declaration of Sentiments," where the concept of sentiment in the title was evoked to remediate the wrongs suffered by North American women. Apart from the directly militant demand issued by the decree, the title of the Seneca Falls pronouncement signals a charge for women's literature in the nineteenth century: from sentiment—a combination of sensibility and an investment in perceptions—to sentiment as a way to approach a political path and a moral high ground from which to correct a nation's wayward path. To be sensible, then, was to be reasonable as the eighteenth-century philosophers proposed, but it was also a gesture imbued with nineteenth-century understandings of one's capacity to receive impressions from the external world.[14] Andrew Burstein notes the Lockean underpinnings of the second definition of sentiment in which human feeling was described as an effect of nerve fibers such that every response of moral content had roots in a physiological source (1999, 7–8). Smith and Hume persisted in this codification of the sentiments according to physical response, with the effect of dominating eighteenth-century discourse. But the novel presents yet another dimension to this debate.

Markman Ellis (1996) notes a split in the sentimental novel defined by the gender system. The masculine sentimental novel influenced philosophy and moral sense; in the hands of Fielding, Richardson, and Sterne, it bespoke cultivation and manners. By contrast, the female sentimental novel in the English tradition (Aphra Behn or Eliza Haywood) stood for indecorous, demotic forces, pushing the novelistic genre toward fashion and popular culture, or toward signs of consumer appetites of a decidedly anti-intellectual stripe. Usually, the sentimental novel, whose design was to move the audience emotionally—hence, moving us to tears—exposed the suffering of the innocent in order to jump-start political thought. Leslie Fiedler situated this convention within the antibourgeois novel. Margaret Cohen takes this a step further and argues, with respect to the sentimental novel, that once the genre assumed a social or political dimension, it came to represent a new individuality that signaled liberation; this separated the female subject from collective customs and norms, and led to something new. In other words, the sentimental social novel of the mid-nineteenth century becomes less concerned with defining inner conflicts (as the eighteenth-century case averred) than with situating individual sense perceptions against the reigning ideology of the day. Cohen calls this a "plot of fracture" (1999, 12). The gendered difference gives the project traction, and here Jane Tompkins is especially direct when she writes that "the popular domestic novel represents a monumental effort to reorganize culture from the woman's point of view" (1986, 124). I don't want to track what Andrew Burstein has referred to as an "emotional history" (1999, xiv) of the nineteenth century or to reproduce Barrán's study of sexuality and transgression in Uruguay, but rather I aim to show how perceptions of women writers lead us to something new: beyond the abstractions of sentimentality, as dramas of interior conflict, their creative texts more importantly capture material culture and record it as part of their reinterpretation of politics and their long-standing grievance against injustice. Material culture and sense perceptions thus become central to the paradigm of novel writing and for reaching for an idea of the future.[15]

Women writers of the nineteenth century were devoted to this expression of sentiment—not only to demonstrate the cost of sexual subordination, but also to denounce the injuries occasioned by tyranny in the new republics. Through sensibility, these women denoted their mistreatment by men and used the decorative aspects of femininity to force submerged feelings to surface. The female body in the literature considered here thus registered the ailments of society though different physical and psychological traumas: through melancholia (Soledad Acosta de Samper), through an obsession with weight and starvation (Mercedes Cabello de Carbonera), through agoraphobia and sexual fear (Juana Manuela Gorriti's "Un año en California"). In these cases, we see that capitalism commodifies fantasies and pleasure; it redirects sexual desire in favor of the acquisition of wealth. But it also triggers female illness, explaining bodily ailments as the result of equivocal choices.

Beyond sentimentality, direct sensual registers—touch and taste, seeing and hearing—expand female expression even further than critics had noted before.[16] Here, the sense work in women's writing not only calls for the experiential notation that gives democracy a body, but it also reveals the limitations of abstract political projects that the founding fathers declared. Exposing the shortcomings of the Federalist plan (in the work of

Gorriti) or objecting to foreign capital as it affected the island economy (Gómez de Avellaneda), denouncing the power of elites in Peru (Matto de Turner) or exposing the crisis engendered by slavery in the United States (Stowe), the culture of sentiment is designed to use female perception as a guide to new ways of thinking: it liberates readers from the constraints of tradition, just as it expands available ethical choices situated in time and place. It also permits the reader to imagine an alternative to cultural norms, starting from the force of perception and a sentient body to guide it. To put it another way, while romanticism with its belief in change required that sensory alertness be the tipping point toward new, unlearned experience, women writers of the same generation also showed the links between perceptions and thought; from there, and not yet set into words, an inkling of political expression began to find its form. Sensual response ran far ahead of reason and verbal expression. Through it, women became not only better writers but also better readers of dimensions of the social. Nevertheless, the literary representation of the senses is not always the same. Thus, if Gorriti brought the ear into play in order to question partisan rivalries and describe the horrors of civil war, Gómez de Avellaneda brought the regime of the visible to press down upon the injustices sustained by the slave economy under colonial rule; Matto de Turner exposed the privileges of elites in a country defined by taste (in its double entendre) that discriminated between social classes while maintaining an unjust culture; and Harriet Beecher Stowe insisted upon the importance of contact, the close encounters of black and white that passed through the human touch.

Sighting Difference

Consider, in this regard, the example of *Sab* (1841), surely one of the most enduring novels of the nineteenth-century Caribbean, a text in which Gertrudis Gómez de Avellaneda (1814–1873) explores the sensibilities defining Cuba under colonial rule. In particular, the perceptual field is used to delimit property lines and to expose the crisis of capital as it emerges in midcentury. In the novel, Gómez de Avellaneda combines her European sensibilities (remember that she wrote the novel in Spain) with a deep nostalgia for the Cuban land and the native intelligence of slaves and criollos who might resist the threat to freedom. This surfaces in her exploration of the world defined by optical discipline and spectacular resistance, visual effects and freedom, and the subaltern knowledge that one might gain simply by watching out.

The opening paragraphs of *Sab* reveal a landscape under surveillance as an anonymous traveler (who we later learn is Enrique Otway) traverses the picturesque landscape and observes the untouched land. The second paragraph offers the following: "Perhaps because of his *scant* knowledge of the road, perhaps because of the *pleasure* he took in *appraising* the landscape before him, the traveler gradually slackened his pace . . . as though to *scrutinize* the places through which he passed. Quite possibly his repeated stops had as their sole object the fuller *savoring* of the richly fertile earth of that privileged country" (Gómez de Avellaneda 1993, 27; italics mine). Notice here the ways in which the countryside is brought under the wing of the traveler. He appraises, scrutinizes, and savors the land as a means to determine its potential value. Pleasure and property assessment go hand in hand; this is the gaze of power. This early introduction to sense work linked with profit becomes the sustaining trope of Gómez de Avellaneda's novel. And indeed, as the book goes on, Enrique Otway, the son of a British investor, will use his keen eye for value to exploit Cuba's fortunes. Gómez de Avellaneda thus critiques the imperial eye and shows an understanding of European power and visual conquest such that sight for the European imagination is shown as a guidepost to knowledge and control.[17] In the process she also endows an alternative visual power to the figure of the slave: *true* knowledge of Cuban soil belongs to Sab, the man of color, and the women to whom he is attached.

Gómez de Avellaneda thus begins her novel with an evocation of the land. Not only is it available for Enrique's appraisal (whose foreign status can be likened to the foreign eye of the author), but on its own, and removed from the concerns for property, the land stimulates in Sab's body a wide variety of perceptions. Continuing on the first page, the author proceeds to tell us of the "brutal sun," the "purple and silver" clouds, the "vigorous . . . vegetation," and the breath of the "gentle breeze" (1993, 27). In the traditions of the romantic picturesque, we are asked to discern the natural environs—to immerse ourselves in the open sensuality of the Caribbean afternoon. That said, we are never far away from the concern for capital, and indeed, by following the seemingly unmotivated descriptions of nature, we soon reach this end ("a fence, which indicated that this was someone's *property*" [1993, 28; italics mine]). Two kinds of seeing are juxtaposed in the text: the unfettered observation of the slave who feels

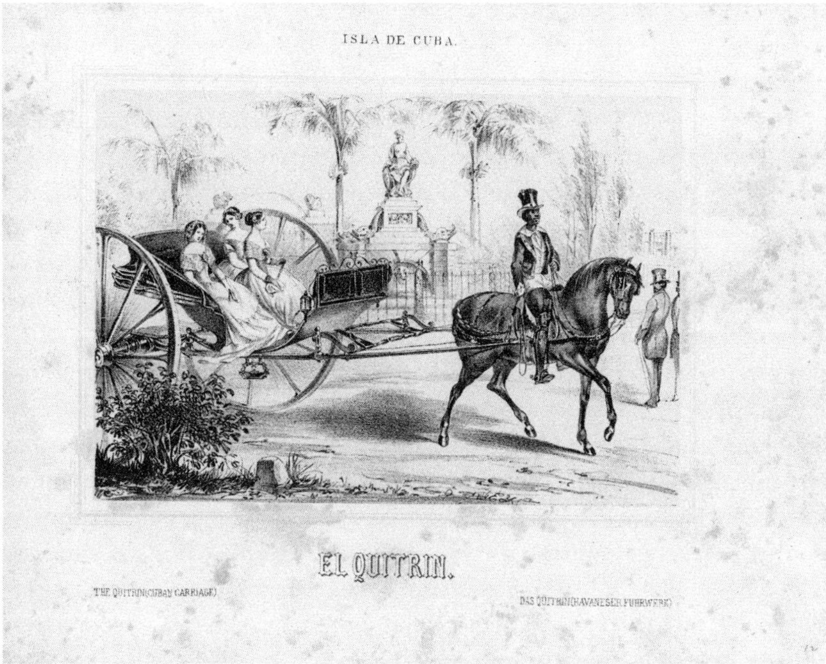

Figure 2.3. Frédéric Mialhe, El quitrín *(Cuban carriage). Plate 12 from* Album pintoresco de la isla de Cuba, *1853. Courtesy of Bancroft Special Collections, University of California at Berkeley Library.*

the weight of nature, and the property-directed eye of the landlord who sees profit in land—signposts of desired freedom or economic power.

In *Sab*, sensual experiences are always surrounded by marks of ownership; they are the center of Goméz de Avellaneda's concern, and allow her to pit the unregulated interactions among subalterns and the surrounding landscape in contrast to the harsh relationships established by laws of property and monied exchange. Sab, for example, refers early on to the effects of the "fiery sky" upon the naked slave and "the weight of the wood and the sugarcane" that "he bears on his shoulders" (29); unlike the slave masters, however, Sab also has an appreciation for the aesthetic values of nature, as we observe in a garden scene describing the flowers that Sab plants for Carlota (56).

Sab and his friends possess wisdom about the land that the English traveler, governed as he is by a drive for profit, can never appreciate or acquire. In effect, in the colonial economy, where land exploitation through slavery is the prime mover of human relations, it is left to others living outside this economy to find an affective experience that leaves them beyond the law. This second group possesses the gift of artful interpretation of what they see. Nevertheless, a problem accompanies their lot: can those who live by the affects enter the realm of history?

"Which eyes are perspicacious enough to interpret a soul?" (36), the narrator asks. Clearly, the foreigners and the landed elite lack the sensibility required to answer. It is left, then, to the experience of the natives—Sab, Teresa, and Martina—to understand through their senses what elites can never see: Martina, for example, is quick to recognize Carlota when she arrives in Cubitas; Teresa discovers the infirm child whom no one notices in Martina's home and, more important, is the only one to grasp Sab's amorous dilemma. Sab, meanwhile, senses the distress of Carlota and homes in on Enrique's deceptions long before Carlota is able to name them herself. Sab, Teresa, and Martina, whose bodies bear the brunt of oppression, rely upon the senses—especially the gift of sight—to reach a deeper reality about themselves and their surroundings. From seeing the world, they then touch feelings that the landed elites can never know. Their perceptions do not speak to property or a desire for advancement; instead, they use the affective space to touch a common truth about freedom and oppression. These apprehensions, however, have no name in the novel and lack a role in Cuba; at least in 1841, the time of *Sab*'s composition, they fail to announce historical change that would guarantee emancipation.

Now of course, one might suggest that the opening scene from which I just quoted coincides with the picturesque of painting, the representation of Orientalism that so dominated visual arts of the European nineteenth century, or the sketches of manners (*cuadros de costumbres*) that were so prevalent in the Hispanic world of that time. Because of their visual interruption, these opening passages pause the narration. With this, Gómez de Avellaneda proposes something beyond the conventional picturesque. Here, the sensory world representing elites and subalterns opens, in the first case, onto cold speculation, and in the second, into a hyperintensity of feeling that cannot be stopped. It forces a contemplation of the truth that flickers behind appearance, inviting us to peer below the surface. The skill in this instance does not distinguish men from women (as in Gorriti's example), but cuts the cloth according to the ranks of social privilege. And in both cases it also shows that sight is connected to a moral origin, to the observer's very soul.

It would appear that Avellaneda reiterates the power of ocularcentric discourse as a way to sustain power and privilege of elites in the colony, yet from this perspective, she tells us, not all truths can be revealed. Another sensibility is required to reroute an understanding of Cuba. This is not different from Gorriti's assessment of the corrupt Federals, where Gorriti stressed the work of the ear, showing the importance of hearsay for the *mazorca* police and for Clemencia's perceptions as well. By capturing traces of words that are inaudible to others, Gorriti melded different tones and voices, she forged an understanding of moral truth that went beyond the lines of Federalist or Unitarian correctness; all of this while the Rosas regime not only worked by visual signs as proof of Federal allegiance—the red ribbon, et cetera—but also prevailed upon eavesdropping and rumor in order to maintain control. To topple this, Gorriti also came to the power of sound; the ear was her mode of responding to the Federalist secret power. By no slight coincidence, then, Gorriti's fictions were usually filled with voices, noise, and music. Recall, then, her repeated citations of musical phrases, especially from opera and dirge. "De profundis," for example, fills the pages of her story "The Black Glove" and is the story's concluding reference, allowing the narrator to lament the loss of love and the tragedy besetting the nation through the vehicle of song. In other stories, she cites Verdi's opera to explain political turmoil at home. Her characters, for example, listen to Ernani both in "Gubi Amaya," where the operatic plot anticipates the masked identities and concealments enacted by rivaling factions in the Argentine civil wars, and in "A Year in California," where characters await the dramatic revelation of identity concealed by the predatory, copper-skinned man. Even in one of her final books, *Oasis en la vida* (1888), the male character, eager to learn of the intimacies of women's friendships, eavesdrops as women practice piano and sing to music. Through her long years of publication, the fine-tuning of the ear serves Gorriti well as she homes in on political conflict and the trials of social clashes.

By contrast, the gaze that is so important in the work of Gómez de Avellaneda fixes the reality of a slave economy; the reader sees the land that begs for manual labor and the master's unrelenting power. It is this situation that Sab cannot hope to thwart. Nevertheless, as Avellaneda makes clear, the power of vision also belongs to subalterns, and although they cannot compete with the master's control, their quick eye focuses on the contrast of truth and deception. Sight, in their case, is used to expose injustice, although without necessarily resolving the crisis of colonial law. It reveals the differences between surface and depths, between physical response and feelings, as it shows a dimension of meaning that lies outside the standard visual sightings that pertain to the profit motive. *Sab*, then, accomplishes two projects in the realm of the senses: first, it shows that the evils of property are not to be resolved through negotiation (this is not a space for advancing the liberal slogan "Let's all be friends"); and second, *Sab* inverts the power of sight by announcing the pervasive blindness of elites and by showing that only the slave can correctly see the truth of social and political life. It is clear, however, that this is not the time to resolve the colonial crisis and the economy it engenders.

A word here about the time of the senses. In Gorriti's case, time is marked by the advance of the Federalist clock, which counts the hours until a bloody slaughter occurs; in *Sab*, time is marked by the calendar, telling us most immediately of the approaching day for the lottery drawing and later of a transfer of land, but also telling us that characters are moving—albeit at a behemoth's pace—toward the time when slavery will end (though it is not in the frame of the novel). But time also affects our understanding of gender and social class: the way we register time sets women apart from men, the gentry from the subalterns, urban foreigners from rural dwellers. It is often expressed through leaps in the novel (see the interlaced stories in *Sab*; see the parallel scenes of Federals and Unitarians who inhabit the works of Gorriti; think of the many spatiotemporal moves that shuttle us through the houses of Matto de Turner's Kíllac; see the juxtaposed scenes in different locations that are set in *Uncle Tom's Cabin*), and it is especially sustained by the "meanwhile," the word that Benedict Anderson (1983) suggested as the way to link the simultaneous episodes of life lived out under the clock of the nation. This "meanwhile" moves fiction from country to city, from the estates of elites to the hovels of peasants, but it also shows that different senses are at work to define the bodies of individuals living different lives under a single flag. From this disharmony in perception, literature acquires its form.

In a recent proposal about temporality in the novel, Fredric Jameson explains time in terms of affective responses, and in particular he makes a distinction between affect and emotion. The affects, he argues, are vague feelings resisting language. These are waves of generalized sensation, something you feel in your bones. Affect is "pure present," not tied to the past; it speaks to an unknown destiny or future. Autonomous, affect counterbalances plot and narration, which carries emotion. Different from feelings, which are diffused and unleashed, emotions have names and meanings; emotions signify something (Jameson 2013, 33). Here, then, we have two categories to help speak about *Sab* and the power of sensory perception. In the novel, we witness the story of Sab, the subaltern women Martina and Teresa, and finally the privileged Carlota who hopes to return to Cubitas and its bucolic world beyond time. Each stands for a different way of managing temporality and each offers a unique proposition for affective experience and reading. We thus have the following narration: Carlota, though at first bewildered, eventually describes her pain, lamenting the baseness of Enrique and her eventual loss of Sab; in the process, she comes to understand the meaning behind her emotion, although she is stuck in a melancholic longing for a past to which she can never return. Acutely aware that she has missed her turn—despite her massive privilege—she is late for the banquet of history. Against this, we have the tableaux of Teresa and Martina, culled from the world of intuitions and sensations, women who are quick to seize their reality without giving it a name. Though they know the course of history, they realize that they are unable to act: one (Martina) chooses to remain in the isolation of Cubitas, where she eventually dies, and the other (Teresa) withdraws to a convent, where she also meets her death. Like the walls of the nunnery—with its structures of enclosure—death imprisons an unnamable grief that cannot be acted upon in history. Neither affectivity nor emotion can lead them to a suitable future. This is considerably apart from Jameson's proposal that works through affectivity as a way to enter historical time. Still under a colonial system with no guarantees of freedom, Gómez de Avellaneda's *Sab* cannot flirt with such speculation.

Looking backward from the novel's conclusion, we see that Sab lets his affectivity explode without giving meaning to the gesture, without achieving agency necessary for the strength of any rebellion. We only learn, after the fact and through his famous letter, of the full gift of his perceptions; only at that time, and because of his entry into print, does he become a subject in history, but by now he is deprived of body, senses, and soul. Like the others, he is indeed too late to contemplate the banquet of civilization. And this is what the novel shows: *Sab* is first, a novel that separates superficial visual appearance from the individual's affects, and second, a novel about the trials and failures of becoming. Sab in his lifetime never earns liberation, and seizes neither freedom nor pleasure; rather, he remains at the level of excess—vigilant, mobile, racing from place to place, always acutely perceptive or, at the time of his death, exploding with blood and bile. All said, in his lifetime, his perceptions come to naught; and as such, he fails to find fulfillment and, no less, his freedom. Similarly, Teresa never gains the love of Enrique, and Carlota, having timorously withdrawn her hand from the burning lips of the slave (Gómez de Avellaneda 1993, 53), is remanded to the earthly hell that is a marriage devoid of love. In this novel, "becoming" is not simply an evolutionary stage with a clear *terminus ad quem* in its path, but it stands still as if an aborted action, a halted physical and psychological presence, a snapshot of frozen human contacts that lack the move toward revolution. And though the landowning classes, frightened because of Haiti, come to fear the sound of machetes and the darkness of the night (75), the native Cuban subjects, who see and hear with absolute precision, cannot marshal their forces to anticipate real transformation or change. And just as the lottery is so important to the novel, the only opportunity for history is found in chance. So imagine, then, that the sensory world—like the scene of gambling the lottery evokes—lies outside of linear advancement; although it is prone to altering the course of events, it lacks root in historical time.

Gómez de Avellaneda works through the disjunction of history and sensory perceptions, using the ocularcentric mode to denote power and oppression just as it stands as a trope for the quandaries of blindness and insight. Writing a half century before the time when Cuba would liberate its slaves, Gómez de Avellaneda captures the inertia of a time in which nothing can be resolved. The novel's motivation, then, is set on "off" as affects and perceptions continue to swirl, disengaged from the law. This is not the celebration of virtue we saw in Gorriti's fiction, but a recognition of absence and the failure to move forward. Sense work proves that we are stuck, as Jameson wrote, in a long perceptual present.

A Touching Tale

In the long conversation about the senses, we are, in the context of Cuba, speaking of a propertied body that engenders, on the one hand, tropes about power and control, and on the other, a dismembering of American personhood and flesh in a timeless frame beyond history. If we move to the slave economy, however, the indisputable presence of marked and visible bodies is accentuated further: the tattoos, brandings, and scars, even conditions of *la mulatez*, are signs of the white man's control over others. Abjection shows itself in human trunks and limbs severed from name and history, broken from the past and from the idea of future. These dimensions of the slave economy were recorded in Cuban literature by writers belonging to the Domingo del Monte group of the 1830s, in the autobiography of the slave Juan Francisco Manzano (1835), and in the novels—in addition to *Sab*—that drove home the abolitionist call (from the cycle of *Francisco* fictions to the magisterial *Cecilia Valdés* of 1882); beyond Cuba, the emancipation cause was also heard in the work of writers as diverse as the Argentine Juana Manso de Noronha (*La familia del comendador*) and the Colombian Jorge Isaacs (*María*), but none achieved the international circulation of *Uncle Tom's Cabin* (1852) by Harriet Beecher Stowe (1811–1896). There are many reasons for the intense popularity of this novel—its appeal to sentimentality, its call for a renewal of Christian faith (Stowe claims to have taken her inspiration for the novel after hearing the voice of God),[18] its moral imperatives designed to awaken compassion among readers, and of course, its enduring effects upon national consciousness in the antebellum years. Despite its oft-signaled flaws—the stereotypical figures, the lachrymose scenes, and the largely paternalist vision that guides Stowe's view of Uncle Tom—the novel remains with us still. Here I want to expand observations about sentiment and sensationalist discourse that occasionally surround the novel in order to think of material ways to reach recognition not just of the terror of enslavement, but of the black and white reconciliation that was so crucial to Stowe's endeavor. Here touch is the feature that gives the "imagined community" its political meaning, a sensorial contact that requires us to reassess the "now."

Uncle Tom's Cabin was of course a masterful document of persuasion, designed to move the passions of readers and awaken them to the abolitionist cause. The details of the sensible world make that awareness possible. By putting the senses on alert, by stimulating audience feelings, by showing up close the physical effects that result from assaults on the body, Stowe gives us a model for reading that depends on perceptual sharpness. In this respect, Stowe's work dovetails with the Latin American women's case for a theory of perceptions, linking the senses to the dilemmas of a nation divided by class, gender, and race. She shows how common perceptions might draw people together.

Again Margaret Cohen gives a useful background about the workings of the sentimental novel at midcentury: "Sentimental social novels all invoke sympathetic community as the response to unequal social division, whatever their stated politics. In answering diverse political critiques of social division with sympathetic community, the sentimental social novel resembles the political and social theory of its time" (1999, 157). In general terms, and as many others have also shown, the sensible world guides popular fiction with its often wild scenes of reckless excitement, dangerous stalking and high adventure, and crossed identities that put in play the gap between appearance and essence, or between authenticity and disguise. Works that are today regarded as high literature—complicated in style and representation, in the mimetic registers of experience, and destined for an audience well trained in the art of reading—also borrow from these conventions. Whether the cliff-hanging adventures offered by James Fenimore Cooper, Poe's bloodcurdling tales of fear and foreboding, or the excesses of gothic fiction that run the gamut from Hawthorne to Melville, the sensible world defines US culture, while in Spanish America the authors of melodramatic novels and the *folletín* sustain an appetite for tragedy or scandal clear through to century's end (when naturalist doctors from Argentina to Puerto Rico—from Eduardo Wilde to Manuel Zeno Gandía—focused on unwieldy bodies resisting science and progress). Sensibility signifies the diversity of populations as well as a desired single community; it arouses suspicions and fears about others, and awakens the terms for bonding. The debate about sentimentality thus pulls us in many directions: Ann Douglas (1976) sees the tears-and-sympathy culture as a midcentury response to the rigors of Calvinism in the United States, but more important, as a strategy to uphold the very qualities that kept women powerless—timidity, religious devotion, and a refusal to compete with others; this, Douglas argues, in a mode unfriendly to feminist thought, is the originating moment of modern mass culture. Jane Tompkins (1986), from a more daring perspective, understands the political power of sentimental literature as a decisive way to challenge fundamental beliefs belonging to the mid-nineteenth century; and Shelley Streeby (2002) explores the popular appeal of sentimental fiction in terms of class and power, or, in more global instances, as a way to read for the effects of empire and territorial expansion. However we regard the impact of the sentimental mode, most can agree that the actions and emotions engendered under its banner bring us into the monstrous present, just as they bring attention to a sense of community urgently in need of repair. In this respect, Stowe's tactile, palpable world (unlike the auditory or ocular focus of Gorriti or Gómez de Avellaneda), was designed to explore the one-on-one black and white *contact* that drove the anxieties of the nation.

Of course, *Uncle Tom's Cabin* awakens sensation and affect: we weep, we lament the horrors of bondage, we accompany the slaves in their ongoing sorrow, we experience the shock of violence. The performance of abjection inspires these responses: Stowe shows us the cruel home of Simon Legree or the scene of the auctions; she shows us the welts and scars that have been etched into human flesh. Certainly, the author draws us in by the *gaze* and, in this regard, through the color of skin, which is always the first visual marker that *Uncle Tom's Cabin* puts on display. The novel is full of intensely visual, almost cinematic scenes, as if the rapid images were to match the seemingly unstoppable movement of bodies on the run. We are thus made to *see* just as we also come to *hear* the creative resistance of slaves. If the traders bark the price of flesh on the auction blocks of New Orleans, the slaves perform their way to freedom. They sing, they chant, they recite their prayers, they read aloud from the Bible, yet no scene begs more attention to sound than the remarkable garret episode in which Cassy and Emmeline perform a ghost show to frighten their horrid master. The whistle of an old bottle capturing the wind, the tapping on the floor of the garret, the human shrieks and cries staged from the hidden rooms above the great house are among the sounds that the superstitious Simon Legree *hears* from the rooms below; they remind us from a lay perspective that the acoustic show is somehow part of a challenge to the master and a resistance against human bondage. Too, the scenes of Aunt Chloe's kitchen remind us of the good *taste* of food that joins the community together. In this respect, the happy home in *Uncle Tom's Cabin* is one in which the senses are sensibly alive. Observe the kitchen scene in the home of Uncle Tom's cabin where Aunt Chloe prepares the evening repast: "Doubt not that is her that you see by the fire, presiding with anxious interest over certain frizzling items in a stew-pan, and anon with grave consideration lifting the cover of a bake-kettle, from whence steam forth indubitable intimations of 'something good'" (Stowe 1981, 67). Here, smell and sound are linked inextricably together, though a pleasant synesthesia suggests quite more than "something good"; Aunt Chloe's bake-kettle reveals the integrity and completeness of the *happy* home. The kitchen of Rachel Halliday similarly excites the taste buds. And in this space, where Eliza has been offered refuge in Ohio, the home is also loud with sound, and even inanimate objects seem to enjoy a felicitous life owing to the kindness and good intentions of the Quakers who reside there. Consider these two passages:

> If any want to get up an inspiration under this head, we refer to our good friend Rachel Halliday, just as she sits there in her little rocking

> chair. It had a turn for quacking and squeaking,—that chair had,—either from having taken cold in early life, or from some asthmatic affection . . . but, as she gently swung backward and forward, the chair kept up a kind of subdued "creechy crawchy," that would have been intolerable in any other chair. But old Simeon Halliday often declared it was as good as any music to him, and the children all avowed that they wouldn't miss of hearing mother's chair for anything in the world. (215)

> Everything went on so sociably, so quietly, so harmoniously, in the great kitchen,—it seemed so pleasant to everyone to do just what they were doing, there was such an atmosphere of mutual confidence and good fellowship everywhere,—even the knives and forks had a social clatter as they went to the table; and the chicken and ham had a cheerful and joyous fizzle in the pan. (223)

Stowe invites us to hear the pleasantries of home and the sizzling of food on the stove. In the field of representations, these passages beg for a sensual dimension that underlies the felicities of family, and they bespeak the idea of a community of individuals all joined as one. This is one way to access the humanity of the others who might remain distant from readers. "I know they *do* feel, just as keenly,—even more so,—than we do," explains one of the white women discussing questions of bondage (200). This is the lesson behind the many scenes through which we are escorted. And *taste* in this instance opens the path to understanding. Simon Gikandi reminds us that sensibility in the age of Enlightenment becomes a way to link culture and commodity (2011, 17), to draw a sensible circle of aesthetic reactions around new objects for sale and commodification. But in *Uncle Tom's Cabin,* the question of taste is centered on the slave; we come to know the desires of white subjects by their sensible relations with human property. This works, of course, in two contrary directions: On the one hand, an awakening sensibility leads the consumer to greater consciousness about her mastery over objects for sale; one sees, tastes, and hears with greater acuity through practice, repetitions of gestures of engagement, and most of all physical contact. On the other hand, through *sensibilité,* one opens oneself to greater feeling (with all the trappings of empathy and commingling that intensified feeling supplies), and perhaps a chance for a political awareness that this second experience awakens. Perhaps it comes as a surprise to think of the sensorial experience, so clearly referenced in *Uncle Tom's Cabin*, as a path toward these two dimensions, but the novel's different strategies for hearing or making sound, for tasting or forming contacts, bring the reader within range of the slaves' world in order that we might share their plight and challenge while also trying to master an aesthetic and political task.

Let me take several scenes to show in detail how this perceptual experiment works. One need only read the exciting, nerve-fraying descriptions of Eliza's escape on the Ohio River as she leaps from ice patch to ice patch on her run to freedom; she is utterly prepared to assume this danger in order to save her son. Her action of leaping over the ice floes is a key moment in the sensorial appeal of *Uncle Tom's Cabin* as Stowe preys upon a rhetorical strategy that deliberately enlivens our feelings and shows her characters coming to terms with the sensational effects that the chase engenders. At the center of Eliza's run, Stowe offers the following passages:

> The frosty ground creaked beneath her feet, and she trembled at the sound; every quaking leaf and fluttering shadow sent the blood backward to her heart, and quickened her footsteps. (104–105)

> In that dizzy moment her feet to her scarce seemed to touch the ground, and a moment brought her to the water's edge. Right on behind they came; and, nerved with strength such as God gives only to the desperate, with one wild cry and flying leap, she vaulted sheer over the turbid current by the shore, on to the raft of ice beyond. It was a desperate leap—impossible to anything but madness and despair. . . . The huge green fragment of ice on which she alighted pitched and creaked as her weight came on it, but staid there not a moment. With wild cries and desperate energy she leaped to another and still another cake; stumbling—leaping—slipping—springing upwards again! Her shoes are gone—her stockings cut from her feet—while blood marked every step; but she saw nothing, felt nothing, till dimly, as in a dream, she saw the Ohio side, and a man helping her up the bank. (117–118)

A rhetorical mechanism is at work to energize the senses. In the first quoted passage, Eliza *hears* the crunch of frost; in the second, we *see* the green bolt of ice; we also *feel* the sounds of the winter cold. And when Eliza becomes so terrified that she can no longer perceive her surroundings ("she saw nothing, felt nothing"), we the readers register the scene through *our own* work with the senses. We thus absorb the onomatopoetic effects of the river ice—as it "pitched and creaked" beneath Eliza's feet—an experience no less important than the short rhythmic phrasings that describe the heroine's escape. As readers, we are also drawn into the scene because the pulsations of our reading match those of Eliza's run. First, the present participles provide a repetitive sound; timeless too, they succeed in locking us in the panic of flight and the pure present of terror. Like Eliza, we are one in a universe of sound and accelerated movement without boundaries or end in sight: the clipped phrases, the onomatopoetic sounds, and the rhythms of rapid flight intensify the movements from which we cannot escape.

Structurally, Stowe sets up the sensorium to signal instances of freedom or hardship; the fork in meanings reminds us, too, that the valence is rarely fixed. In fact, as readers we should remain wary of a possible error that might confine sensory expressions to a fixed set of interpretations. No, sense work is not the same across temporalities and nations, nor do the modes of sensorial responses correspond to an unalterable chart of political opposition or protest. In other words, sound is not always about eavesdropping (as in the case of Gorriti), nor is the power of the gaze (as we saw in *Sab*) a steady indicator to point out the discrepancy between unequal powers, nor is a sense of taste always a vehicle to signal conflict between social classes (to be traced in Matto de Turner's *Aves sin nido* in the following pages). The example of Eliza's flight allows us to think of the uses of sound and movement as they are designed for particular *effects* belonging to the antebellum years in the United States; it is organized around the slavery debate and the call for reform of the law. And in this respect, it calls for reader engagement of physical and aesthetic perceptions, as well as a sense of justice.

Although the full range of the senses is available for reader consumption, *touch* is at the novel's center, setting a trope for Stowe to drive her political message home. Indeed, it is *contact*—starting with the "touch of those warm arms . . . [that] seemed to add fire and spirit to her movements!" (1981, 105)—that carries us away. Contact is the abiding inspiration that gives Eliza and her audience of readers their power. On the ice floe, Stowe registers Eliza's feeling as emotion "pour[s] into her in electric streams" (106) and urges her to protect her child. Stowe prevails upon the jolting technology of the time in order to describe this frenzy: contact is electrical, like lightning; it carries a magnetic energy that seems almost as miraculous as an aesthetic experience or as powerful as beholding the new machinery that surrounded Stowe and her cohorts in North America at midcentury. Yet this electrical boost is not disconnected from the workings of the mind. Continuing a reflection on the senses, Stowe writes: "Sublime is the dominion of the mind over the body, that for a time, can make flesh and nerve impregnable, and string the sinews like steel, so that the weak become so mighty" (105–106). Note here, in the connection between bodily contact and maternal mission, that moral purpose inspires courage. The body yields to the power of thought. Stowe thus links physicality to spiritual inspiration; from sensation, she marks the push toward rebellion, but also tells us that without the mind and soul in concert with the body, reform and Christian redemption can never be achieved. *Contact* and desire lie at the center of this frame.

Designed to secure an identification of black and white that begins with a common body—in this case, the body of the mother, and the contact between mother and child—Stowe insists on contact throughout the body of her text. The story of Eliza's flight is told three times in the chapter, each time narrated differently through the voices of characters who find excitement and pleasure in the tale. Each intervention comes through a highly animated voice, inflected with Southern tones and peppered with exclamations, but above all, it comes as a rush to shock the listeners and readers. In this way, the story of Eliza's escape not only spreads like rumor, but the body of voice belonging to the teller acquires a palpable form. And because it is repeated in so many voices and different styles, it very clearly reminds us of the materiality of telling.

To summarize: telling is the substance of pleasure, but it is also the basis of *contact*. The dyad can be read as an aesthetic achievement as well as a political force. Stowe thus reaches out to touch the readers of *Uncle Tom's Cabin* as the characters touch each other. The author's purpose is undeniable and we understand it when, after so many affective appeals, after so many demonstrations of the creaks and cracks of flight that Eliza and Harry endure, and along with the breathless race against time for a mother to save her child, Stowe turns to her audiences and writes: "If it were *your* Harry, mother, or your Willie, that were going to be torn from you by a brutal trader … how fast could *you* walk?" (105). Or later, when a desperate slave woman whose child has been taken away to the auction lots drowns herself in a river, Stowe turns to her reader and asks, "Have you ever lost a child?" (148). The point is to have the experience and then find the meaning in the soul, to frame the moment of contact as a shared perception that goes beyond races; in this line, and enclosed in Stowe's project of persuasion, we are asked, however subtle the message, not to leave the exaltation of the senses without placing them in a field of social rituals that can be recuperated by intellect and spirit.

This is a groundbreaking way of engaging sentiment. It is not an appeal to emotion alone, as in the many tear-jerking scenes belonging to sentimental fiction. Rather, Stowe recruits the senses in order to expose shared experience and perceptions among her readers, and to point to the missteps that have kept black and white races apart. She reminds us that there is no limit on feeling. Through Eliza's example, she directly tells us, "Feel too much? Am not I a woman,—a mother?" (133). Is the novel merely awash in emotion or is something else stirring about? Ultimately, the goal is to prove that our human experience is one.

Stowe, in fact, is concerned with awakening white readers to antislavery causes and rarely strays from the idea of finding a source of identification between black and white people. To achieve this, she introduces *experience* as a category of evaluation. And though it produces different perspectives about the world of bondage ("[T]hat's been my experience," says the evil slave catcher Haley in defense of his trade [47]), she tries to signal a common path that might join the enslaved and the free. Perhaps this is naïve, as Saidiya Hartman observes. She offers a stinging rebuke of the kind of argument that, applied to fiction, would elicit reader empathy for slaves without altering their general status of abjection. Empathy, observes Hartman, gives the reader a swell of emotion that does not promise necessarily to ameliorate the condition of the other (1997, 22–25). In other words, ties of sentiment reinforce black bondage, allowing white readers figuratively to occupy the black body without any obligation to alter history or to suffer the consequences of real oppression; in the process, black pain becomes a pleasure of white mastery, as Hartman observes (21). But if we stay with Hartman's assessment (and her view is shared by many),[19] we miss the broad appeal of *Uncle Tom's Cabin*, which is based not only on the reader's pleasure taken from the lachrymose scenes, but also on the author's recruitment of readers to acknowledge our common perceptions.

What interests me is the persistence with which Stowe establishes this singular narrative thread based on a unity of perceptions: we all see, hear, and touch the world in similar terms, proving in the long run, that black and white bodies should be considered as one. This route for understanding perception is placed in evidence even in the book's subtitle: *Uncle Tom's Cabin; or, Life among the Lowly*. It leads us not to *observe* the lowly and to *study* their dreadful lives but to situate ourselves *among* them, to partake of their experiences as our own. We might recall here that the original title planned in 1851 was *Uncle Tom's Cabin; or, The Man That Was a Thing*.[20] The shift in title allowed a turn of direction, inviting the reader to participate directly in the lives of slaves, to share their feelings and perceptions. Moreover, if black men are things as the slave traders portend, then Stowe's final objective goes a step beyond, bringing the sensuous, affective realm of these men within close range of readers, proving despite slaves' status as property that they indeed have perceptions and feelings worth knowing. In order to keep common perceptions alive, shared between characters and readers, Stowe takes the next step, awakening reader compassion in order to turn the political tide. By contrast, deadened perceptions can only be met with death. This, then, is Stowe's recipe for abolitionist thought, as much as it is a lesson for reading.

A shared sense of rhythm extends through the pages of *Uncle Tom's Cabin*. It sustains the movement of the text and exists as the pillar that gives the novel its strength. In this regard, while the text claims a moral stance, it also offers a proposal for reading. Singing and hearing hymns and songs and tasting different foods are placed in evidence in order to teach us how to interpret, to use the senses to achieve the pleasant life, but more important, to understand the span of moral purpose that encircles the happy home and the contact among people therein. Perhaps it is less surprising to think of the sensorial experience, so clearly referenced in *Uncle Tom's Cabin*, if we remember the work on this topic inaugurated by Stowe's sister, Catherine Beecher. In a treatise of 1831, *Elements of Mental and Moral Philosophy Founded upon Experience, Reason, and the Bible*, Beecher offers a panorama of sense theory as it was understood in her day. Revealing herself to be especially in tune with the work of sensationalist thinkers (Locke is her principal referent), she escorts her readers through a variety of experiences triggered by the senses and applies to them the importance of reason and consciousness, which then would sift out our sensations and assign them moral reason. This crucial but largely overlooked document situates sensation and perception as the principal guidelines for teaching first good judgment and writing skills and eventually the virtue of the Bible. It is all the more significant since, in the hands and imagination of a woman writer, the text takes the political discussion of sense experience to a moral dimension not necessarily held by the very sensationalists whose influence she cites. In the process, she also surpasses the so-called sentimental men whose politics and intellectual drive were at work in the United States in the first half of the nineteenth century.[21]

In the present context, I am particularly interested in Catherine

Beecher's ideas on interpretation through language. One of her principal modes of apprehension is conveyed through the vehicle of sound and audition: "The sense of hearing is one more connected with the intellectual and moral powers of man, than either taste or smell, as it is through the medium of this organ that both music and speech operate on the human mind" (Beecher 1831, 21–22). Beecher insisted that her students learn to *hear* the rhythms of the phrase; after all, for Beecher hearing was not only a central experience of literature and life but also the underlying basis of one's approximation to the truths of the Bible. Almost in the lines of Saussure nearly a century later, Beecher went on to explain: "We first learn the *sounds* that recall ideas, and then by means of a frequent union of these sounds with some visible sign, the power once possessed simply by the sound, is conveyed to the sign.... These arbitrary signs are called letters ... [and] by the almost infinite variety of combination, of which these are capable, every idea ... can be expressed" (21–22). Beecher was interested in the power of *sound* as part of her education of the senses; harmony, rhythm, melody, and tone carried the effects of a word "to heighten social, patriotic, and devotional feeling" (23). Language without the sensual component was incapable of sustaining attention, while an ear trained for rhythms of phrase could help an individual aspire to both a moral life and democratic practice. Hence, the value of song. Celebrating the power of patriotic hymns, Beecher chose the "Marseillaise" as her example insofar as she claimed that it "produced more effect than all the eloquence of orators or machinations of plotting statesmen" (23).

Like her older sister, Harriet Beecher Stowe also makes us aware of the rhythms that drive the text, though she sought through other sense perceptions to establish a common ground among readers. In that regard, the sense of touch principally guides her work.[22] We already saw that Eliza was electrified by contact with her son. Her emotions were swayed; her commitment was alerted by the sense of touch between them. Nonetheless, other encounters demand instruction. Through touch, one learns to correct the perils of grave social flaws, to build a fraternal bond. Touch helps remember social injustice as well as a horizon of love.

In *Uncle Tom's Cabin*, though the slaves are often on the run, Stowe points out the asynchronies of black and white contact that need remediation. We are thus told of the whippings to which Legree subjects Tom; we see the auction block where prospective buyers mishandle the bodies of slaves; we see a thwarted contact that augurs sexual abuse (remember

Cassy's refutation with her famous "touch me, if you dare!" [Stowe 1981, 504]). While these scenes present unwieldy peril as a result of human contact, other scenes of contact in the novel anticipate a politics to come. In this respect, the narrative of Miss Ophelia and Topsy briefly deserves our attention.

Ophelia travels south from her New England home in order to assist her cousin Augustine St. Clare, a slave owner who represents bad management of the plantation. By contrast to her cousin, Ophelia is the hand of moderation; she stands for industry, order, and prudence. In addition to straightening the disheveled home, her good abolitionist politics reveal her initially as a character of some appeal. However, the arrival of the slave girl Topsy puts this hypothesis to a test. While St. Clare volubly defends his slaves and refuses to use the lash against them, he also engages in a black/white exchange that denies his slaves a future. Physical encounter in this case exploits a strange success: despite his fearless contact (he embraces the slaves, he holds their hands, he lets his touch and gaze meet theirs), St. Clare never sees the need to set his subjects free. Ophelia, by contrast, gives another dimension to this tale. At first, Ophelia is repelled by Topsy's touch and voice. Assigned (with some degree of malice by her cousin) to care for the unruly child, "Ophelia stood silent, perfectly paralyzed with amazement" (352) and "approached her new subject very much as a person might be supposed to approach a black spider" (354). To touch Topsy seems impossible; her "shrill voice" is cacophonic; her toilette is "too great a shock to the nerves" (355). In short, Ophelia cannot withstand the close presence of Topsy. She rejects her touch, she withdraws from her company; in the presence of the child, she is guided by only principled "endurance" (355). The experience that puts them face-to–face lets us see the breadth of fear that cross-racial contact inspires. The course of the ensuing ninety pages in the novel diminishes that dread: "She was more diligent in teaching Topsy, . . . did not any longer shrink from her touch, or manifest an ill-repressed disgust, because she felt none. She viewed her now through the softened medium that Eva's hand had first held before her eyes, and saw in her only an immortal creature" (443). Reconciliation of the flesh is Ophelia's greatest gain; only then can she find the strength to offer Topsy a guarantee of freedom.

We see how politics sustains itself through perceptions and sensations, reaching the light of reason only when backed by legal contract. But there's another point: obviously, the senses cannot be free of the contingency of time. In other words, contact is made important insofar as it is linked to the "now." Note the following exchanges between St. Clare and Ophelia:

> "I don't want you to joke, but to reason," said Miss Ophelia. "There is no use in my trying to make this child a Christian child, unless I save her from all the chances and reverses of slavery; and, if you really are willing I should have her, I want you to give me a deed or gift, or some legal paper."
>
> "Well, well," said St. Clare. "I will;" and he sat down, and unfolded a newspaper to read.
>
> "But I want it done now," said Miss Ophelia.
>
> "What's your hurry?"
>
> "Because now is the only time there ever is to do a thing in," said Miss Ophelia. "Come, now, here's paper, pen, and ink; just write a paper."
>
> St. Clare, like most men of his class of mind, cordially hated the present tense of action, generally; and, therefore, he was considerably annoyed by Miss Ophelia's downrightness. (445)

> "Always practical and to the point!" said St. Clare, his face breaking out into a smile. "You never leave me any time for general reflections, Cousin; you always bring me short up against the actual present; you have a kind of eternal *now*, always in your mind."
>
> "*Now* is all the time I have anything to do with," said Miss Ophelia. (450; emphasis mine)

In general, Stowe's novel works through multiple temporalities: the time of the North, the time of the South, the scenes occurring in different houses, the many spaces that span the novel in the course of a single moment, and, to be sure, the time of the senses that expands the present time of description and links us in a singular "now." Once again I refer to Benedict Anderson (1983), who observed the "meanwhile" of the nation, the simultaneity of clock time that is demanded by big expanses and the many localities that constitute a single law. The "meanwhile" seen in the work of Stowe also introduces the power of the present, which belongs to bodies and sensations throughout the land; together they voice an urgency for *immediate* abolitionist action. Here politics and sensation are joined: the time of contact is for awakening, to set the machinery toward change in law.

Tasting Modernity

The representation of the senses in nineteenth-century fiction is not restricted to sight, audition, or touch. As Stowe indicates to us in *Uncle Tom's Cabin*, even taste works to give identity to communities that convene throughout the novel. By the *fin de siglo*, however, when good taste defines elites, the palate expresses new modalities of social life and proves the barriers between the classes. This is significant in Clorinda Matto de Turner's writing where the culinary conversation deliberately shows how Peruvians manage the country's bounty. In *Aves sin nido* (1889; *Torn from the Nest*), an aggressive narrative denouncing the excesses of the Catholic Church and the avarice of the gentry, Clorinda Matto de Turner (1852–1909) paints a world that separates creole privilege from the abjection of rural peasants. The dividing line in this case is set by technology and taste. Several details give evidence of the breadth of this literary proposal.

In his foreword to the novel, Antonio Cornejo Polar refers to *Torn from the Nest* as an attempt to represent in literature the details of lived experience, revealed to us through the geographic spaces (Lima and the Peruvian highlands) and "essential aspects" of a national scene (in Matto de Turner 1998, xxii). Cornejo speaks grosso modo of Matto de Turner's overarching national project, but here I want to focus on the sensual life that registers conflicts in material culture. Perceptions work as a first step to understand the divisions of race and class, and to show that gendered difference counts in order to make sense of the world. This is tested first in the literary representation of new inventions and devices—the material objects of modernity that punctuate the fiction and celebrate the rising industry of the middle classes; the second test is found in the offerings of the kitchen table, marking the binaries of scarcity and abundance, and of regional and cosmopolitan traditions.

To bring in the sensual connection, Matto de Turner reviews the technologies and fashions that fill the modern world: a Davis sewing machine (66); Barry hair dye (85); cigarettes galore; Lucía, the protagonist, in her "elegant riding habit" and her "Russian leather gloves" (147). Matto de Turner also carries promotional material in her novel and refers to the Bank of Arequipa (171) and the Grand Hotel Imperial, which welcomes the characters when they arrive in Lima from their starting point in Kíllac (165). The hotel offers the travelers "fine Belgian carpets," furniture upholstered in "dark blue napped silk" (165), and Chinese porcelain vases (168). There are several readings at stake here. On the one hand, the imported fabrics and Oriental details anticipate the passions of the *modernista* poets who would soon be on the rise; they surround the characters with sensual temptation that awakens the gaze and touch. On the other, an emphasis on material culture also reminds us of Matto de Turner's deep commitment to enterprise, industry, and profit, a turn away from the landed oligarchy in order to support new forms of mass production endorsed by capitalist investors. Beyond this, there is her understanding of the double life in Peru: rural and urban, premodern and new are in dubious coexistence. Here the railroad is central to her sharp critique. Of course, modernity would not be complete without the "puffing of the locomotive ... and the whistle that announces progress, brought by the rails to the place where Manco Capac stopped to found the empire of the Incas" (151). Yet paradoxically, for its dizzying speed (156), the train later derails and crashes (158). A sign of modernity's dangers, a caveat to those who, like Sarmiento, tied Latin America's advancement to the construction of the rail lines,[23] the wreck in *Torn from the Nest* stops the narrative clock and reminds us of the *other* temporality that governs the *fin de siglo*. After all, the train collides with a herd of cows and nearly falls into a river. A collision of different worldviews? A stance against modernization? Matto de Turner is too clever to oppose the new (and indeed she supports it), but she once again sets modernity alongside traditional life. In this way, she guides our attention to the untouched past, in this case rural agriculture or the folk creations of the people of Kíllac. But in the process, she is able to skip over the corruption that guides business in the regional *fin de siglo*. Matto de Turner, in short, turns to a premodern time before the proverbial fall. The novel is littered with signs of this enduring culture, among them the handcrafted chairs made in Colombia and Bolivia forty years before the novel was written (which "are now museum pieces in the cities of Peru" [80]) and the primitive merchandise that Indian women offer to travelers from the mountain ranches (156). Two worlds are thus set in juxtaposition: the city world of Lima with its latest inventions versus the premodern life of the inhabitants of Kíllac who stand outside of history. In all of this, what is most striking, however, is Matto de Turner's world division based on the sense of *taste*, and for this she skips the metaphorical trope of taste as refinement of *gusto*, but focuses quite literally on the appetites for food.

Food occupies a grand space in the narrative system of *Torn from the Nest*, separating the indulgences of creole elites from the starvation of Indian populations. Because the contrast of the classes is put in opposition, the noted emphasis on taste stands out all the more. Taste, then, in its double meaning of good choice and good palate, becomes a way to separate the palate of elites from the palate of the masses. Taste also speaks for wealth and poverty as much as it appeals to the ways in which the body—the palate, the taste buds, the mouth—will intervene to evaluate past and future, tradition alongside progress. See, then, how Matto de Turner condemns the Indian's modest diet of turnip leaves and beans (58) insofar as it endangers the health and longevity of natives; see her delight as Doña Peronila bakes fish in an earthenware pan and prepares chicha for the house (57); follow her exposure of the priest's gluttonous pleasures in local dining fare, especially the "pigeon a la criolla" (63), which he covers from a parishioner's view in order not to share it, and which he sniffs with disdain as the last visitor leaves because his repast is no longer warm. The novel is littered with references to food and eating, from the meals of the humble to the "gastronomic tournaments, alias banquets" (85) of corrupt officials and elites of Kíllac. For their extremes, she denounces the excess of alcoholic drink among the clergy and Kíllac elites (85, 139, 146) and condemns the Huachipairi tribe for their anthropophagous rituals (74–75).

Matto de Turner also traces with delight the "steam [that] rose from the soup," focusing on its aroma (17); the rich scents of coffee and *chuño* (19); and the delicacy of "roast stuffed guinea pigs, chicken almandine, ... green beans and a stew" (109). This festive tone culminates in the final banquet that Fernando and Lucía Marín prepare for their neighbors in order to lean on the Kíllac gentry and secure a political favor. The gathering is described for its extravagant cost (141), for its lavish offerings at the table, and the exquisiteness of the platters (143). Abundance is in clear view just as taste undoubtedly drives this scene (while the native populations, by contrast, are left with little to eat). A secondary message points toward the culinary independence of Latin America in the late nineteenth century, where despite the urge toward progress, the humble local food is still the repast of preference. The nation finds its flavor in local cuisine and through the native cultures that have suffered the indignities of colonization. Clorinda Matto de Turner thus presents a political conflict organized around a dispute about taste. Here, the enticements of food on the palate are central to defining a sense of self in late nineteenth-century Peru—taste as a sign of class division, taste as a sign of traditional life set against the modern.

Women reiterate a concern for taste as a century-long obsession, of a national scene pointing to divided experiences about the common palate, while taste signals a national identity formed beyond European standards.

Thus while Brillat-Savarin in France published *The Physiology of Taste* (1825), American women broke away from Paris in order to elevate local cuisines. As in Matto de Turner's case, a strong political message is offered that centers on home economies as the basis of class distinction. If the women of the United States promote frugality and prudence (see especially the texts of Lydia Maria Child and Catherine Beecher), Latin American women such as Clorinda Matto de Turner offer an equivalent when they speak of domestic economy, thrift, and food.[24] But when it comes to taste, the worlds are divided: while Matto de Turner takes the domestic table to show the harsh divisions of classes, other Latin American women identify with the dining of elites and only rarely consider those who might be restricted to a leaner table. Taste shows the gradations of power and wealth defining South American culture without necessarily supplying an attendant critique of the divisions between social classes.[25]

Consider briefly a text by Matto de Turner's contemporary, Juana Manuela Gorriti. *Cocina ecléctica*, in its simplest version, was an assembly of recipes by Latin America's elite women, señoras from Mexico to Chile and Argentina under the sway of Gorriti, who by 1890 was securely established on the Spanish American literary landscape. Gorriti's collection of recipes was a way to govern taste, to find its literal meaning in its gustatory, olfactory, and visual components of edibles for the palate. Her book also seized upon and promoted cuisine as a defining mark of modern culture. Gorriti's experiment is playful, but also bespeaks a Pan-American commonality among Latin American elites. The contributors to Gorriti's cookbook promoted the bounty of the American table, celebrating local cuisines that were decidedly different from the European model (although, it should be noted, Mercedes Cabello de Carbonera borrowed a recipe from a Parisian cook, and a woman from Montevideo took a recipe from a transatlantic chef who registered as his claim to fame a culinary preparation for the famous Italian soprano Adelina Patti!). Despite these minor deviations from American ingredients and dishes, the recipes of *Cocina ecléctica* showed a variety of temptations, putting emphasis on forming good taste through Spanish American and Brazilian cuisine. Combined with Gorriti's editorial interventions ("Nowhere in the world do they know how to prepare rabbit as well as in Bolivia" [1977, 255]), taste defines a local direction for the senses. Within this framework, an emphasis on taste serves not only to uphold the class distinctions that Matto de Turner stressed in her novel, but to find a community in the Americas that could appreciate a common meal.

This focus on taste is yet another way to reach the objectives of Matto de Turner's vision: the need for ecclesiastical reform, the correction of those government leaders given to theft and crime, the failure of education to train the native masses. But good taste underlies it all; a way to forge once again a version of Peruvian identity through the experience of nourishment and food, a way to present the regional sketch as a debate about appeals to the palate.[26]

A Sensible Conclusion

I opened this chapter with reference to Bacle's prints, which gave a lighthearted rendition of women's place in the Argentine public sphere during the early years of the Rosas regime. Using the sensations of airiness to propel bodies in flight or showing the weight of the *peinetón* that would hold female figures down on earth, Bacle portrayed his women as vacuous creatures lacking grander thoughts about anything other than haberdashery and high fashion. Far more serious, however, nineteenth-century women writers offered a detailed tutorial for the senses, training citizens for a political life of action and ethical choice. This was introduced by their overriding attention to a different kind of material culture—not just fabric and combs, but devices such as telephones and transatlantic cables, sewing machines and stoves, kitchenware and plumbing—and related these to the enhanced perceptual skills that these novelties seemed to awaken. Technology expanded the range of sensory perceptions; hearing, sight, taste, and touch acquired wider dimensions. All of this allowed the modern citizen—regardless of gender—to participate more fully in the new experience of modernization. The human body occupied center stage to capture this expansion; sense perceptions registered novelty, political and social change.

The works of fiction discussed in this chapter provide a frame for sense work to be captured in present time but also within the specificity of local political struggles. Recall how Carlota's dilemma is set when she eschews the "coal hot lips" of the slave in Gómez de Avellaneda's *Sab*. Fear of passion, fear of contact, and fear of freedom are linked in a single trope. Carlotta misses the advantage of present time to take significant action, just as Sab, with his expert gaze, comprehends the politics behind land grabs and colonial invasion but refuses to act in the moment. The result, then, is that Gómez de Avellaneda's novel expresses melancholic reflection, since everyone has missed the opportunities that the "now" might provide. Similarly, in Gorriti's stories, the present moment is always under inquiry as the divided forces in the civil wars refuse to act in time to save liberty and lives. Only Clemencia puts her body on the line in order to act for political justice, while the others are left in states of grief and clamped in the bondage of regret. By contrast, Clorinda Matto de Turner's solution works through the "now" of present time just as taste is instrumentalized in a move toward political explication. And in Harriet Beecher Stowe's work, we see that the "now" of action is the only acceptable course for ending the legacy of slavery and bringing change to the republic. The "now" that is the time of the senses is the course of perceptual acuity and experience in the world, but it is also a time for action.

Is this the moment to think of the first step of Hegelian self-consciousness as an alertness to one's body? Or is it the time to call attention to the writings of Karl Marx, who in the *Economic and Philosophic Manuscripts of 1844* wrote that the "forming of the five senses is a labor of the entire history of the world down to the present" (1964, 141)?[27] What Hegel and Marx overlooked was the wide panorama of *gendered* actions that would direct a history of the senses from the margins. Indeed, they failed to imagine that their story could be rescued by "scribbling women" (so demeaned with these words by Hawthorne), nor could they imagine that sense work would be traced through a narrative of female labor. Through the pressures placed on the flesh of the hand, through appeals to sound and taste, through conflicts between what is observed and what remains occluded, these women found in sense work a radical understanding of politics and daily life; a sense work that anticipates history.

CHAPTER 3

Collective Synesthesia

The 1920s Avant-Garde

The world enters through my eyes.
It enters through my hands and my feet.

VICENTE HUIDOBRO

The sinister old man walks through a cardboard landscape. He marches east and west, over hill and dale; he zigzags through city and country. He follows dazzling and narrow paths where everything is artificial. Yet a plot soon emerges: we learn that the man goes in search of a carnival where he hopes to perform his magic. Once there, and in order to enter the big tent, he cajoles local officials, among them a resistant town clerk who is found dead the following morning. A murder mystery thus lingers as the performer secures a role in the circus and begins his enactments on stage. We are about to witness the work of an illusionist who will awaken his puppet from a deathlike sleep; responding to his master's calling, the dormant creature arises to take his place at the old man's side. Astonished spectators are enthralled as the captive's senses come alive; he is now prepared to open his eyes, to see, to hear, to touch, to move, and finally to act. The master taunts the innocents who behold this incredible performance—"Cesare knows every secret—between the past and future"—and with this, he incites the crowd to pose a question to his Frankensteinian monster.

These uncanny aspects combined with murderous crime lie at the center of *The Cabinet of Dr. Caligari* (1920), the inaugural film of the horror genre that captivated viewers worldwide, dragging them between a desire for revelation and a bald indulgence of the senses. With so much ambiguity about the unstable boundaries of fear, *Caligari* touched the nerve cells of the viewing public, while it also served as a metaphor for the intricacies of avant-garde art. After all, the film is not simply about madness and murder; it is also about the craft of narration, parading a cast of readers and tellers who compete for the right to tell and then to interpret their stories.

The allure of this German expressionist film was not lost upon Argentine readers. *Crítica*, the newspaper of largest circulation in Buenos Aires in the 1920s, posted an advertisement for the film: "What is Caligari?" ("¿Qué es Calegari?" 1922). Anticipating the film's debut in Buenos Aires, the publicity drew readers in with the following lines: "Caligari excites you with a strange sensation. Caligari frightens you with horrifying tragedy.... Caligari grabs your senses, Caligari is very impressive." In effect, when the famous silent film reached the capital city, it was promoted as an experience of strangeness, a jolt to the nervous system. By 1922, the film had not yet received the range of political commentary linking Caligari's control over his subjects to the rise of the authoritarian state, but in its time, it stood as a bizarre example of art that excited the affects and senses.[1] Fear, trembling, movement, and shock seduced the moviegoing public eager to see something new. This lasts in the film up to the final frisson, revealing Caligari the mountebank as a cunning man of science and Francis the narrator as a psychiatric patient lacking the resources to flee.

Let me stay with this film for a moment in order to flesh out the details that help us think about the articulation of the sensate world starting in the decade of the 1920s. Under Robert Wiene's direction, *The Cabinet of Dr. Caligari* was a special event that proposed a scare attack on the nervous systems of cinema audiences worldwide. Consider the scene at the carnival when a man asks the monster a question: "How long do I have to live?" The question startles spectators within the film who watch the illusionist's show, but it also affects film viewers, touching a nerve in those who wish to know the anguished answer. As the man is told he will live till dawn, his body registers shock: he trembles, he shakes, he loses his grounding, he falls into convulsion. Like the stuff of the tabloids that filled readers with "shock and awe" responses, the film shows the gyrations of the actor's body and captures what we feel as well: we feel his terror in our bodies. We thus experience a shock of recognition, and from there, things only get worse.

The exposé of the monstrous and the horrible in *Caligari* points to other aesthetic conflicts: the "art cinema" feel of expressionism collides with the thrills designed for the masses. Through the impact of perceptual stimuli, mass culture meets the avant-garde.[2] Artistic experiments of this kind signaled new directions taken by the creative imagination, and insofar as they throw their weight toward the value of intersubjective connections (mind control of the weak by the strong or an intuitive bonding among equals), they suggest the basis of political thinking as well.

I am intrigued by the example of *Caligari* insofar as it brings into contact the concerns for hypervigilance along with vague suggestions of interconnectedness that are related to avant-garde projects. Boundaries and flow, borders and sweeps: these are the conditions for knowing that direct the inquiries of mass and popular cultures as well as high-art endeavors. They allow the collision of the sensual "real" against the calculations of reason.

In this regard, a visual artist like the Argentine Xul Solar or a novelist like Roberto Arlt (I will turn to them later in this chapter) accompanied the interests of the German filmmakers: they invented expressionist dreamscapes and recruited extrasensory perceptions to cut through the course of their work. The point is not whether these artists themselves believed in supernatural forces (Xul Solar apparently endorsed these beliefs, whereas Roberto Arlt, in an early essay, attacked the esoteric practices that flooded Argentina in the first decades of the twentieth century), but that their visual works and literary texts were pitched to an audience eager to be thrilled by bewilderment or fear. Here, phantasms behind the work of art prey upon our attraction to irrational powers, ranging from delusions of authoritarian control to our private faith in the working of magic. These instances of nonreason subvert the boundaries defining organized thought, but they also introduce alternative types of community budding outside the state. While in some cases, this may seem like a continuation of the vogue of occult sciences that pervaded elite and mass cultures from the mid-nineteenth century, in others, it remains a way to investigate the limits of knowledge in times of rapid modernization. It also supplies an aesthetic and intuitive basis for intersubjective connection. For this work, it required an awakening of affects that began by disturbing the field of perceptions.

I will address the question of spiritualism in the decades of high modernism, but suffice it to say at this point that trances and séances, crystal visions, and automatic writing—all depending on faith in the unconscious mind and the connections that the performance could engender in reaching for contact with the dead—were the topics not only of psychoanalysts and philosophers from Jung to William James but also of leading artists and cultural critics in the teens and twenties.[3] They relied on sensory responses, incited by mechanical devices, to forge these interconnections linking the living and deceased. In fact, many inventions of the late nineteenth century, from electricity to phonography, were pursued not because of their domestic convenience but because of their intrapsychic potential, allowing the living to remember those dear ones who had gone before them. We might recall, in this regard, the ways in which Edison's discovery of the light bulb initially served less a household use, illuminating homes at nighttime, than the magnetic experiments that were conducted by occultists and psychics. Too, the phonograph was first designed to record the voices of the dying; only later, when spooked away by its too-morbid function, people began to use it to listen to music. Capturing the border zones between the living and the dead was a goal engaging both practitioners of the occult and modern inventors, but it also drew in writers and artists exploring avant-garde form. Electrical shocks, violent movement, and synesthetic crossings of sounds and color brought individuals close to a spiritual path while they also aided others in pursuit of artistic innovation. Witness only the magical forces at work in Vicente Huidobro's *Cagliostro* (1923), a novel written with future cinematic adaptation in mind; though it was modeled on an Italian occultist and set in ancient Egypt, many claim that it was inspired by the *Caligari* film (see De Costa's foreword to Huidobro [1981, 27]). A highly experimental poet and spiritualist, Huidobro took the lead in the Spanish American 1920s, but he was not alone.[4] Too easily we tend to forget about these trends that informed 1920s culture; I wish to bring them back in order to show how the conflicts between extrarational inquiry and logic were set to shape the general outlook of artists and thinkers who got their start in this decade.

By now, the avant-garde has been subjected to countless modes of interpretation and analysis. From the Americanist perspective, many critics have taken it as a moment of competing modernizations in which North and South American nationals contested the authority of Europe. Others have seen the avant-garde as a defiant imposition of regional interests, as in the case of Brazil, where painters and writers demanded a founding modernist expression based on autochthonous roots. In my earlier work, I also saw the local Argentine avant-garde immersed in a struggle for self-affirmation and power (Masiello 1986). From another angle, Vicky Unruh has come to understand the avant-garde as a form of activism, a "communal enterprise," as she puts it, that runs through South America. In particular, she reads the avant-garde through its regional distinctions in order to locate what she calls—in contradistinction to Ortega y Gasset—a "rehumanization" of art (Unruh 1994, 23).

Here, I want to revisit those early decades of the twentieth century not to echo their timeworn claims to originality and disruption, but to touch a founding contradiction that shapes the cultural movements of those years emerging from a debated experience about embodied perception. While the sensationalist press was eager for market and sales and tried to scare us to death, avant-garde artists considered a synesthetic, collective knowledge that combined aesthetic novelty with intermingled perceptions. The 1920s, then, as a hinge moment that carries forward the lessons of nineteenth-century artists and thinkers regarding the use of the senses, also anticipates an understanding of the sensorium that will shape discussions of experience into the twenty-first century. In this direction, creative works cross intuitive, affective states (and spiritualist dimensions in the extreme) with material bombardments of sensation that affect perceptions in the "now." The tensions between the two guide 1920s-era writers and artists.

A Theater of Conflicts

In their voracity to possess experience firsthand, to give it a name and meaning, modern writers and artists of the twenties went beyond a strictly encoded path of inquiry. They were not set on a single path with a clean and simple agenda. Rather, their art absorbed an ongoing pressure between demands for absolute knowledge (anchored in a specific time and place) and a desire for unbroken flow; it was traced in crossovers between reasoned logic and sensual instincts; it was even performed in a theater of new technologies in which the human sensorium challenged the groundings of reason and history and sought otherworldly ideas. In this context, artists even turned to esoteric sciences to nurture distant fantasy and indulge communitarian beliefs.

Not only did sense experience put artists and writers in contact with newly found objects, it allowed them to record the technologies of the day, to experience velocity, to explore radiophonic sound, and to track changing representations of space, time, and movement. Through scents and tastes, through tactility and somatic awareness, artists represented the full experience of modernity in the twentieth century and conveyed the excitement of sensual contact with new objects in the perceptual field. A more mystical version of this narrative feasted on the alchemy of sense and matter. Stated alternatively, one witnessed the performance of the marvelous reality of daily life through new technology and inventions; in more complex terms, some artists moved to find a materiality in the untouchable spirit. At the center of both pursuits was a project to conquer distance.

Along the first lines, Vicente Huidobro wrote in the prologue of his novel-film *Cagliostro* (1923): "Why should we consider [it] impossible that alchemists invented gold? Why is this so extraordinary? Aren't we surrounded by extraordinary things? Isn't it extraordinary to put a record on the gramophone and hear ... the power of human voice? Is it any less extraordinary that a single cable can transmit the necessary strength, from a distant dynamo, so that hundreds of streetcars can run through a city?" (1942, 15). Huidobro signaled a magic that sutured the gap between direct experience and knowing: he was also attentive to technological mediation that shortened distance between objects and perceptions. Of course, we hear a faraway voice; we are moved by mechanical means. But there's more. A new blending of the senses apprehended the extraordinary field of objects; "things" and sensations were brought in close, distances were cut short. To capture this, Huidobro remembered first that our knowledge is by necessity embodied; the body is the first line of contact for extraordinary material force. This would bring Huidobro to a spiritualist philosophy that allowed him to communicate with other worlds and not alone the sphere of the living. Less spiritual in their approach, other artists celebrated form and physique. This appears, for example, in Horacio Quiroga's observations at the turn of the century about velocity, energy, and the nervous system:

> One of the new characteristics of the century is our body's capacity to acquire abnormal speed. This happens, first, by electricity. Its nerve center ... transmits sensation in a single minute. A formidable hyperesthesia, whose secret is found in an insignificant chemical reaction, and whose transcendence delivers, in an hour, the same impression over five continents.... And then the locomotives, torpedo boats, and transatlantic lines, all the means of locomotion produced by what their iron bellies digest in kilowatts, and whose vital force cuts through lands and sea, and through bolts of progress or destruction. (Quiroga 1967a, 61)

Quiroga's enthusiastic reception of machines is quickly transferred to his interest in the energies of the body; he thus goes on to praise the human physical power demonstrated by exertion and sport. With respect to the bicycle, he writes: "The great merit of the bicycle is its capacity to transport, to let you arrive by yourself, to devour distances, to surprise the chronograph records, and to exclaim at the end of the race: *my strength got me here!* This is the triumph, this is the satisfaction. I am the Force, the Motor, the only being who deserves all the applause" (62–63). This Nietzschean show of prowess has a second major benefit: through exercise and exertion, I can shorten the lengths that keep me from distant places; I can control my reach. The examples cited show a fascination for new technologies of the early twentieth century and express a desire of writers and artists to overcome insuperable distance. In this respect, an emphasis on the human sensorium, so important in its modernist heyday (the Dada noise poems, the cinema of sensation, the frisson of avant-garde public performance with its parades, demonstrations, and noisy cabaret scandals), pulls us in two directions: we read for the (kitsch) spirit of cultural production, appealing to the masses through sensation, or we read for a salvation of the individual (artist) against the rising forces of capital expansion.

This tension in art and literature comes about as a way to challenge the rapid dehumanization that is often associated with the logic of clocks, the alienation of factory work, and the imposing technologies of war. Seen in this context, a "sensate turn" restores the illusion of an individual's power, allowing one to claim a *direct* control over experience, events, and contact; it also reminds us that human encounter lies at the source of representation. And let's not forget the dialogue with the dead; I'll return to this as the chapter advances.

In general terms, a marvelous materiality becomes the focus of the moderns, and with it, a new way of allowing the senses to shape the meaning of our lives and grasp the scope of history. This expands from the field of mass culture to the poetry of the avant-garde. In this regard, consider the images of the magazine *Caras y caretas*, a weekly Argentine publication that ran from 1898 to 1941. Humor, inventions, everything new, a who's who of freaks and moderns, *Caras y caretas* brought Argentina up to date with its images, gadgets, and stories. This was mass-market publishing for the middle class, promoting new technologies that improved individual perceptions. Enhancements to the body—creams, pills, diuretics, cures for edema and hair loss—accompanied a pressing desire to acutely sharpen the senses. Hence the attention to audio devices, eyeglasses, radios, and record players; the comparison of the senses of animals to the

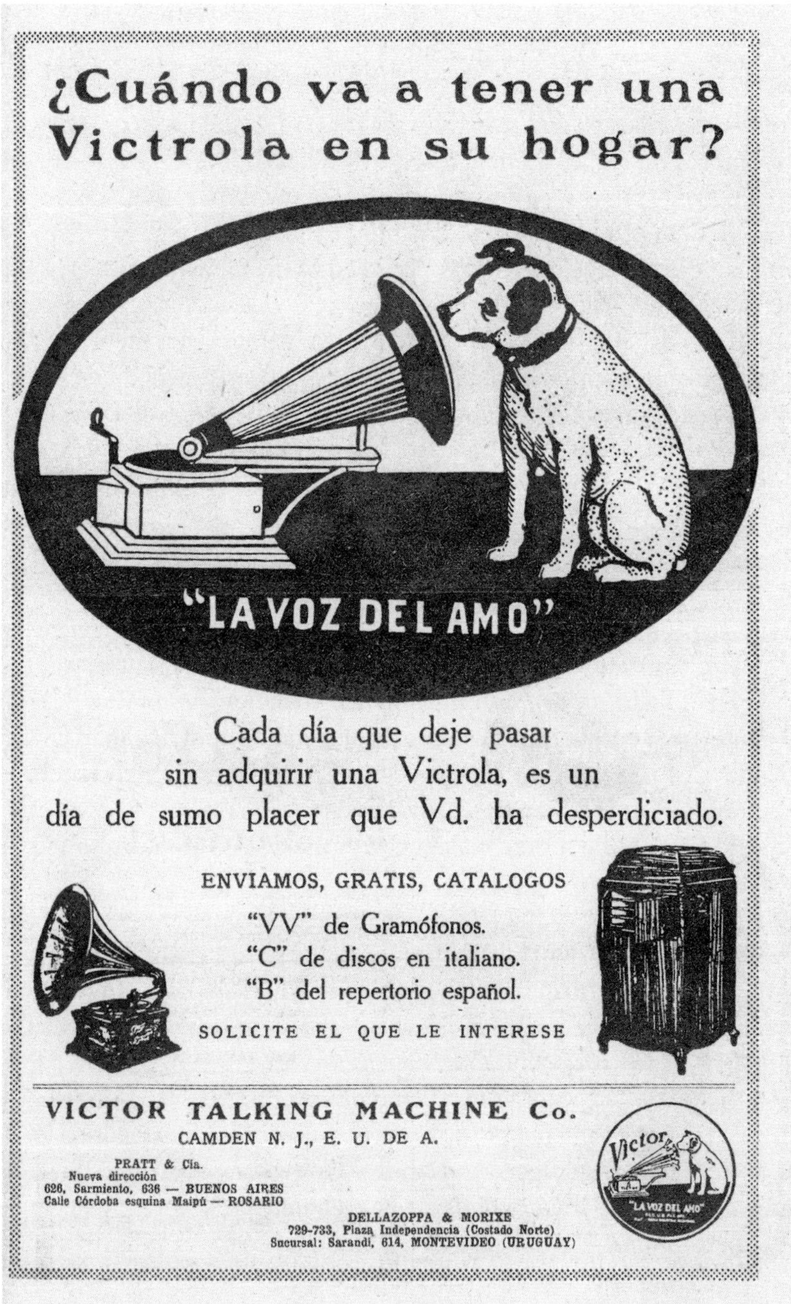

Figure 3.1. Advertisement from Caras y caretas, *no. 1340, June 7, 1924. Courtesy of University of California at Berkeley Library.*

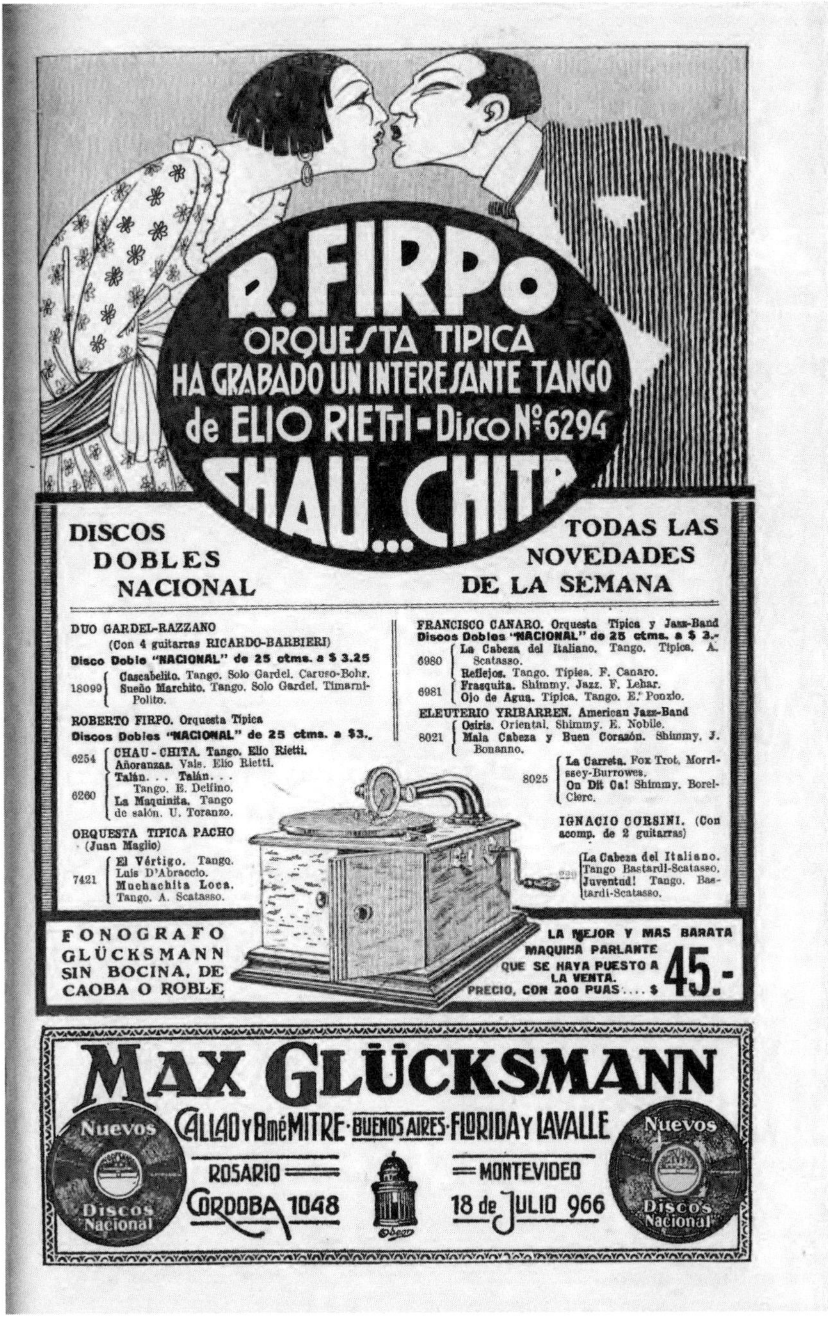

Figure 3.2. Advertisement from Caras y caretas, *no. 1358, October 11, 1924. Courtesy of University of California at Berkeley Library.*

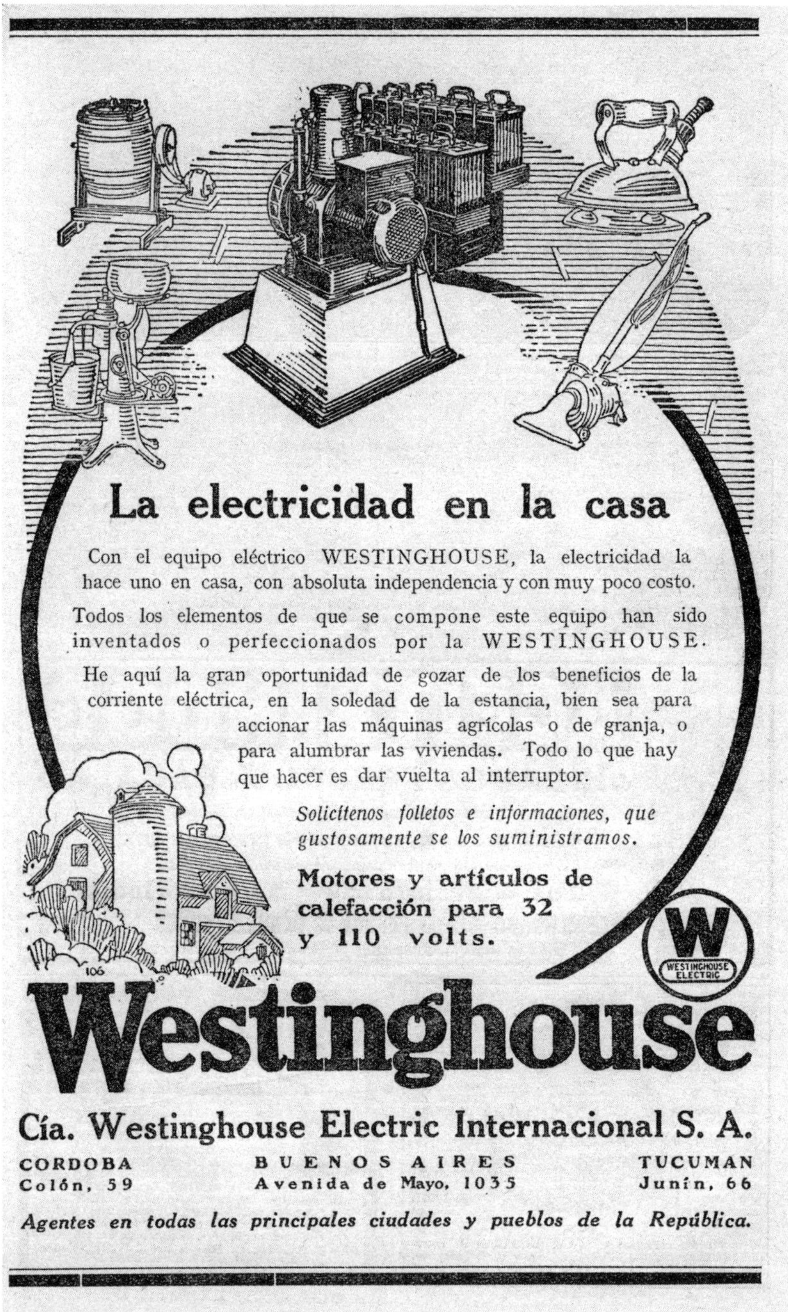

Figure 3.3. Advertisement from Caras y caretas, *no. 1529, January 28, 1928. Courtesy of University of California at Berkeley Library.*

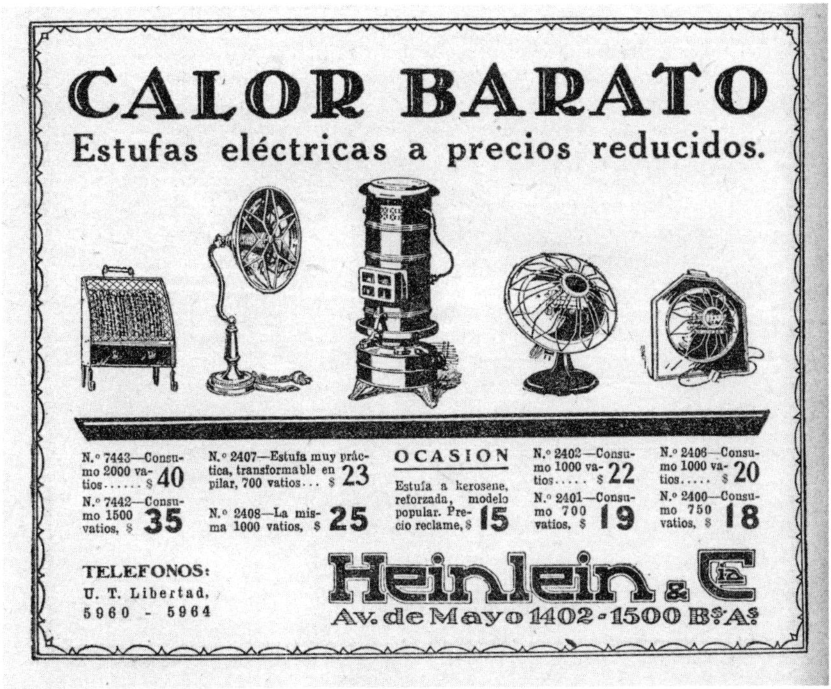

Figure 3.4. Advertisement from Caras y caretas, *no. 1340, June 7, 1924. Courtesy of University of California at Berkeley Library.*

perceptual habits of humans; and the ways to improve taste and touch. All of this formed part of the visual and narrative feast of this modern review. It paralleled the literary attention that was given to the sensual body.

From the time of the *modernistas*, writers couldn't help notice the available sensory devices designed to enhance natural perceptions. Rubén Darío's attention to sound and voice, a defining feature of his poetic breakthrough, is only brought back to earth when we think of the surrounding inventions that touched his lyric world. The news of the phonograph in 1878, the introduction of Edison's gramophone in 1899, the electric lights that dazzled the Fueguian Indians, and the wax cylinders that Lehmann Nitsche used to record the voices of Argentine natives (starting in 1905)[5] are but a small part of the technological repertoire that fascinated the public and promised to augment hearing and vision at century's end. And while scientists measured the quality of voice, charting decibels and tones of transmissions, *modernista* poets measured the timbre that the lyric line conveyed. Herrera y Reissig, for example, registered the sound of a

RADIOTELEFONIA

RECEPTOR A GALENA DE MUY BUENOS RESULTADOS

No obstante la gran cantidad de aficionados que en la actualidad utilizan receptores a lámpara para escuchar las transmisiones de broadcasting, los hay aún, y en gran cantidad, que, por una u otra razón, no pueden adquirir o construir uno de dichos receptores y deben conformarse con un simple receptor a galena, que la mayoría de las veces, por habitar en lugares próximos a alguna estación de broadcasting o de aficionado, no pueden escuchar la estación de su agrado a causa de que la mala selección del circuito no lo permite. En tales casos, recomendamos a los lectores de CARAS Y CARETAS el circuito que publicamos con estas líneas, llamado Renart, y cuya selectividad es satisfactoria, aún en aquellos casos de vecindad de alguna estación molesta.

Lo primordial para que un receptor a galena funcione correctamente y no desperdicie la poca energía que recibe de la antena, es que su construcción sea cuidadosa y *bien soldadas todas sus conexiones.* (En las soldaduras utilizadas en la construcción de receptores radiotelefónicos no debe jamás usarse ácido como mordiente. Lo mejor para estos casos es la siguiente preparación: Un trozo de resina pulverizado y diluído en un poco de alcohol. Antes de soldar, se aplica con un pincelito un poco de este líquido en el sitio necesario).

Otra de las cosas que deben cuidarse en esta clase de receptores es el cristal galena que se elija, que debe ser de muy buena calidad, natural y sintético. En plaza pueden encontrarse cristales sintéticos de gran rendimiento.

Los materiales necesarios para la construcción son: Un juego de bobinas (ver detalle de su construcción); un portacristal con su "bigote de gato"; un condensador variable de .0005 de microfarrario (23 placas); 4 bornas y alambre para conexiones. Un pequeño trozo de ebonita servirá para armar el receptor. Se adquirirá, además, un trozo de galena de buena calidad.

DETALLE DE CONSTRUCCION

Juego de bobinas. — Las tres bobinas o inductancias necesarias pueden hacerse del tipo solenoide, o a espiras juntas, o del tipo de las llamadas "Perry", cuya construcción conocen bien todos nuestros aficionados. El primario es la inductancia de 5 espiras, tipo solenoide, de nueve centímetros de diámetro, de alambre forrado de 1 y ½ milímetros de diámetro; el Secundario es la bobina de 40 espiras, tipo solenoide o Perry, de alambre forrado, de 1 y ½ milímetros de diámetro, siendo el diámetro interno de la misma diez centímetros; el "Tickler" es una inductancia de 30 espiras de alambre forrado, de 1 milímetro de diámetro; es del tipo solenoide y con un diámetro de nueve centímetros. Todos los bobinados se hacen en el mismo sentido y son fijos entre sí. El Primario y el "Tickler" van fijos, dentro del Secundario, uno en cada uno de sus costados. La manera de mantenerlos fijos queda a criterio del constructor, que puede hacerlo ya sea con pequeñas cuñas de madera o atando los bobinados entre sí. Una vez armadas las inductancias, se procederá a fijarlas al trozo de ebonita que servirá de frente al receptor. En la parte anterior de la ebonita, se colocarán las cuatro bornas y el portacristal.

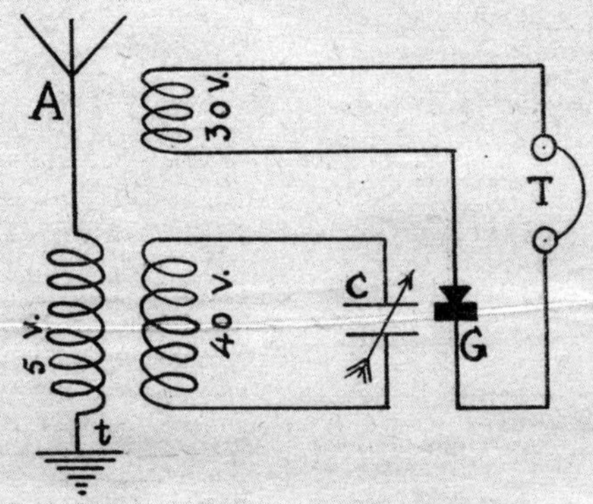

Circuito del receptor: A, antena; T, tierra; C, condensador variable; G, galena; T, teléfono.

Lo más separado posible de las bobinas se colocará el condensador variable. Las conexiones a hacer entre los elementos son las marcadas en el grabado.

FUNCIONAMIENTO

Un receptor con tal circuito es susceptible de detectar ondas de broadcasting en un radio muchas veces superior a 80 kilómetros, no pudiendo ser más simple su manejo: basta con girar el "dial" del condensador y fijar el "bigote de gato" en un punto bueno de la galena. La sintonía del receptor es exacta, debiendo variarse muy lentamente el condensador.

Una antena de un conductor, de 20 metros, basta para este receptor. Si se tuviera una antena demasiado larga, colóquesele en serie un pequeño condensador fijo de .0001 ó .00025 de mfdio.

RAUL BORDENAVE

Figure 3.5. "Un record argentino de radiografía." Caras y caretas, *no. 1340, June 7, 1924. Courtesy of University of California at Berkeley Library.*

sneeze; Asunción Silva studied his exhalations as precursors to the emission of sound. I am not referring to the ways in which the *modernista* poets praised the international expositions and fairs for their novelties and inventions; I'm considering instead the ways in which technologies determined the poem. Musical transmissions, double visions, the feel of new fabrics and dress made their way into the poetry that emerged at the turn of the century. By the avant-garde years of the 1920s, this materialist obsession with sense perceptions continued to guide the canonical poets.

Pablo Neruda's desire to bring "things" within his line of vision, thus cutting distance between himself and the world (and thereby awakening the senses), sets the pace for his *Residencia en la tierra* (Residence on earth). Not simply in his celebration of sound—the basis of the poem—but also in the senses of sight, taste, and touch that his verses often convey, Neruda repeatedly described the landscapes of city and country, the textures of clothing and shoes, and the taste of the salty sea. The world became his sensual possession whose form and substance he conveyed to his readers through the undulant rhythms of his phrases. Remember, in this respect, not only his "Arte poética" from the first *Residencia* ("[poetry] asks for the prophetic that resides in me . . . / and a blast of objects" [2005, 135]), but also his manifesto "Toward an Impure Poetry" (1935), in which he described the need for a poetic experience of *contact*, a personal awakening to the multiplicity of stimuli and events that covered the globe:

> Let that be the poetry we search for: worn with the hand's obligations, as by acids, steeped in sweat and in smoke, smelling of the lilies and urine, spattered diversely by the trades that we live by, inside the law or beyond it.
>
> A poetry impure as the clothing we wear, or our bodies, soup-stained, soiled with our shameful behavior, our wrinkles and vigils and dreams, observations and prophecies, declarations of loathing and love, idyls and beasts, the shocks of encounter, political loyalties, denials and doubts, affirmations and taxes.
>
> The holy canons of madrigal, the mandates of touch, smell, taste, sight, hearing, the passion for justice, sexual desire, the sea sounding—willfully rejecting and accepting nothing: the deep penetration of things in the transports of love, a consummate poetry soiled by the pigeon's claw, ice-marked and tooth-marked, bitten delicately with our sweat drops and usage, perhaps. Till the instrument played without

> respite yields us its solacing surface, and the wood shows the thorniest suavities shaped by the pride of the tool. Blossom and water and wheat kernel share one precious consistency, the sumptuous appeal of the tactile. (Neruda 1961, 39–40)

Neruda describes a materiality whose palpable form is rough and jagged; he reaches out for an environment populated by contrasting sights and sounds, tastes and rhythms that beg to be touched but that often elude the poet's powers to grasp it all in words. The flare-up of the sensational world always demands the poet's attentions, though he lacks full capacity to behold it. Here, we are not in the terrain of *Caligari*'s shock and terror, but stand at a crossroads where sensual beings awaken, declaring that they are alive. In short, we could say that the direct perceptual experience of intellectuals of the early twentieth century allowed them to center their bodies to receive both wonder and horror. For some, this was an irritant—the realization of a "for-profit" pathway of immediate stimulation sustained by the yellow press; for others, it was a chance to attain deeper consciousness and reach for intersubjective ties.

Across the board, the senses were supposed to "do the thinking for us," installing the body as a register of borderline experience between the material world and our spirit. Recall the high-culture figures and popular-science fans alike attempting to locate the connections between sensation and the unconscious—the séance leaders, the theosophists, the magicians and psychoanalysts; everyone from the heirs of Mme Blavatsky to the followers of Carl Jung were driven to make use of perceptual aids to reach the life of phantasms—while at the same time, the sentient body gave proof of our presence in the world.

Sense and Experience

Martin Jay (2005) alerts us to the debates about experience that run from antiquity to current times. Repeatedly, the question is about accessibility: how we balance the relationship between experience and knowledge; how we might identify what is "authentic"; and how we might close in on direct experience and find a way to define it. Without necessarily returning to Descartes and Leibniz, the observations of Hume or Condillac, or taking up the frenzied sensuous encounters that were sought by the romantics, let me turn here to the question of experience as it was understood in the early twentieth century and, with that, the chance to enter in discussion about the links between embodied perception, spirit, and reason in avant-garde literature and art.

The debate about experience, whether managed through sense impression alone or as a first step to cognition and judgment, occupies both art practitioners and writers in the early decades of the twentieth century. Georg Simmel observed in "The Metropolis and Mental Life" (1903) that individuals living in modern times were subjected to overwhelming forces: noise, speed, movement, the excess of urban clamor (1950, 409–410). The solution—a way to calm the nerves—was found in intellectual pursuits, preserving subjective life against the stimuli of the city. Such pursuits allowed us to keep things at a distance (418). From a text published in 1907, Simmel continued his explorations when he wrote of his intention to "pursue the meaning that mutual sensory perception and influencing have for the social life of human beings, their coexistence, cooperation and opposition.... That we get involved in interactions at all depends on the fact that we have a sensory effect upon one another" (1997b, 110). He goes on to see sensory impressions as the common basis of social relationships, with each sense impression as a bridge to reach the object desired (111). Although he separates the senses (the sense of smell from sight, for example), he understands that they are interrelated, and in all of this, the *face* is the center and site of this conjoined knowledge (113): we need to see each other. Finally, Simmel observes in a statement crucial for the later avant-garde: "In general, with the increase in culture, the long-distance effects of the senses become weaker and their local effects become stronger; we become not only short-sighted but short-sensed in general; yet at these short distances, we become that much more sensitive" (119). Simmel reintroduces the question of *distance*, and in this respect, he inquires about long- and short-range experience over time: how we might bring things closer within our reach through the alertness of our senses, how we might situate knowledge. Many of the writers and artists of modernism sought to restore the power of the senses to get in direct touch with a reality that was quickly fleeing from their immediate control; this obsession became their guiding aesthetic and social banner, and, indeed, as a result of it, tropes of *distance and nearness* were everywhere to be found.

Years later, Walter Benjamin, whose reputation was founded by early and sustained attention to these questions, rethought the relationship of the senses to individual experience by focusing on the bombardments of stimuli that came within our reach. Equally important, he attended to the strange effects of dissociation that modern technology supplied and pointed to the distant voices that were brought near through telephonic communication, the finger that snapped the shutter spring of a camera to retain a permanent image of the "now," the blaring advertisements of newspapers and billboards that tempted us every day and never let us rest. These were among the many ways to assault the perceiving subject, dislocating the fixity of past and present and of distance and closeness. In this respect, Benjamin famously observed, "[T]echnology has subjected the human sensorium to a complex kind of training" (2006, 191). Benjamin would keep his eye on these questions as he inquired about not only the long-distance effects of telephony, cinema, and radio, but also the close-up shocks that occurred on a daily basis, offering the potential to shape individual consciousness or cause great alienation. He thus revived the highly contested Enlightenment distinctions between *Erlebnis* and *Erfahrung*, the former referring to lived experience and the latter referring to the type of wisdom that comes from the journey—*Fahrt*—of thinking, an accumulation of memories that have been processed soulfully and with the commission of our deepest intellect. The shorthand for this would result in a spectacle of immediate sensation versus a protracted life of the mind; empiricism versus metaphysical abstraction; the flesh-and-blood body as a vehicle of knowledge versus abstract claims for universal truth that can be retained and transmitted from generation to generation. The shock of lived experience is key to Benjamin's concept of *Erlebnis*, and it is also particularly important for the ways in which it pervades and deforms the deep experience of *Erfahrung*. This concept appears throughout Benjamin's career: from *One-Way Street* (1928) to his important discussion in "On Some Motifs in Baudelaire" (1939). And although Benjamin, during his long consideration of this topic, recasts his definitions of *Erlebnis* in relation to *Erfahrung*, the shock value that is found in literature and art (whether in Breton's *Nadja* or Baudelaire's *Fleurs du mal*) continues to be central to his reflection. Indeed, it is the red thread that runs through these essays that were written through the course of a decade.

For Benjamin, Baudelaire's poetry absorbed the shocks of modern experience and allowed us to make sense of history, albeit in vague, intuitive ways. Translated to the modern era in which the avant-garde of the 1920s emerges, the crowds, streets, and technological innovation appealed to both the senses and the inner consciousness that received them. Rueful of those forms of mass entertainment that spoke merely to gratification and perturbed by the roar of the crowd, Benjamin sought a contemplative register that integrated sensational effects and spirit. In this way, he never disregarded the regime of sensation; rather, he came to terms with it by studying the ways in which modernity's shock effects were absorbed by the sentient body and then processed over time.[6] Baudelaire's poetry becomes a starting point not only because it is situated on the cusp of modernity, but also because it strikes out at a new kind of reader—the one who prefers sensual pleasure to intellectual pursuit; the one who is guided by appeals to the spleen over appeals to the mind. Here Benjamin salutes the work of Baudelaire for its intense awareness of a new experience afloat that needed to be recorded. From here, Benjamin speaks of his own moment, noting that when the aura surrounding the work of art begins to fade, likewise our appreciation of art threatens to disintegrate into "immediate shock experience" alone (2006, 210). He thus sought to go beyond jarring events (the impact of loud music, the thrust of the urban crowd, the fanfare of avant-garde spectacles that were meant to jostle the senses) and paid considerably more attention to traces of direct experience that had the capacity to affect long-term memory (the perception of a scent that stays with us, our tactile memory of a work of art). Akin to an "afterimage," these residual effects for Benjamin are the most enduring.

With some loose thread of affinity, this was translated by Bergson's concept of *durée*, a way to track the mind's retention of this afterimage of the real, fixing itself (in Benjamin's assessment) as a "permanent record" (Benjamin 2006, 172); memory, then, as a storage bin of perceptual representations that overrides the long-held distinction between matter and spirit. This narrative continued as "involuntary memory" in the novels of Proust, who was more concerned about long-term recollection rather than direct sensation alone. Through a different route, it resembled William James's idea of "pure experience" as a melding of subject-object distinctions that gave material for our conceptual thinking.[7]

The Hispanic world was not absent from this debate. Also in the first decades of the twentieth century, José Ortega y Gasset (1883–1955), modeling himself on the phenomenology of Husserl during the years that he studied at Marburg, made a case for the primacy of objects and events on the formation of subjectivity; this later evolved into Ortega's defense of a "vitalist reason" (*razón vital*) in which he replaced the Cartesian pure reason with an explanation for consciousness that depended on the merger of subjective life with external reality.[8] As he wrote in his posthumously published text on Leibniz: "What we have is the reality of who I am opening to and suffering the reality that is my environment, and that the assumed description of the phenomenon of 'consciousness' is resolved in the description of 'human life' *as* the co-existence of the 'I' with surrounding things or with circumstance" (Ortega y Gasset 2009, 1119n2).

It would be erroneous to define Ortega as a sensationalist in his early work; nevertheless, he defends the primacy of the body as a sensual receptor that awakens the human spirit. Rejecting tout court the idealism of neo-Kantian thinkers, he aims for a middle ground, somewhere between a phenomenology of perception and a systematic approach to experience that leads to an understanding of the inner self. It is perhaps in this idea of "leading to the spirit" that two moments in perception are evoked: in the first, one relies on the senses to see, to hear, to listen; in the second, one reflects on that moment of perception as an event that occurred in the past. We come to knowledge only after the fact, after the moment of sensual encounter.

This becomes apparent, for example, in his essays on Proust, texts which appeared in several installments in the Argentine newspaper *La nación* starting in January 1923. Celebrating Proust's remarkable novel, Ortega praises *À la recherche* as a work of memory and impression, but he also praises the ways in which Proust alters distance and perspective. Ortega thus likens Proust's verbal experiments to the work of the impressionists in art, locating external realities within the internal strategies for apprehension belonging to the perceiver: "We have [in Proust] a genial abandonment of the conventional external forms of things, obliging Proust to define them by their inner form, by the structure of their interior weave. But this is of microscopic condition. That is why Proust approaches things anomalously and practices a poetic histology. His work approaches the anatomical inquiries that the Germans call, for instance, 'Uber feineren Bau der Retina des Kaninchens'" (Ortega y Gasset 1923). Ortega was attentive to the minute details of perception; he reviewed the impact of stimuli and our relationship with sensible matters: colors, sounds, odors, and forms, and the way they come into our presence through observation and then remain with us through memory. Reconsidering the priority assigned to vision, he insisted on a shift and turned to tactility as the basic sense from which all other experience derives:

> It seems every day more plausible that touch was the first sensory experience and that all the others were later defined from it. From our more radical point of view, it's clear that the decisive form of our relationship with things is, in effect, tactility. And if this is the case, then touch and contact are the most pervasive experiences in the structuring of our world. . . . In it, two inseparable factors are always present: the body that we touch and our body with which we touch the other. (1964, 105–106)

In *Meditaciones del Quijote* (Meditations on the Quixote, 1914), Ortega takes a notable detour in this discussion, identifying the realm of sensuous art with the southern or Mediterranean temper, which he claimed was contrary to the apodictic thinking and meditation that the northern personality sustained. In the eighth chapter of the *Meditaciones,* he is especially critical of the sensuous impulse: "Because we should definitely call the aptitude of our interior being, sensualism. We are merely the frame for the sense organs: we see, we hear, we smell, we touch, we taste, we feel organic pleasure and pain. With a certain pride, we repeat the expression of Gaultier: 'the external world exists just for us'" (Ortega y Gasset 2004, 780). Ortega thus reveals a sliding assessment of the sensate experience: at times, he turns to sensuality as the fundamental basis for approaching art regardless of our cultural location; on other occasions, he repudiates a literature of sensation as a reduction of human experience.

When it comes to avant-garde experiments with embodied perceptions, Ortega often voiced skepticism regarding the very public manifestations of new cultural movements in Spain, where visual-surprise poetry left its mark on the 1920s and where new media technologies such as cinema attracted the mass viewing public. Although he insisted on a performative mode of exchange between subject and object (his word here is *ejecutividad*),[9] Ortega—like Benjamin—was nonetheless quick to condemn those artistic endeavors that depended on the sensorial shock alone. He particularly opposed the rapid, even sentimental, responses that seemed to bypass reason:

> All artistic style that lives off mechanical effects obtained by repercussion and contagion in the soul of the observer is naturally an inferior form. Melodrama, *folletín,* pornographic novels are extreme examples of an artistic production that lives off mechanical repercus-

> sions triggered in the reader. Note that for the intensity of effects, its power to enrapture, nothing else can compare. This helps correct the error of believing that a work is measured by its ability to enrapture, to violently penetrate its subjects. If this were true, the superior artistic forms would be small tickles and alcoholic imbibement. (qtd. in de Torre 1925, 276)

In a similar vein, Borges also entered the debate on sensation. During his early adherence to the *ultraísta* group, Borges wrote against a literature of sense stimulation:

> Lyric poetry hasn't done anything but bounce between a hunt for audio or visual effects, and the itch to express the personality of its maker. The first of two attempts is tied to painting or music, and the second to psychological error since personality, the "I," is only a wide collective label to name with one word many states of consciousness. Any new condition is added to the others and forms part of the essential identity of the "I" and says the same goes for the *individual* or the *other*. Any event, any perception, any idea defines us with equal virtue: that is, it can attach itself to us.... [It is a] useless obduracy that tries to verbally fix a wandering "I" that changes at every moment. ("Anatomía de mi ultra," 1921; qtd. in Fernández Moreno 1967, 493)

In "La nadería de la personalidad" (The nothingness of personality), Borges is even more adamant, turning against the sensualists who would define the self by its contact with the external world:

> There is no composite "I." ... Those things from which I can note a beginning or an end are not my "I." ... I, for example, am not the visual reality that my eyes apprehend, for if that were the case, all darkness would kill me and there would be nothing left of me either to desire the spectacle of the world or to forget it. Nor am I the sounds that I hear because if that were the case, silence would erase me and I would go from sound to sound without any memory of the previous sound. A similar argument could be built from olfactory, gustatory, and tactile senses, which allow us to prove not only that I am not the world of appearances ... but that apperceptions leading to the world neither are my "I." That is, I am not my activity of seeing, hearing, smelling,

> tasting, touching. Nor am I my body, which is one more phenomenon among others. (Borges 1925, 94–95)[10]

The goal was to override the sensorial games (and deceptions) enacted by the avant-garde and find the sobering point where a perceiving subject might be awakened ethically and intellectually. Here Guillermo de Torre enters the discussion when he advocates "a genuinely personal subjectivity, made objective by the surrounding elements of a live reality ... loaning our 'I' to things and reciprocally shaping an affective state that things have shaped in our being.... [T]hanks to the *Einfuhlung*, according to Lipps, subject and object, the 'I' and the 'non-I' coincide and identify with one another" (1925, 282–283). Borges, de Torre, and Ortega y Gasset sustain varying opinions about the sensate "I"; if one factor links them, it is in the idea of overriding the shock-driven experience belonging to modernist frenzy.

James Joyce was in line with the thinking of these Spanish-language writers. Remember, for starters, the scene from *A Portrait of the Artist as a Young Man* (1916) in which Stephen reflects on the dangers of kinetic approaches to art: "The feelings excited by improper art are kinetic, desire or loathing. Desire urges us to possess, to go to something; loathing urges us to abandon, to go from something. These are kinetic emotions. The arts which excite them, pornographical or didactic, are therefore improper arts. The esthetic emotion ... is therefore static. The mind is arrested and raised above desire and loathing" (Joyce 1992, 222). Joyce would struggle with this problem in *Portrait*, showing Stephen's intransigent defense of beauty as an abstract concept that refuses to be contained by any map of immediacy. Yet a paradox quickly emerges since so much of *Portrait* was forcefully anchored in the materiality that Stephen sought to reject. In a larger framework, *Portrait* thus drives us to see Stephen's struggles to understand art and beauty as they are constituted by sensual experience both in the artwork itself and in the perceptual acumen of the beholder. The whole project of this novel, then, is to explore this specific dimension: from the consequences of blending the senses to the effects of their differentiation (chapters 1 and 2); from attempts to define the relationship between flesh and spirit and the role of sensory perception as mediator between these two spheres (chapter 3); from the Christian mortification of the senses to the epiphany that might be achieved through sensuality in art (chapters 4 and 5). And in *Ulysses* (1922), for all the debate that Stephen again sustains regarding the "Ineluctable modality of the visible" (Joyce 1986, 31), the novel is impossible to read without taking into account the full extent of the human body as an organizing structure of fiction. We only have to read Joyce's famous schema, proposed to Carlo Linati, in which he indicates how each chapter of the novel corresponds to a particular bodily organ; remember also his comments to Frank Budgen in which he spoke of *Ulysses* as "the epic of the human body" (Budgen 1960, 21). But there's more: *Ulysses* offers the metaphor of the body as the basis for transformation of art. Transubstantiation, that miracle moment of the Catholic mass when the wine and wafer are transformed into the body and blood of Christ, is the basis for Joyce's foundational metaphor for the miracle of representation, when we allow the power of the word to convince us of the reality of flesh, when words cease to be simply glyphs on the page and lead us to accept the viability of image, setting, character, and story as embodied figures sustained by belief. Under this lens, *Ulysses* will never let us escape the bounds of corporeal readings, although Joyce, through the voice of Stephen, will consistently seek the merits of abstraction.

From the debates that ensued regarding sensation, it becomes clear that the thinkers and writers belonging to the modernist cohort could not settle on a single opinion regarding the relationship between sense stimulation and interior life. The goal for many was not to repress the shocks of the era but to link them to an inner awareness. Freud, for example, considered that when the effect of shock expired, what remained was expressed in the "phenomenon of becoming conscious" (qtd. in Benjamin 2006, 175). What's more, he understood that as consciousness protected itself against the threat of intense sensation, it could avert a traumatic effect; inner consciousness found a coping mechanism to cushion against shock for the long term. In this way, shock when pushed to an extreme could even be regarded as a therapeutic force. And this is where literature comes to the rescue with its capacity for transforming the horrors of the present into the deep experience of "profane illumination," as Benjamin preferred to describe it (1979, 239).[11]

Synesthesia

By stimulating new associations, by transferring the power of technology to the "image sphere" of representation, by provoking what Ortega y Gasset had seen as a "pulverization of reality within itself" through the unreality of art (1975, 147), the separate registers of the sensorial regimes often seem to conflate or cross. Our unconscious self brings forth these unclear or illogical deconstructions of the familiar world; and when they come to life, as Benjamin proposed, they offer the possibility of not just profane illumination, but indeed a revolutionary praxis. Much of modernity is defined by this inquiry, but in particular in the age of heightened technology belonging to the early twentieth century, the focus on sensate life is crucial to art and culture. In this context, synesthesia as technique often fulfills a role.

If, as Jonathan Crary has noted, the early nineteenth century marked the individuation of the senses, by midcentury a poet like Baudelaire began to find advantage in working with sensory crossovers that perceptions often supply. This was especially seen in Baudelaire's "Correspondances," whose techniques earned Benjamin's praise, where synesthesia appeals to rituals and repetitions from the "data of prehistory" (Benjamin 2006, 298). In other words, synesthesia allows the past to wedge its way into the memory of experience; the double aesthetic moment sustains two spatiotemporal flows in one. To this effect, Benjamin also cites Valéry, who described this longtime confusion as a way to prolong desire: "We may inhale the smell of a scent-smelling flower as long as we like; we cannot rid ourselves of the fragrance that has aroused our senses and no recollection, no thought, no mode of behavior can obliterate its effect or release us from the hold it has on us" (qtd. in Benjamin 2006, 203). This results in a lasting aura of an object, overriding time and distance. It is imprecise, but nonetheless fully present; it appeals to our senses far beyond reason. With this discussion, Benjamin marks the place for the phantasmagoria of modern experience—the hunches, the guesses, the collective unconscious—that lead to the ritual appeal of unspoken sensation and archetypal constructions of meaning. In this instance, the work of poetry, which crosses immediate sensation and memory, opens up hidden realities that were quietly awaiting revelation beneath the flow of daily life. And if this is the space for the development of that long journey of experience known as *Erfahrung* (Benjamin 2006, 210), the experience of synesthesia will lead us to the kind of inseparable merger of materials that in the most extreme cases can lead to the indissociability that collective experience affords.

In his essay on surrealism, Benjamin observed that profane illumination can come to a collective body and serve as an entry into a revolutionary practice that is directly in line with Marx's proposals: "The collective is a body, too. And the *physics* that is being organized for it in technology can, through all its political and factual reality, only be produced in that image sphere to which profane illumination initiates us. Only when body and image so interpenetrate that all revolutionary tension becomes a set of collective innervations and all the bodily innervations of the collective become revolutionary discharge, has reality transcended itself to the extent demanded by the *Communist Manifesto*. For the moment, only the Surrealists have understood its present commands. They exchange, to a man, the play of human features for the face of an alarm clock that in each minute rings for sixty seconds" (1979, 239). Known as the "dialectical image," this powerful encounter that Benjamin pursued may be likened to a politicization of the artistic practice of synesthesia. Let me see if I can find my way through this association and relate it to cultural production.

Intersubjective Thinking

A fusion of sensorial experiences, synesthesia is analogous to the crossover that is aimed for in intersubjective thinking. This melding of sensory perception was of deep concern to modernists, and was debated with heated intensity. For example, Wagner's synesthetic project in music, which depended on the presubjective affects aligned in a single moment, inspired the indignation of Adorno. Focused on totality, on expressiveness over signification, Wagner's drive toward integration depended on unifying the fragments, and thus issued a challenge to institutions that would catalogue and divide experience. Adorno was hardly enchanted with this proposal, arguing that in bourgeois existence, a combined sensorium was hard to imagine; instead, the separate senses told a history of reification that we should never disregard.[12] Yet creative modernist writers were nonetheless lured by synesthetic appeal. In this vein, Proust sought the synesthetic moment that was designed to be absorbed by the body, capturing the flow between past and present, melding private and public time. The merged sensorium is the aesthetic basis of *À la recherche*, registering fresh perceptions over the confining aspects of intellectual abstraction; synesthesia becomes the route of access to a hitherto unavailable past.

Let's look more closely at synesthesia. In crafting the artwork with fused stimulations in mind, writers and visual artists upset traditional categories of meaning; they dissolved the singularity of perceptions and upset the archives of sensations. Screeching landscapes, tactile visions, or a colored auditory field formed new correspondences for culture. In short, the ensemble of crossed experiences delivered to us in those years depended on a wide range of effects, eluding both strict commercial and institutional control. Liberated thus, crossed sensory effects, the stuff of both high art and mass culture, engaged the total artwork in multiple ways at once, connecting rational and unconscious levels of experience, registering distance and nearness, and in its most radical expression, leading us to think of a collective community whose experiences of reception melded with ours. The body inscribed, receiving this onslaught of sensory knowledge, was both a brace against dehumanization and a bridge to communal endeavors. William James also saw in this sensory overlap a natural feature, harkening back to infancy and what he described with a certain delight as "one great blooming, buzzing confusion" (1918, 488). The senses here are entangled with one another in the world of lived experience, one in which perceptions cannot be divided neatly into discreet parts.[13]

But what, then, is synesthesia for those who belonged to the modernist cohort? Access to the sensorial melding of twentieth-century art and literature is quite different from the experience of writers in the age of antiquity, where authors such as Aristotle and Lucretius thought that each sense perceptor corresponded to a specific type of encounter or to a clearly marked targeted stimulus.[14] Beyond the ancients and more in keeping with the eighteenth-century philosopher Condillac, who, through the figure of his famous statue, outlined a chance for multiple sensations originating from a sense of touch, the avant-garde tracked perceptual experience as multiple and materially based. Jonathan Crary (1990) notes the ways in which the senses first meld and then fall back into discrete units with the rise of modernity. With respect to advances of the nineteenth century, he leads us to ways in which a single sense—ocularcentric power—finally comes to triumph. Yet against Crary's trajectory, early twentieth-century culture seems *not* to do away with sensory melding; rather, in its effort to evoke the quandaries of nearness and distance, it continues to blur clear distinctions. Kandinsky pursued his quest for "yellow sound," as he wrote in a letter to Schoenberg, as part of an effort to find the core of sensations that crossed the boundaries of isolated perception. The Dadaist Raoul Hausmann, also seeking to cross music and color, considered "space time" as the sixth and most important of our senses. His invention of the optophone in 1922, based on his "optophonic letter poems" (similar to the calligramatic efforts of writers like Huidobro), was designed to transform sound signals into light and eventually color, a kind of televisual invention that was also supposed to stimulate teletactility.[15]

In modernist and avant-garde art of the twentieth century, the combination of sound and color harmonies was much more complicated than previously imagined by Rimbaud, and before him, Schlegel. Thus the Argentine visual artist Xul Solar linked colors to the musical scale, while Jacobo Fijman, the Argentine poet whose madness would lead him to assume the role of the mascot poet of the *martínfierristas*, wrote of the merger of color and voice or color and sense of smell. In his inaugural book, *Molino rojo* (1926), a collection of forty-one poems, Fijman likened the arid site of the asylum to a palette lacking pigments of sensual arousal. Deforming syntax and logic in order to convey incomplete thoughts, reversing the hierarchies of logic and transforming the natural world, he used primary colors to express the emotions that uniquely belong to the poet: "Green silences of the red woods / squeezed by pleasure and joy" ("Mañana de sol"; Fijman 1926, 13); "Yellow scents ... / A blue and white smile" ("Requiem"; 1926, 34). The colors that appear in these texts map a poetic consciousness conquering the whiteness of institutional confinement. Smell, silence, and joy emerge, each with its corresponding color. Equally important, this synesthetic call frees the poet from the discipline of the library and the catalogues of reason:

I am free of the four cardinal points
and from good and evil;
From the science of my library,
From my small dreams of a civilized orangutan. (1926, 89)

Synesthesia in this instance defies the archive of organized thought. Roberto Arlt took a different approach to these material exchanges when in *Los siete locos* (The seven madmen, 1929) he tried to explain the passage of time as a "drop of sound" (1978, 151). The image links sonority and touch, crossing materiality and abstraction. In this context, time acquires a footprint in space and sound, allowing Arlt's characters to experience the full dimensions of temporal flow through mixed sensory registers.

There is also a case to be made for a crossing of touch and audition. Baldomero Sanín Cano, a Colombian author who defended the craft of the worker, praised the beauty of manual labor and the centrality of the hand: "All sensibility is concentrated in the hand," he wrote in his book *La civilización manual* (1925, 48).[16] Manual work reaches out for contact; it is the primary access of sensual data, more important than vision or hearing. In this respect, Sanín Cano not only defines the human hand as our point of outreach to civilization, but he also explains it as our tool of memory, our assistant in absorbing culture. Finally, Sanín Cano proposes a largely metaphoric blending that has consequences for the synesthetic culture that I have been attempting to describe: "The hand has become a new sense capable of replacing all the other organs of contact" (49). The hand replaces the sensory nimbleness that belongs to the ear; it allows the crossing of work and pleasure. Civilization, more than an exercise of listening or thinking, is driven by the art of touch ("Civilization is more than cerebral; it is first of all radically manual" [48]).[17] Is this a proposal for the sense of touch as central to our engagement in the world? Does touch merge with other senses in order to guide us through the traffic of modernity? Or does touch substitute for thought, bypassing logic and reason? The idea above all is to create a merger of senses in which the hand performs the sensory work of the other bodily organs. A kind of synesthetic displacement, the attention to the hand leads Sanín Cano to an eventual politics of contact and engagement. Replacing the work of the brain, the hand—in the art of contact—takes on a civilizing mission.

Finally, in the extreme avant-garde of the early twentieth century, Filippo Tommaso Marinetti insisted upon tactility as one of the basic premises of the futurist movement. His "tactile tables" were intended to teach the public to become sensitive to plastic impressions, designed "to achieve tactile harmonies and to contribute indirectly toward the perfection of spiritual communication between human beings, through the epidermis" (Marinetti 1971, 111). He goes on to write: "The distinction between the five senses is arbitrary. Today one can uncover and catalog many other senses. . . . Tactilism promotes this discovery" (111). Marinetti's colleague, the musician Luigi Russolo, also followed along these lines. Russolo brought street and salon together, as his manifesto *The Art of Noises* (1913) proposes. His idea was to avail himself of the sounds of the entire world as they might fit in musical composition, but at the same time insisting that tactility also be crossed with sound. We can feel music, he wrote, through the *intonarumori*, noise instruments that produced different sounds and pitches: among them howls, crackles, metallic scrapings, motor hums, and gurgling of water; but he also gave us synesthetic sounds such as a rustle, to evoke leaves falling or fabrics rubbing against each other, or a burster that reminded us of dishes as they tumbled from heights and shattered (Russolo 1986, 12).[18] Russolo later created a *rumorarmonio*, a noise harmonium that combined in a single device all the noise instruments that he had previously invented, and also devised machines that would reproduce the noise of war.[19] "Futurist composers," he wrote, "should continue to enlarge and enrich the field of sound" (1986, 28). Perhaps Shklovsky was right when he wrote in 1925 that "art exists that we may recover the sensation of life; it exists to make one feel things, to make the stone *stony*. The purpose of art is to impart the sensation of things as they are perceived and not as they are known" (1975, 12). In the years of modernist innovation, synesthesia as technique expressed these blended perceptions and signaled the moment at which cognition awakens.

A good deal of recent scholarship has tried to home in on the meaning of synesthetic crossings. Steven Connor, for example, recently observed that this device foregrounds the idea of "commixture" and "complexions" (2004a). The blend erases the idea of a nodal point as the beginning of all experience and instead brings us closer to the kind of rhizomatic thinking suggested by Deleuze; synesthetic effects spread without control, eluding precise mappings and identities of the kind that we habitually know. Rather than occupying a place in time, the intersensorial experience resembles an uncharted route or uncertain passage; it approaches Bergsonian *durée*. No wonder, then, that synesthesia often served the modernist cohort; it produces a vague, undifferentiated feeling that unsettles our claims of certainty. Yet as scholars like John G. Gammack remind us, synesthesia prompts us toward a noetic or all-inclusive approach to knowledge; less a contrivance than a neurological response, he insists, the synesthetic experience triggers an intuitive cluster of associations that a general audience might grasp as a whole (2002, 163).

Today's neuroscientists claim a preference for this literary trope, bringing it into the discourses of the medical field.[20] In this respect, Reuven Tsur helps us think about the value of undifferentiated experience when he compares neuropsychological synesthesia to its creative literary expression. For Tsur, neuropsychological synesthesia follows regularly predictable patterns such that the element of chance is diminished; literary synesthesia, by contrast, escapes orderly boundaries. The effect of this "sense mixing" in the cultural sphere underlines an ongoing tension within the body of the beholder, but it also points out a general crisis of understanding, calling into question the limits and advantages of representation. Thus printed texts, through metaphor and other verbal tropes, appeal to audition and touch; visual images bring forth the experience of the haptic and elicit a sense of movement; musical texts evoke time and color. In all cases, synesthesia offers what Tsur calls a "double-edge" device, producing in some instances emotional effects and in others witty discordance, but what he calls "chaotic overdifferentiation" may trump those perceptions (2007, 37). Nonetheless, we face the paradox of it all: verbal representation is used to account for a process that cannot be named in language; visual representation evokes objects and moods that we cannot see; the auditory realm appeals to plasticity and our sense of touch.

Modernist initiatives following this route of experimentation challenged the idea that language had a predictable basis of meaning or a single focus of representation. Shouting, screaming, dabbling in nonsense, expanding and contracting the fonts on a page, crossing vision and tactility, mixing audition with sense of taste: this is a central part of the avant-garde stock, and it is repeated through the genres. The crossover of sound and meaning in its simplest case might be found in onomatopoeia. We perhaps best remember the optophonemic poems of the Dadaists Raoul Hausmann and Hugo Ball, the bruitist onomatopoeia of the futurist Filippo Tommaso Marinetti, the preoccupation with sensory dendrites that appears in the poetry of Leopoldo Lugones, or the sensory distortions of Oliverio Girondo's *Veinte poemas para ser leídos en el tranvía* (Twenty poems to be read on a streetcar, 1922), in which the poems carry somatic prompts that invite multiple readings: "The curtain, upon closing, looks like a curtain half open," he wrote famously in "Café concierto," as if to signal the ambiguity of the visual field unlocking a static image. But there is also a crossing in the sensual landscape, a merger of objects and places with the body of the observer. "One breathes the breeze of a postcard" (*Veinte poemas*); "A silence distracts our pupils and opens up our nose!" (*Calcomanías*, or Decals) (Girondo 1999). Despite the snapshot visions that he claims to put forth, Girondo appeals to a field of sensations that is wider than the strictly visual. By the time he reaches *En la masmédula* (In the mostpithy, 1957), words shed their links to conventional signification and become a "scat" of pulsations, onomatopoeia, and rhythms in which combined syllables create meaning from unconscious associations ("Sobracanes / pregárgolas sangrías / canes pluslagrimales / entre bastardos roces contelúricos de muy ausentes márgenes" [Excesshounds / pregargoyles indentation / plustearing dogs / between orphaned contelluric grazings by very absent margins]). We hear, touch, and inhale the voluble expanse of his poems.

A more complicated instance might be seen in the hundred-letter "thunderwords" that appear in *Finnegans Wake* (1939), through which Joyce leaves us on a tightrope somewhere between signification and raw noise. These ten famous (and incomprehensible?) phrases, which on the surface look like nonsense in sound, help move us to the mind of the character as he drifts into sleep; the letters and sounds seem to drill intensely into the depths of a preverbal mind without regard for the order of syntax. Joyce tells us that he is seeking the reverberations of words, starting—in the first example of the *Wake*—with the sound of thunder and moving forward to the sounds that fill the electrical environment of technology that defined Joyce's culture in the 1930s. Tactile, sonorous, and ever elusive, these morphemes and phonemes break free of signification yet remain in our unconscious. Is Joyce engaged in an act of sense-crossing beyond the realm of reason?

The *bulla*, or racket, whose origins César Vallejo tries to find ("Who is making such a racket?" opens his volume *Trilce* from 1922), is attached not only to the sound of poetry but to the very body of verse. The body speaks and the body receives; it contains the disparate elements that are the sensory materials of the world. Note, then, the synesthetic devices that Vallejo assembled in *Trilce,* a book that begins with bird droppings that coalesce in a viscous, palpable landmass and advances to descriptions of human waste that links all of us in natural cycles of growth and disintegration. Vallejo makes us feel the merger of senses through the impact of these events on the body. Often this impact is confused, as when Vallejo writes of the "estruendo mudo" (silent roar), printed in reverse as "odumodneurtse," so that silent cacophony is sustained as a visual experience; we *see* the power of sound.[21] The neologisms, the apostrophes, the crossings of touch and sight, the onomatopoetic invasion of sound on the page (who can forget *Trilce* XXXII?—"999 calorías. / Rumbb . . . Trraaprrrr rrach . . . chaz / Serpentínica u del biscochero / engirafada al timpano" [999 calories. / Rumbb . . . Trraaprrrr rrach . . . chaz / Snakey or out of the cookie bin, stretching its giraffe neck up to my ear])—all these allow energy to be experienced through the body, through sound, pulsation, and sight. What is obvious, here, is that the calculation of numbers and basic math are not going to help us. Rather, we must learn to think from the body, putting our heads aside.[22]

The prevalence of noise is a dominant feature of Vallejo's important book. As an example, in *Trilce* IV, he writes: "Rechinan dos carretas contra los martillos hasta los lagrimales trifurcas" (Two carts grind against the hammers reaching three-pointed tears). Whose cart grinds and whose eyes tear upon hearing a grating sound? Does Vallejo describe the cart as it meets the blow of the hammer, or does he describe the human response to such obnoxious noise? In this poem, finally, we learn that people are only organs, sensory functions lacking a capacity for love. In *Trilce* XLIV, Vallejo considers the somatic and emotional resonance of the sound of a piano:

> Este piano viaja para adentro, . . .
> Arrástrase bajo túneles,
> más allá, bajo túneles de dolor,
> bajo vertebras que fugan naturalmente. . . .
> Oh pulso misterioso.
> [This piano travels to the inside, . . .
> It runs under tunnels
> and beyond, under tunnels of pain,
> under vertebrae that naturally flee. . . .
> Oh mysterious pulse.] (C. Vallejo 1993)

We cannot explain the impact of sound and tune, or even give it a name. This is the point at which the artistic experiment assaults the body, reminding us that corporeal sensation is always crossed by undefinable rhythms that also invade our most basic perceptions far before logic awakens. We are animal if we live by the senses alone, but when, as Vallejo asks us, will we press past the *bulla*, or racket, to reach our capacity for love? Throughout *Trilce*, Vallejo prompts us to think that in our shared responses we can locate the center of the ineluctably human. It is often remarked that these letter and sound combinations, a sense mixing of the most radical order, refuse to take us to the site of reason. Like bolts of lightning or peals of thunder, their crossed sensorial appeals sweep away conventional understanding and appeal to an unspoken collective grasp.

Writing about optophonemics in 1962, Raoul Hausmann linked sound to the larger community of readers when he explained that "phonetic poetry employs hybrid sounds of language drawn from the depths of the *mega-mneme* . . . whilst simultaneously seeking to open up possibilities for a language of the future." His perspective is not unlike that of Paolo Virno (2010) or Hannah Chapelle Wojciehowski and Vittorio Gallese (2011), who in recent years have come to see the aesthetic experience as a mediated form of intersubjectivity, a cognitive archaeology of the human community plumbed from the depths of our perceptual capabilities and based on our shared reactions to stimulations that refuse to be ordered by reason. It is here that we reach back to an almost archaic premodern time, bridging the distances that keep us apart, finding in the melded forms a way to override disjunction.

Many have tried to draw a hierarchy among senses, yet this insistence on synesthetic melding prevails: under the sign of the Spanish baroque, Calderón de la Barca linked faith with audition; San Juan de la Cruz referred to his "soledad sonora" (resonant solitude) in *El cántico espiritual*; and Saint Teresa of Ávila described her union with God as the ecstasy of the body. Later, the synesthetic experience became linked to human beginnings, to infancy or childhood. Rousseau, for example, in *Émile* (1762), proposed to rescue the nature within us (the primitive, undifferentiated sensations that define infant experience) and make certain that early childhood training carried an education of the senses lest the child, grown to adulthood, find himself like a monster, hopelessly confused and inept. Critics have called attention to the weight of Rousseau's description upon Mary Shelley, whose invented creature in *Frankenstein* (1818) comes into being with a mass of undifferentiated sensations. Birth is related to the onslaught of perceptions, as the monster tells us in chapter 3: "It is with considerable difficulty that I remember the original era of my being: all the events of the period appear confused and indistinct. A strange multiplicity of sensations seized me, and I saw, felt, heard, and smelt at the same time; and it was, indeed, a long time before I learned to distinguish between the operations of my various senses" (Shelley 2007, 105). To get here, the monster's good doctor followed not simply the normal course of scientific research, but also the fields of alchemy, galvanism, and electrical response.

Echoing the plot of Mary Shelley's novel, the Uruguayan Horacio Quiroga wrote "El hombre artificial" (The Artificial Man, 1910), a novella serialized in *Caras y caretas* about a group of laboratory scientists who attempt to create human life. Falling sway to the power of electricity and other newfound technologies, they thus bring to life a creature of undifferentiated sensory perceptions.[23] The scientists' goal is to endow their creation with substantial "life experience" and help it learn to distinguish the senses in order to survive in the world. They thus attempt to awaken the being by the inaugural experience of torture. Stimulated by electrical prods, their creation quickly comes to understand anguish and suffering; he learns thus to use the senses with discrimination and finally to speak his discomfort. The laboratory inventor, upon seeing the full extent of the other's pain, falls into despair and takes his own life (Quiroga 1967b). However we take the metaphors of *Émile*, *Frankenstein*, or the story by Quiroga, it is inevitable that we come to think of these narratives as tales describing the birth of the senses along with a moral imperative to discern their separate functions and keep them *irreversibly apart*.

The later modernist example turns against narratives of this kind, blurring the lines between the senses without any attempts to restore their uniqueness. Indeed, the work of synesthesia upon the senses sustains a formal irresolvability; it appeals to the deeply personal responses of the spectator or reader while also pitching toward the interpretive and emotional reception of the community as a whole. Moving us along the surfaces, synesthetic devices paradoxically reach for communal depths. At the same time, practitioners of modern synesthesia confess that it is impossible to locate a "genuine" experience in the text. In other words, among modernists, there is no equivalent return to the birthing moment described by Rousseau, Shelley, and Quiroga; there is no subsequent separation of the senses that is seen as a path toward progress.

Avant-garde artists and writers of the twenties instead put forth a concept of body that refused to single out modes of perception or to register them one by one, and presented as an aesthetic issue the *blurring* of indistinct forms. In some ways, this mode of representation anticipates the proposals of Merleau-Ponty, who, in his quest to "re-establish the roots of the mind in the body" (1964a, 3), sought to grasp hold of "spontaneity which gathers together the plurality of monads, the past and the present, nature and culture in a single whole" (11). He projects his idea of ambiguous sense experience that points to a "world that is . . . an indefinite and open multiplicity in which relations are relations of reciprocal implication" (1962, 1). The first impact of mixed sensation thus determines consciousness and thought; transferred to the literary and artistic domain, it becomes modernity's theme.[24] For modernist writers and artists, embodied thought becomes a guiding principle and banner: it marks the double time of the archaic and the modern; it cuts through distances sustained over space and time; it overcomes the gap between sense perception and judgment. It produces, as Merleau-Ponty indeed observed, a "miracle" in which sense derives from apparent non-sense (1964b, xvii); among the common manifestations of this magic within the artistic text is that of synesthesia.

Jean Epstein and Guillermo de Torre: "A New State of Intelligence"

I want to read together several authors of the 1920s avant-garde who bring into contrast the question of direct experience and interior life, who draw attention to the crosscurrents of sensation and intellect, and resolve them through synesthesia: Jean Epstein and Guillermo de Torre. A filmmaker and early theorist of cinema, Jean Epstein (1897–1953) made incursions into contemporary poetry by seeking out the aesthetic disposition that guided his generation. His slim volume *La poésie d'aujourd'hui, un nouvel état d'intelligence* (1921), a work that spoke to aesthetics and generational inclinations of his time, found its way into de Torre's writing and eventually reached Spanish America. Epstein focused on what he called "a new state of intelligence," which he based on the kind of free association without order that is often produced when one is in a state of fatigue.[25] We feel before understanding; we have the capacity for recognizing objects, he claims, without beforehand going through the process of deep assimilation that requires historical knowledge: "The tired spirit tends . . . to see resemblance, to recognize more than to know. Memory's fatigue is there all the time. It invites the most extraordinary analogies, the least believable. It tends toward invention" (Epstein 1921, 198). Basing his ideas on emergent physiological science, on theories of sensation and cognition, Epstein wanted to explain a general excitement of the nervous system as the equivalent of a "generational psychosis" (the term belongs to Blaise Cendrars, who in the afterword to Epstein's book defines this excitement as a collective expression [in Epstein 1921, 213]). In this instance, analogy and metaphor replace deduction, logic surrenders to the rapid imprint of sensation, and a general quasi-religious fervor, refusing order and often turning to mystical abstractions, infiltrates our daily condition. Above all, Epstein claims, we live in a time in which we tend to confuse conscious and unconscious regimes (84). Like the experience of superstition and intuition, we thus enter the discursive regime of what he first calls "coenaesthesia," that combination of organic sensations that composes an individual's awareness of bodily existence, and with it, the perceptual chaos that inhabits a subject as she defines her relation to the world. This is the vital and interior state that surpasses the sum of individual senses; it allows for the merger of discreet sense experiences and speaks to the totality of common feelings that express our being in the world. In art, the uncontrollable fervor of coenaesthesia emerges as something like a religious experience; things and objects appear mysterious, coincidental, and illogical, the result of an embodied response that on the surface excludes the bounds of reason (86). It is akin to the ineffable "sixth sense" that Aristotle sought to define in *De anima*, an oblique approach to the world that is ineffable and formless. Even science, in the hands of poets, bends to this impression and resembles a spiritual quest: "The majority of writers, infinitely more intelligent than the masses, no longer dream of science as a way to happiness.... What they ask of science, their constant concern, are for vague astonishments, imprecise marvels, the transformation of coenaesthetic feelings into horoscopes, in prophecies of truth; in short, these are the new aesthetic possibilities" (Epstein 1921, 90–91). The main effect of coenaesthesia, Epstein tells us, is to *feel* before comprehending.[26] In a sweep that rejects formal logic and acts instead on the shocks sustained by the nervous system, it carries a general excitement, not unlike sexual stimulation; it provokes hallucination and movement, mental rapidity and ultimately attention fatigue. In this condition, thought proceeds in fragments, in rapid succession; analogy replaces deduction. And since there are only situations, *story* counts least of all. For Epstein, cinema is the key artistic example to capture this disequilibrium, to register unstable and rapid movement and multiple sensations at once; cinema develops this high-reflex performance in order to produce an *effect*. Epstein's observations about cinema explain the newness of the medium and, as we will see shortly, provide a parallel for avant-garde poetry.[27]

Guillermo de Torre (1900–1971) expands upon Epstein's proposal in his *Literaturas europeas de vanguardia* (1925), a classic introduction to avant-garde art in the international arena of the early twentieth century. Despite the obscurity to which it has been relegated today, de Torre's remarkable book became a gospel for Spaniards and Latin Americans subscribing to the cause of the avant-gardes; it was a mainstay for a coterie of fans who followed modern literature in the Hispanic world on both sides of the Atlantic.[28] A poet and leading proponent of Spanish *ultraísmo*, de Torre was the first Iberian writer to take an overarching look at the avant-garde movements in which he was immersed in those years. In the style of Max Nordau, whose celebrated study of French avant-garde movements set the tone for approaching these literary activities for many years to come, de Torre focused principally on the "isms" and on the writings of Blaise Cendrars, Jean Cocteau, Paul Morand, and Max Jacob. But he also celebrated Huidobro and Marinetti, situating them within a line of influence whose source text begins with Whitman. De Torre's volume of poetry,

Hélices (1923), a tome that suffers from all the avant-garde excesses that we have come to identify with visual poetry in the 1920s, is also inscribed in his critical overview. Poetry in the calligramatic style of Apollinaire; cinematic influence and movement; an indebtedness to new technology, especially the automobile and the airplane; a simultaneity of spatiotemporal experiences and an irreverence for tradition; a passage from the idealism of the romantics to a bold materialism of form: de Torre took these now-classic events of avant-garde writing and produced in his *Literaturas europeas de vanguardia* what we might consider a reader's guide to the literary currents of the early years of the century. Centering his discussion was the impact that Jean Epstein's work held for the avant-garde. Read together, Epstein and de Torre give us a gateway to understanding the ways in which the sensorial world was apprehended in the 1920s and allow us to enter in dialogue with major expressions of intellectual thought of the time. The key here is the link to a "sensorial intellect" (de Torre 1925, 130) first proposed by Jean Epstein.[29]

De Torre begins with a critique of those avant-garde subscribers who follow a literature of sensation: shock, surprise, and mechanical effects top his list. He notes in the new generation "a lyrical obsession for materials" (1925, 246), although he goes on to set limits to the problem and, on the surface, questions the merits of a uniquely sensual approach. Citing Plato, he writes: "[T]he senses only perceive events; sentiment is what endures" (277).[30] De Torre's solution, then, is to seek a melding of exterior and imaginative worlds through the mediation of art. To reach this point, however, he proposes a concept of reality that is divided in intellectual and sensorial regimes. Initially appearing to reverse the claims made by Jean Epstein, the Spanish critic defends an aesthetic practice that depends not upon exterior realities but upon a collision of interior and exterior worlds captured by the work of art: "[T]he subject of a poem secures its expressive autonomy not by reflecting external reality, but by its interior reconfiguration, by its poetic equivalent that is captured by the spirit. It's a case of the prevalence of intellectual realities over the realities perceived by the senses that cubist art has tried to defend" (129). But Guillermo de Torre is quick to remind us that the sensational world of the cubists (he takes his examples from Apollinaire, Max Jacob, and Vicente Huidobro) should not be abandoned; keeping their work in the foreground, he seeks to find a melding of sensation that reaches for new intellectual depths. De Torre looks at the superposition of incongruous forms, juxtapositions of sensations and images, the simultaneity of visual and verbal planes, and the threads of vibration sustained by human antennae leading to the world of ideas (129). If it is true, as de Torre claims, that when narrative is abandoned, only the project of sensation remains, then de Torre seeks new objectives. The goal here is to awaken interiority in the reader or viewer. The techniques for achieving this are commandeered by a sensorial intellect in dialogue—albeit in disordered fashion—with the fleeting images and events that pass before the observer; we are anchored in a pure present: "In this way, the spontaneous impulse, velocity, the unconscious flow and coenaesthesia—all signaled by Epstein—rise up to a single intellectual plane. And above, an abounding 'sensorial intellect,' finds a satisfying art and lyric in what I call 'intelligent senses'" (130).

Seeking to conceptualize avant-garde literary form, de Torre begins with a two-step approach to the perception of matter: "The senses give us the material, understanding gives us the form" (277). Here, an interior psychological mechanism is at work with embodied perception; synesthesia is the term he uses to name this internal response: "Synesthesia is the group of notions that sensibility expresses at any one time over vegetative life" (290). Against the rigor of immutable form, he demands the merger of images with deep experience, a blending of conscious and unconscious apprehensions of material form that evoke psyche and physis.

Jean Epstein offered a defense of coenaesthesia from its first iteration in the nineteenth century to its defining practice in modern times. But de Torre was even more emphatic when he insisted that coenaesthesia was the basis of all aesthetic events belonging to the avant-garde; he defined this not only in terms of the physiological response, but also as a rhetorical move: coenaesthesia—and its analogy in *synesthesia*—speaks to the heart of the literatures of the early twentieth century that de Torre observed and studied. From the crosscurrents of sight and sound, touch and taste, image and words come forth; synesthesia is shorthand for this magical blending in the field of perception, triggering an internal response in which the senses are fused. Sense associations are crossed; sympathies are extended; synesthesia leads us toward the dynamic process behind the avant-garde text. De Torre focuses on specific instances of technique within the poem and in particular on the capacity for condensation that synesthesia affords: "[P]erception of the outside world is not reflected in a new poem by a single sense, but by the concurrence of all of them at once" (1925, 292). This simultaneity of sensorial perceptions, each with its own combinations, produces a mosaic of experiences that is unique to each writer. "Each synesthetic sensation . . . favors reflection and remembrance that do not rest on intelligence, but on a synesthetic unconscious. Everything from religion to scientific inquiry that writers demand of the cult of newness ... even the horoscope, all share this characteristic" (290). De Torre elicits a connection (most likely borrowed from Epstein) to astrology, linking the avant-garde to spiritualist pursuits, tying coenaesthesia to the experience of otherworldly regimes.

With these observations, Guillermo de Torre allows us to focus on the transformative moments sustained by sensory mixture. With synesthesia (before metaphor, he adds), we are seeking out the "unstable and fleeting connection, a blip of intellectual movement, a collision, a circumstance, a conglomeration" (302–303). Above all, the new aesthetic proposal puts the qualities of instability and the transmigratory movements between inner and outer worlds at the center of the avant-garde text. It brings about a sense of mystery and coincidence, doubt or potentiality; we are in the space of sensory excitement, a momentary suspension of the reason of law. For de Torre, literature and art of the 1920s assumed this monumental challenge. The decade was faced with the hard realities of postwar times: the transformation of labor, the emergence of mass culture, the dramatic growth of urban centers, the alienation caused by rapid modernity, and the ferocious monitoring of human lives by the factory clock and by the colorless nature of the monied economy that eschewed quality for flat indifference. The culture of the avant-garde allowed us to embrace this disturbing scenario following a different course.

In de Torre's terms, the avant-garde was to find a point of connection among a community of artists and the public, and to overcome the threat of alienation that the metropolis sustained. Like Simmel, who found in the rural town an ideal space for interconnectedness,[31] de Torre saw the members of the avant-garde in search of a lost community, seeking the "communicating vases" that were so important to surrealists like Breton. His hope was pinned to finding in poetry the Whitmanesque collective soul. A quest reiterated throughout the early decades of the twentieth century—whether in Jung's pursuit of a collective unconscious or in William James's concept of "flow of life," through which consciousness was seen as continuous with the surroundings, or even in Yvan Goll's celebration of the fraternal cosmic bonding among poets of the world that he proposed in *Les cinq continents* (1922)—de Torre's search found this communal spirit in the daily experience of coenaesthesia, and in literature, synesthetic merger (1925, 335).[32]

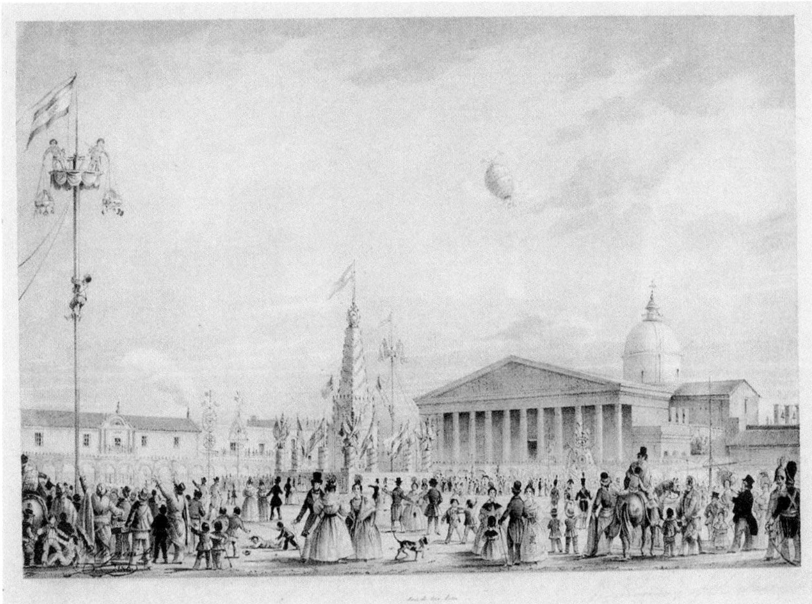

Plate 1. Carlos Pellegrini, Fiestas mayas, *1841. Lithograph. 21 × 30.7 cm. Museo Nacional de Bellas Artes, Buenos Aires.*

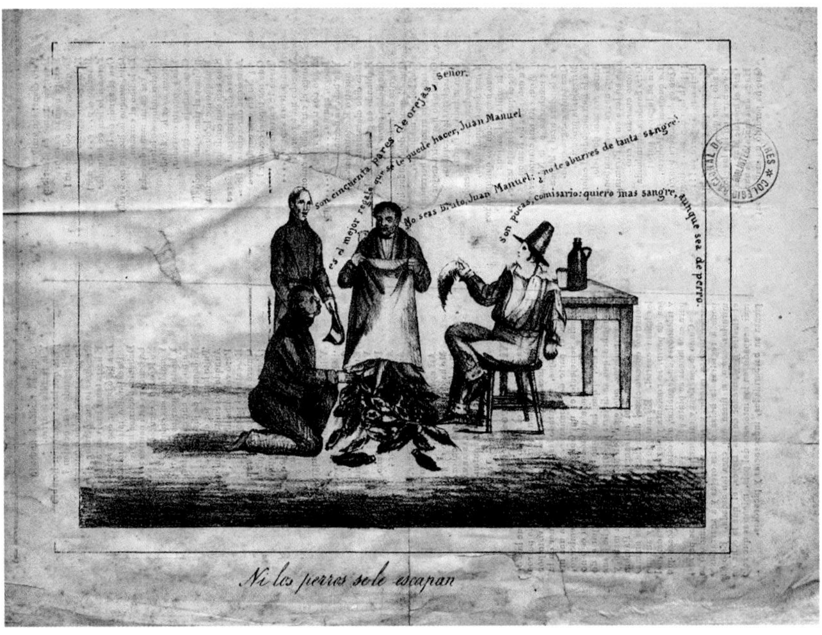

Plate 2. "Ni los perros se le escapan." El grito argentino, *no. 33, June 30, 1839, Montevideo. Courtesy of Mariano Moreno National Library of Argentina.*

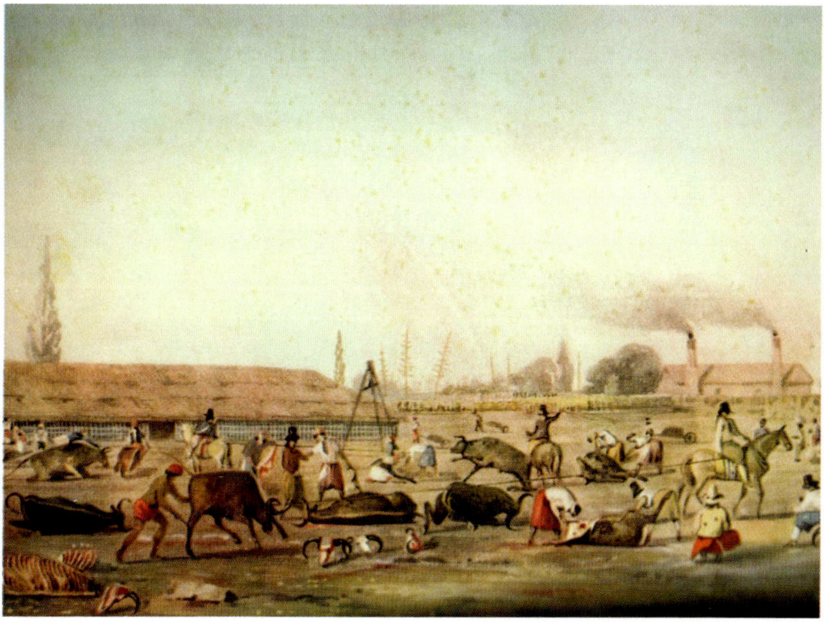

Plate 3. Carlos Pellegrini, Impression of a Buenos Aires Slaughterhouse, *1829. Museo Nacional de Bellas Artes, Buenos Aires.*

OPPOSITE PAGE

Plate 4. César Hipólito Bacle, Peinetones en casa, *from* Extravagancias de 1854. *Courtesy of Museo Histórico de Buenos Aires "Cornelio de Saavedra," Buenos Aires.*

Plate 5. César Hipólito Bacle, Peinetones en el paseo, *from* Extravagancias de 1854. *Courtesy of Museo Histórico de Buenos Aires "Cornelio de Saavedra," Buenos Aires.*

C.o 5. Extravagancias de 1834. N.o 1.

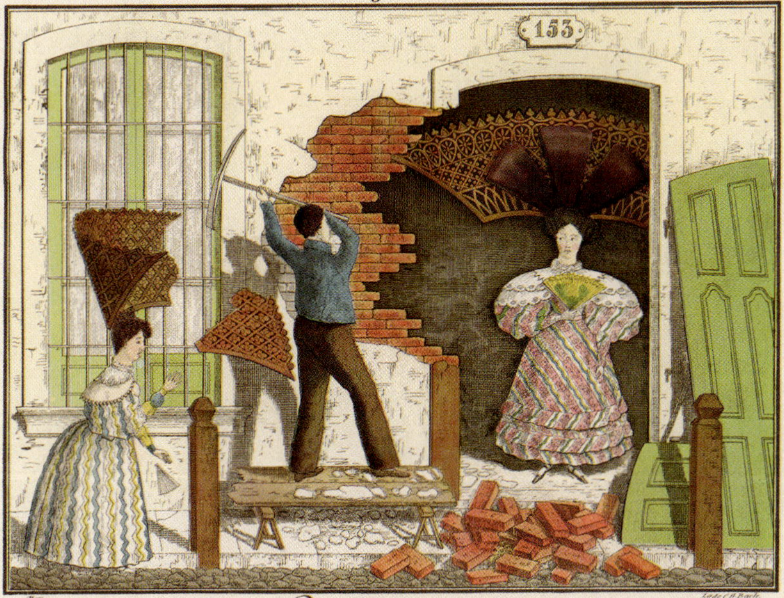

Peinetones en casa.

? Todavia mas, Señora¿ — No: basta: ahora del otro lado.

C.o 5. Extravagancias de 1834. N.o 3.

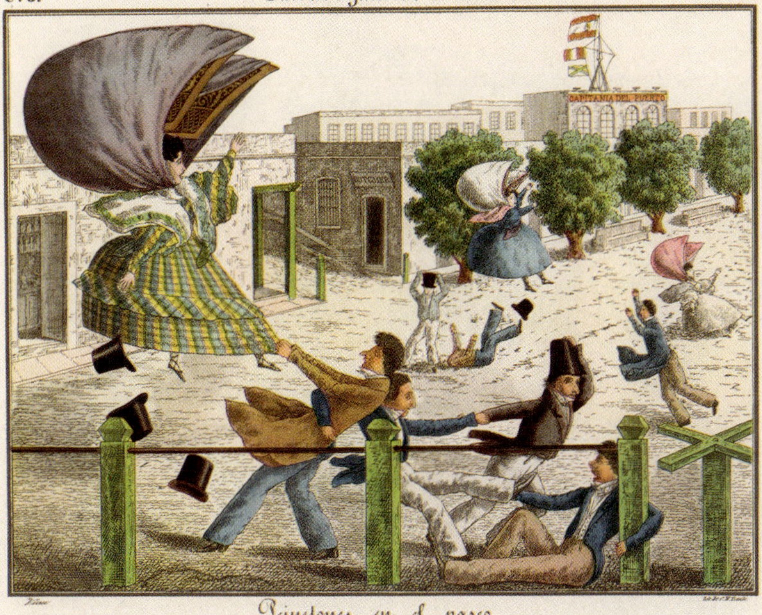

Peinetones en el paseo.

¡Auxilio: que el ventaron se arrebata a mi Señora!

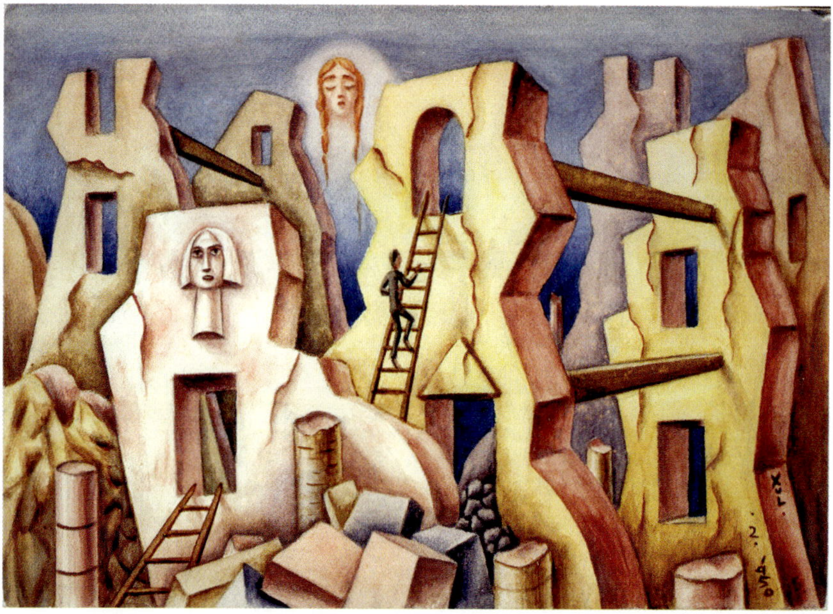

Plate 6. Xul Solar, Ruinas, *1950. Courtesy of Fundación Pan Klub—Museo Xul Solar.*

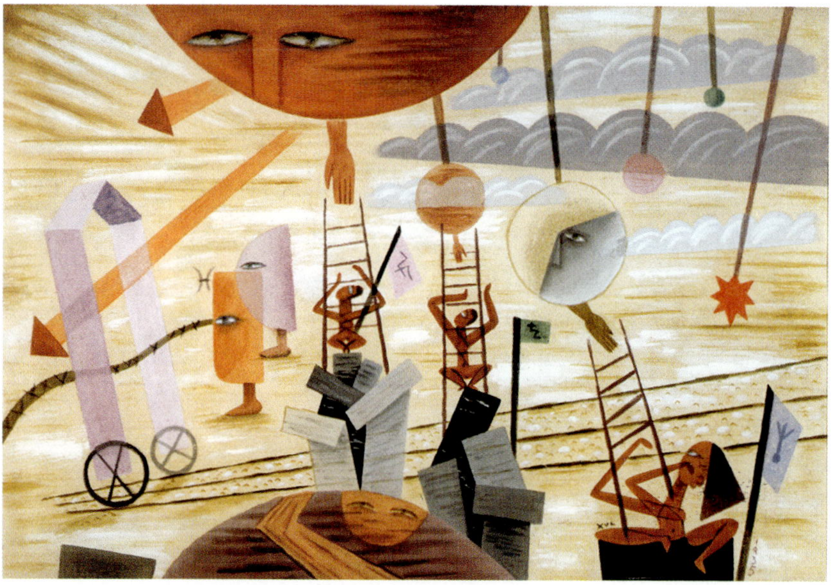

Plate 7. Xul Solar, Puerta del este, *1935. Courtesy of Fundación Pan Klub—Museo Xul Solar.*

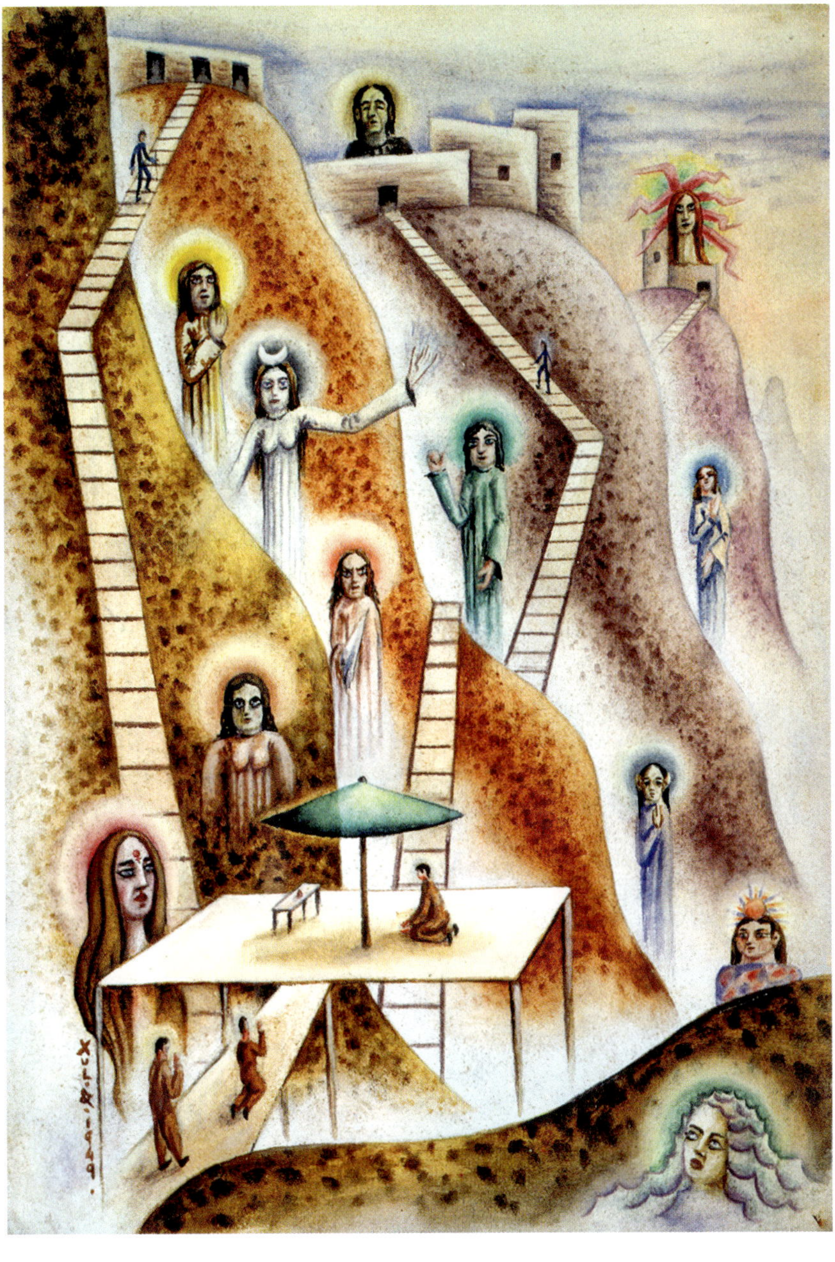

Plate 8. Xul Solar, Zodíaco, *1949. Courtesy of Fundación Pan Klub—Museo Xul Solar. All rights reserved.*

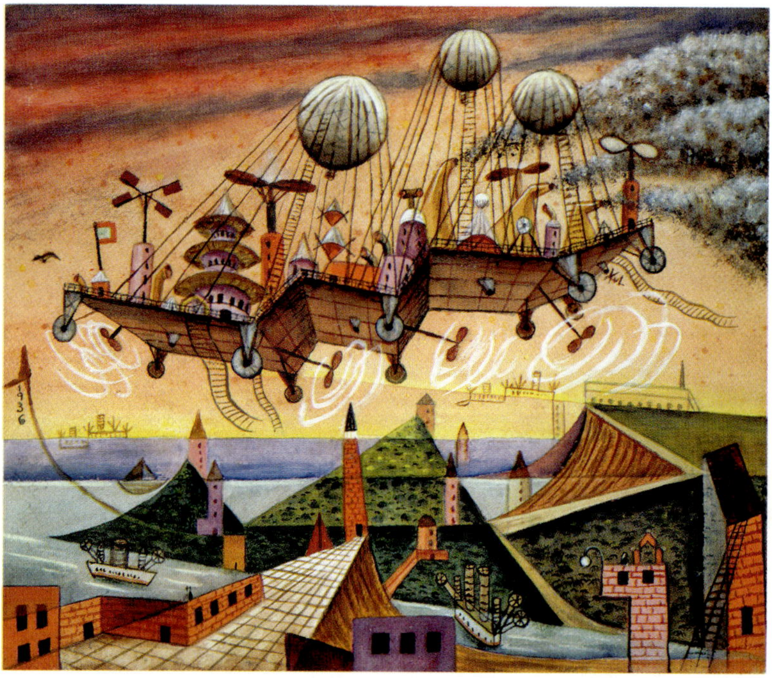

Plate 9. Xul Solar, Vuel villa, *1936. Courtesy of Fundación Pan Klub—Museo Xul Solar. All rights reserved.*

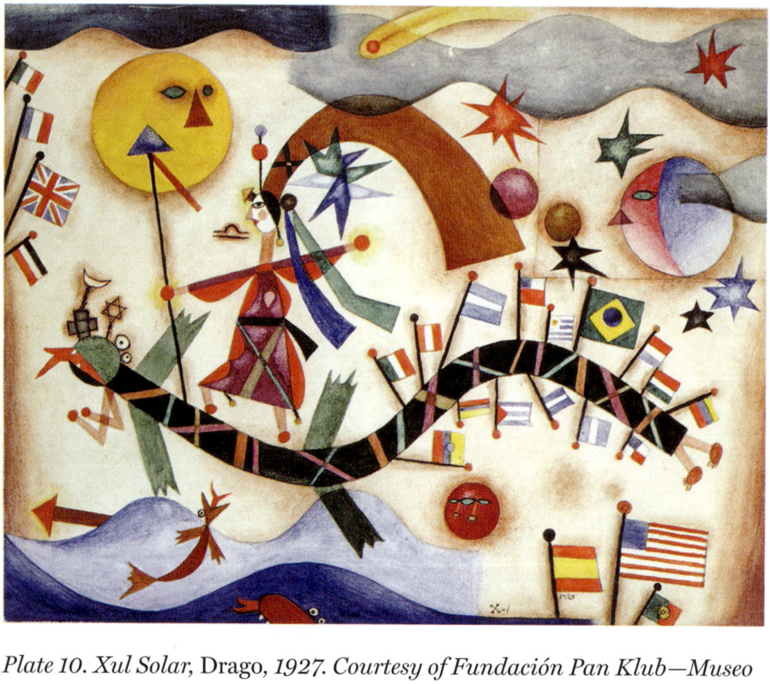

Plate 10. Xul Solar, Drago, *1927. Courtesy of Fundación Pan Klub—Museo Xul Solar. All rights reserved.*

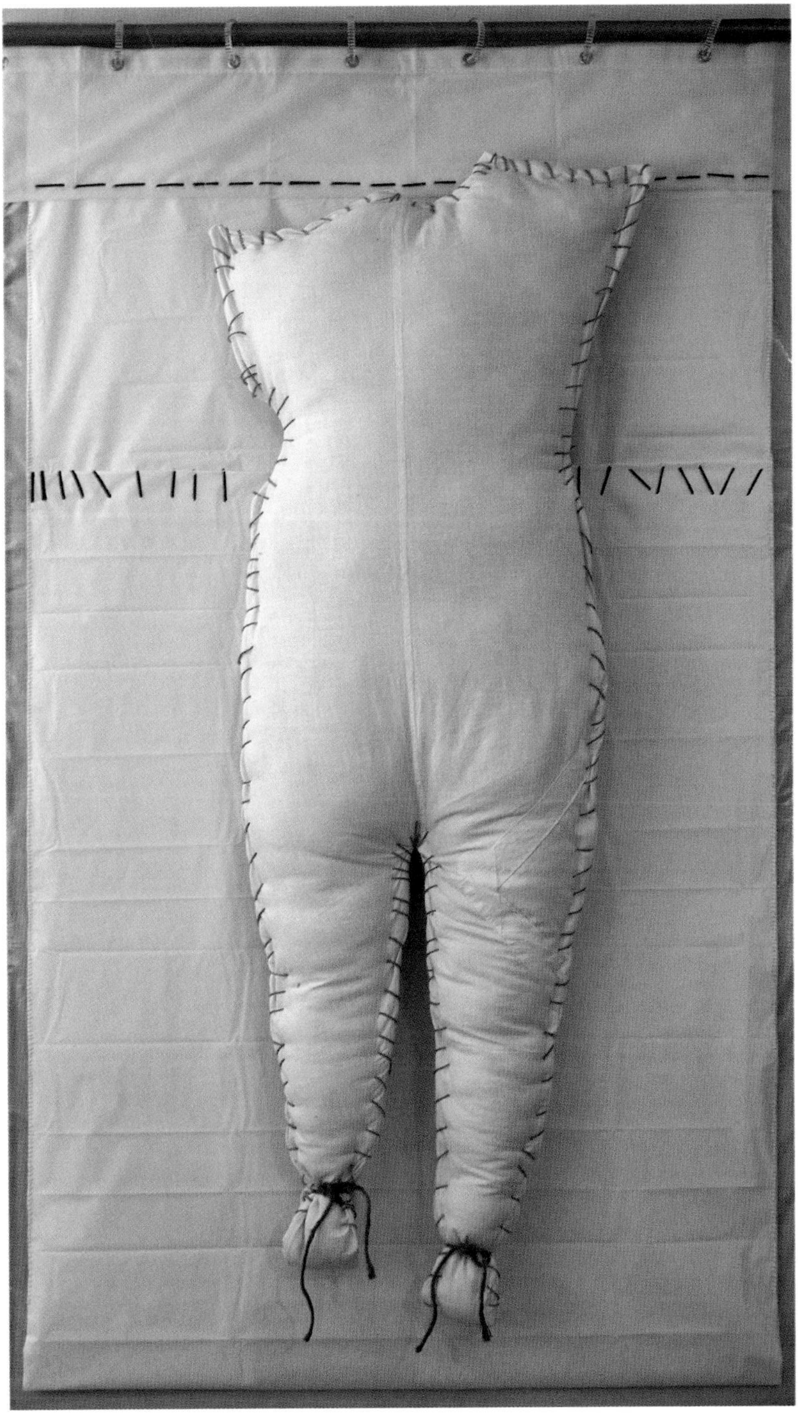

Plate 11. Catalina Parra, Imbunche gigante, *1977. Sculpture. Photograph by Isabel Soler Parra; image courtesy of the artist.*

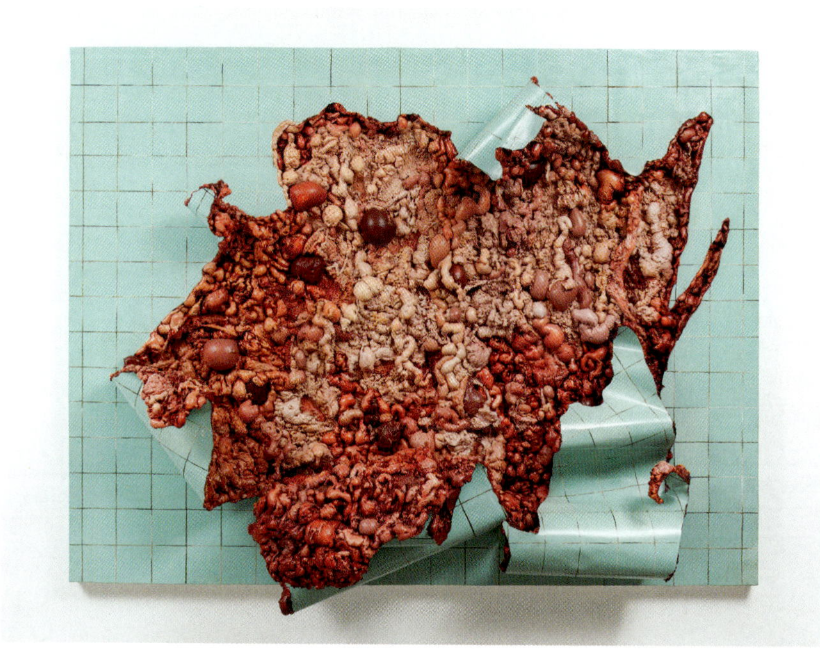

Plate 12. Adriana Varejão, Green Tilework in Live Flesh, *2000. Oil on canvas and polyurethane on aluminum and wood support. 220 × 290 × 70 cm. Collection Tate Modern, London. © Adriana Varejão. Courtesy of the artist.*

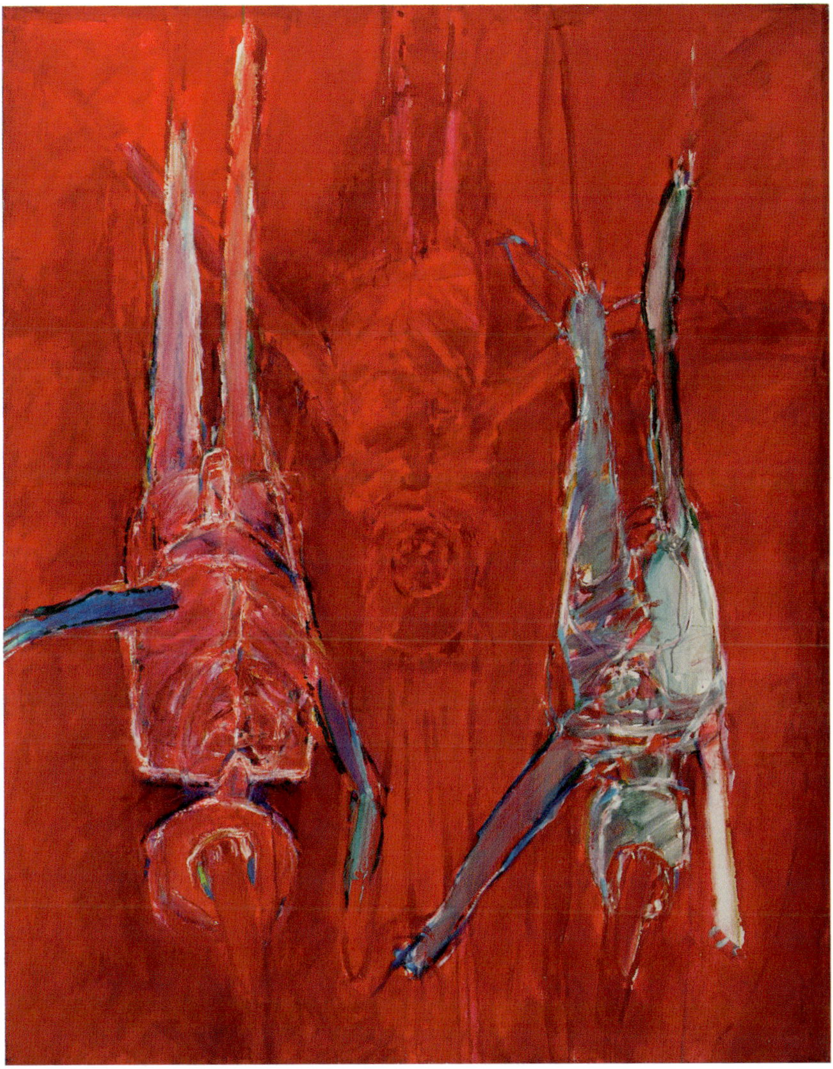

Plate 13. Guillermo Núñez, from the series De le déjeuner sur l'herbe, *1989. 162 × 130 cm. Courtesy of the artist.*

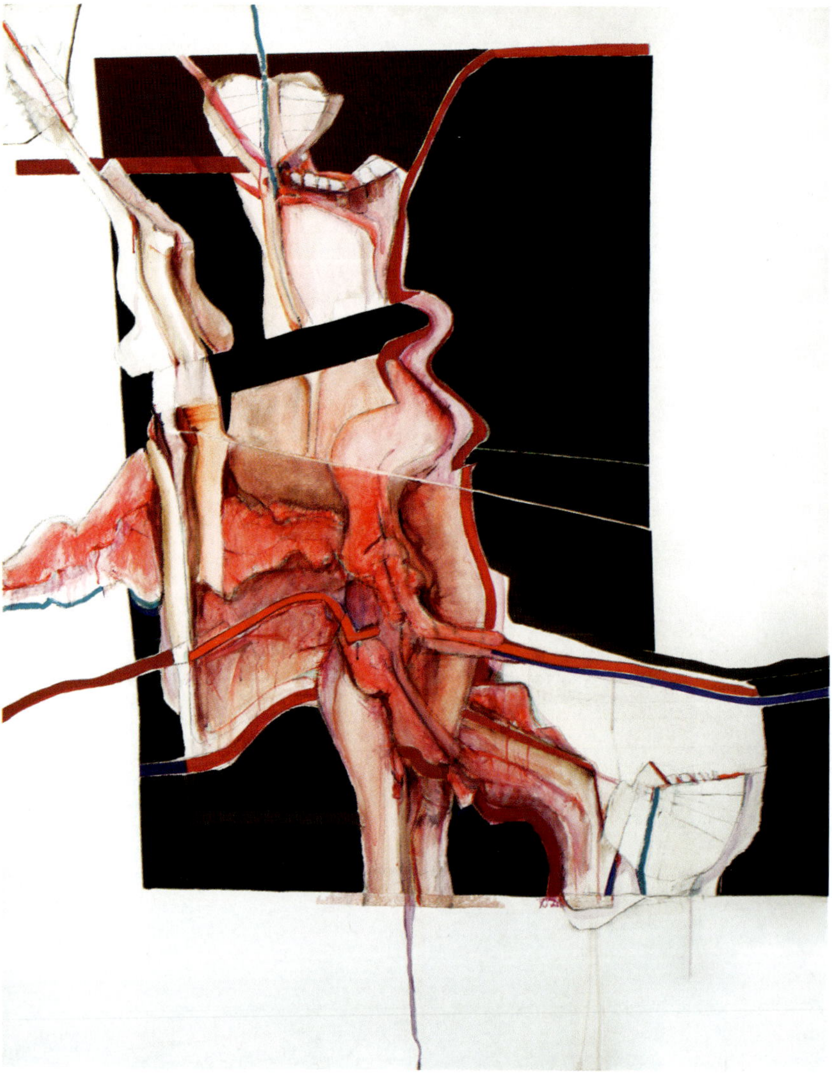

Plate 14. Guillermo Núñez, Esculpir con el dolor, un tremendo grito de esperanza, *1976. 163 × 130 cm. Courtesy of the artist.*

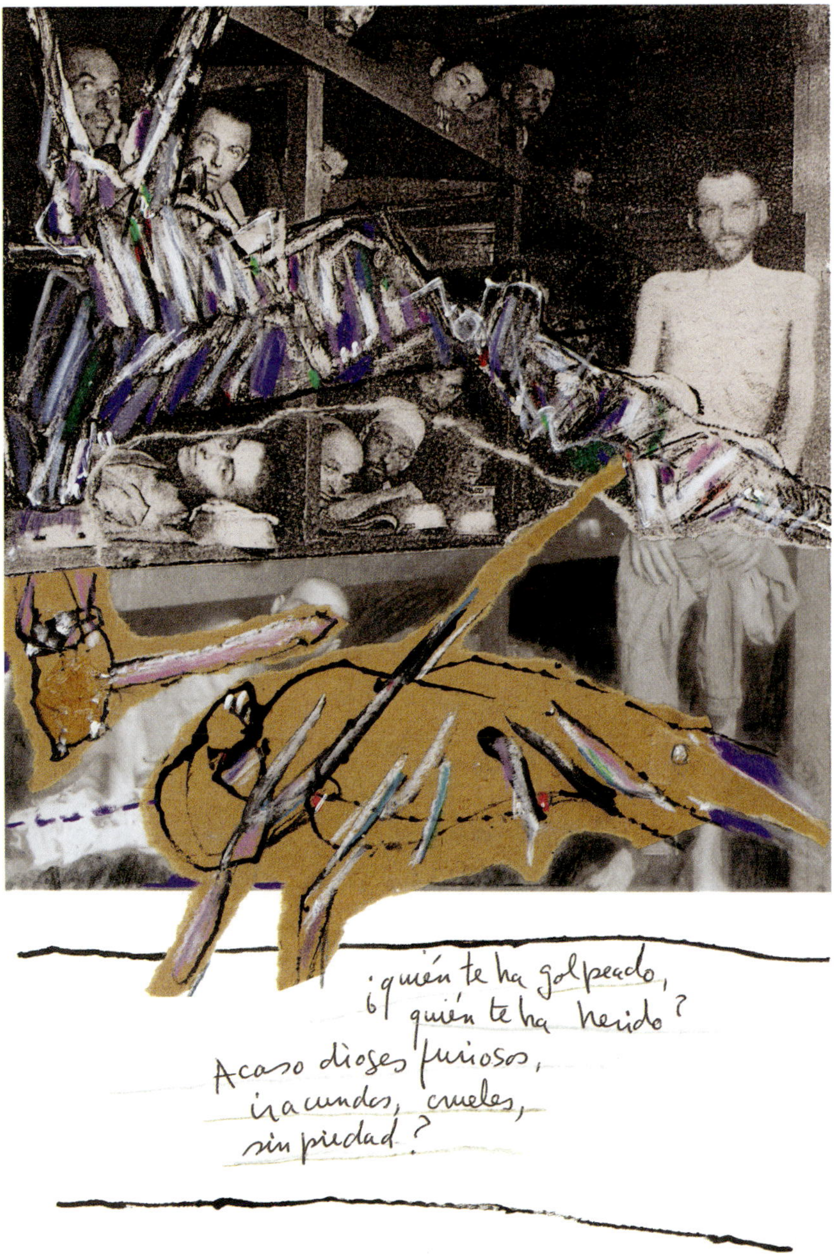

Plate 15. Guillermo Núñez, Galaxia, *2000. Serigraph and collage. Included in* La quinta del sordo, *exhibition held at Centro Cultural Matucana, 2003. Photo by Andrea de Simone; image courtesy of the artist.*

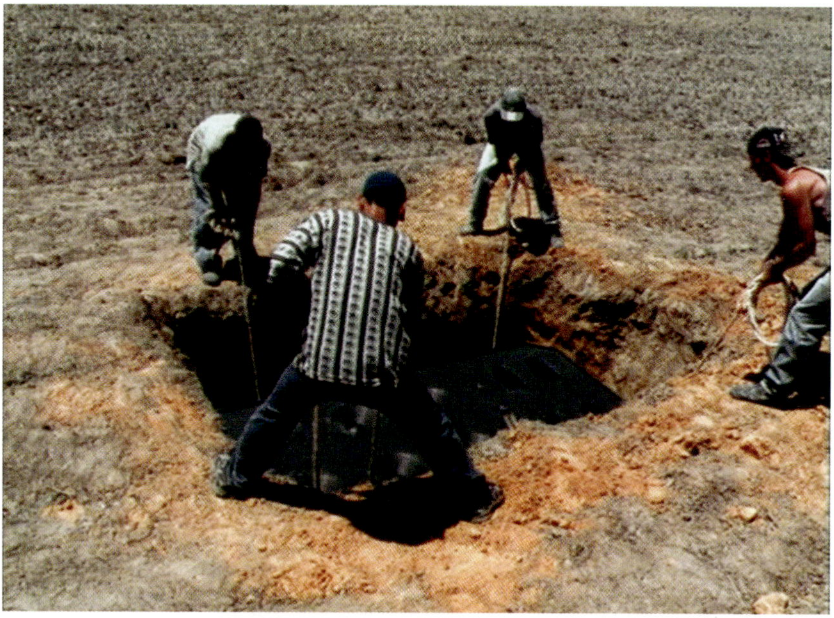

Plate 16. Luz Negra, *2002. 16 mm, 11' 45". Directed by Nuno Ramos and Eduardo Climachauska. Script by Nuno Ramos. © Nuno Ramos; used by permission.*

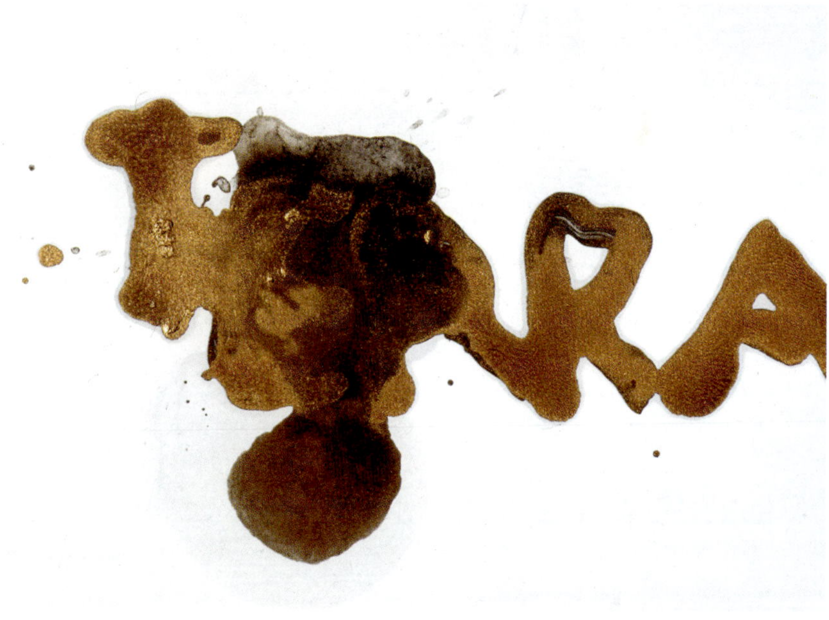

Plate 17. Nuno Ramos, Terra, *1990. Gold paint and turpentine on paper. 20.5 × 29.5 cm. From the series* 90 palavras douradas, *1990. © Nuno Ramos; used by permission.*

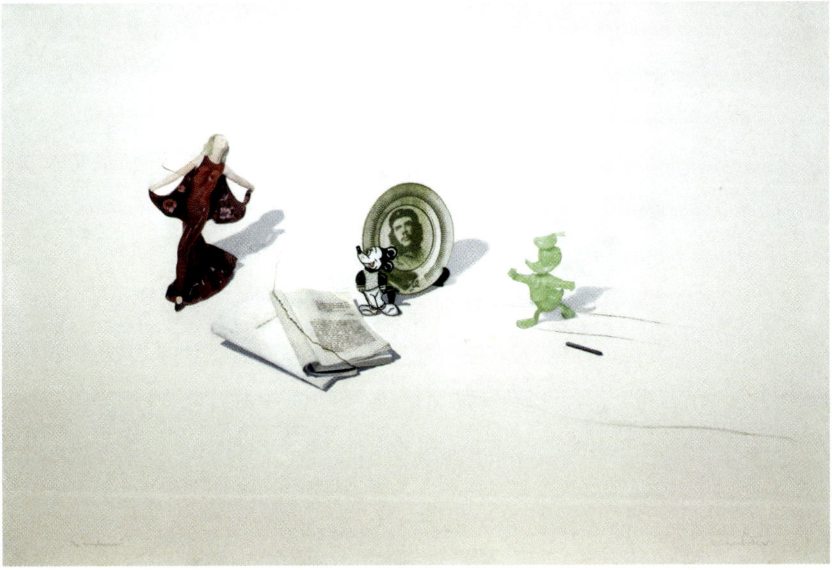

Plate 18. Liliana Porter, The Simulacrum, *1991. Synthetic polymer paint, silk-screen, and collage on paper. 40 × 60 in. Private collection. Courtesy of the artist.*

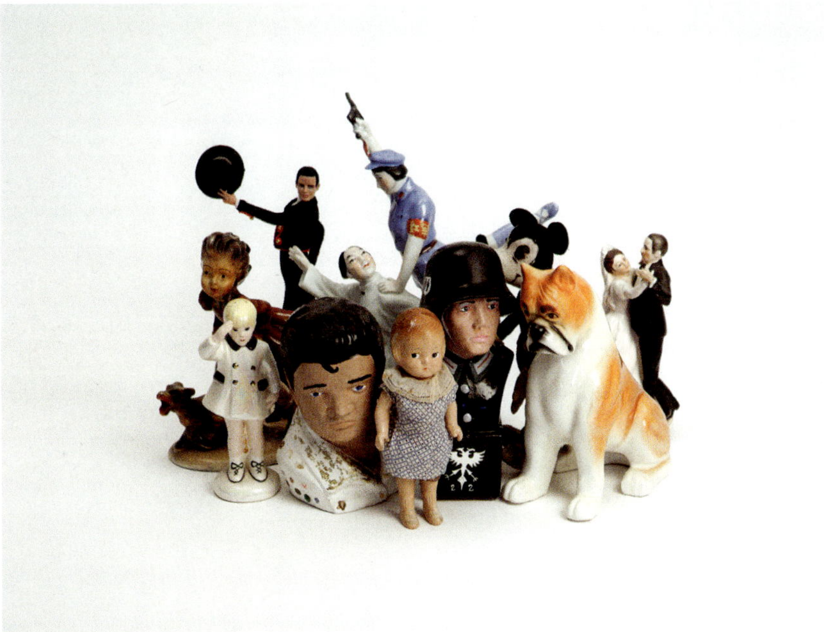

Plate 19. Liliana Porter, Them with Nazi, *2011. Digital Duraflex. Limited edition of five. 20½ × 27 in. Courtesy of the artist.*

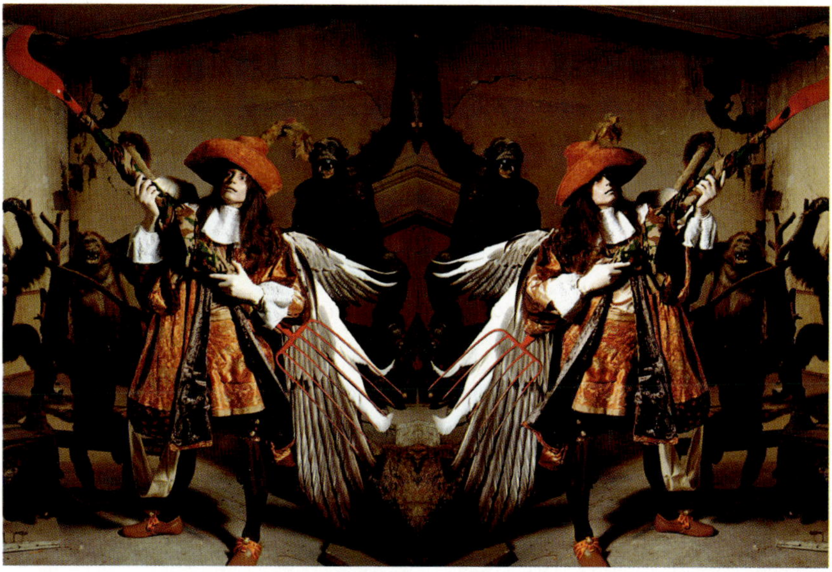

Plate 20. Demian Schopf, Asiel timor dei, *2001. From the series* La revolución silenciosa. *Courtesy of the artist.*

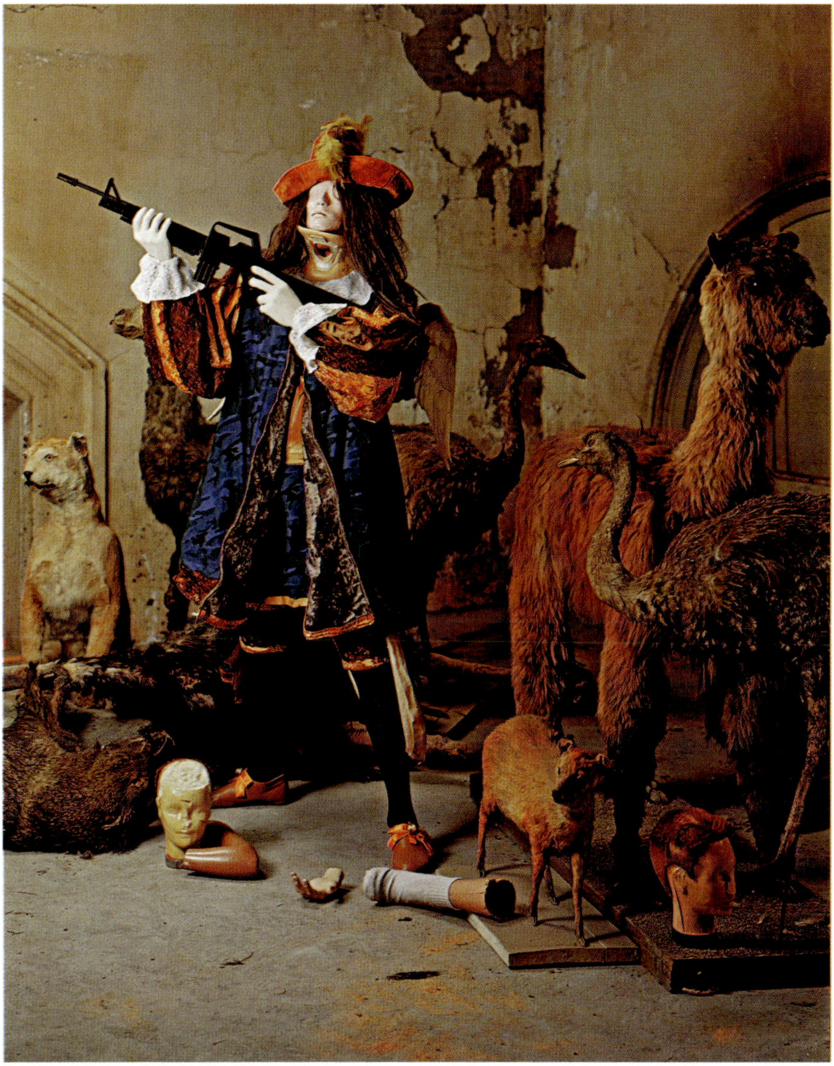

Plate 21. Demian Schopf, Asiel timor dei, *2002. From the series* La revolución silenciosa. *Courtesy of the artist.*

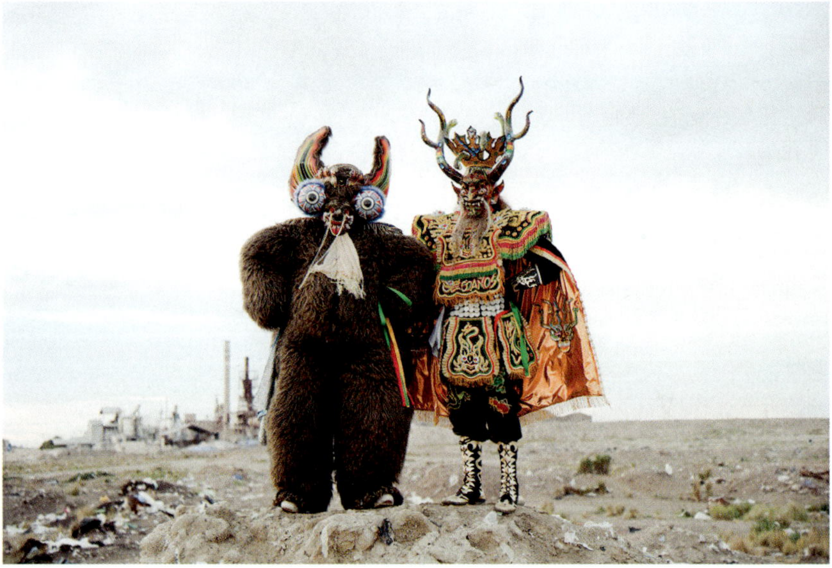

Plate 22. Demian Schopf, The Minor Choirs, Jukumari and Supay, *2011. Courtesy of the artist.*

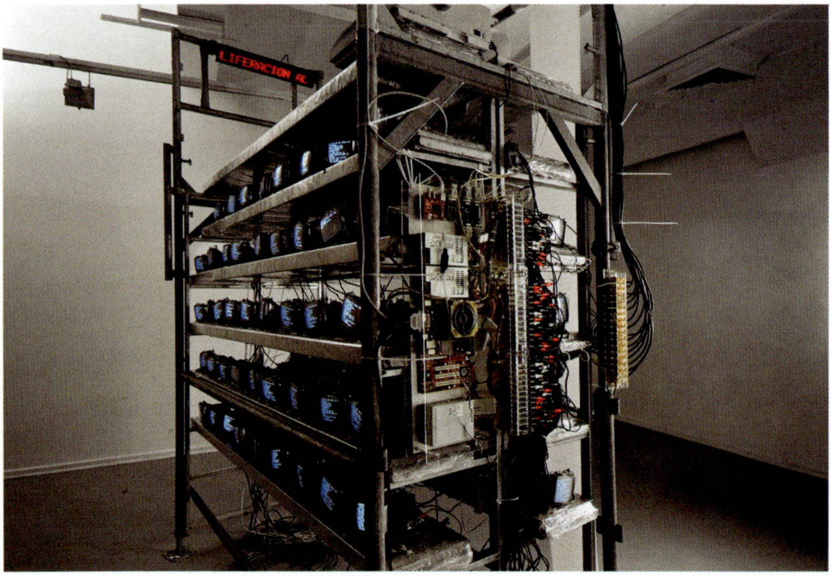

Plate 23. Demian Schopf, Máquina Cóndor, *2006–2016. Courtesy of the artist.*

Tantalizing Terror

We come to a point of divergence here: while a phenomenological approach guided modernist thinkers to reconsider the role of the sensate body, restoring to the individual a certain power over modernity's thrust, other factors intervened, which in general terms resulted in divided opinions about the effects of sensorial perception. On the one hand, the yellow press indulged the shock and thrills demanded by readers, leading audiences to modern scandals and earthshaking scenes of calamity and destruction that benefited a hunger for *sales*; on the other hand, for moderns of a spiritualist stripe, the sensate world was the initial step toward *collective understanding*. Apparently pulling in opposite directions, these frenzied projects for embodied knowledge circulated among both highbrow elites and popular readers. As such, they prompted one writer in *Martín Fierro* to speak of the decade of the 1920s as a modern "collective synesthesia" (A. Vallejo 1926, 97).

Let's look first at the sale of sensation. The "terror in the aisles" that drew mass audiences to the movies has been well documented; Tom Gunning (2004) has called this an aesthetic of astonishment through which the shock of the moving image left a palpable imprint on the public and created a demand for more. Similarly, freak shows and roller-coaster rides cropped up in Coney Islands around the globe, shaking us to pieces. At the same time, the popular press indulged the desires of a public with its nerves on edge; reports of urban shocks or phantoms and ghosts linked sensation to our deepest fears. The stories embraced questions of distance and nearness, they suggested danger and safety, and they occasionally crossed animal and human; when tossed and tumbled in a narrative stew, they yielded a popular fiction that could be readily sold to the masses. Ranging from the "crónica roja" of crime stories to strange accounts of extrasensory experience, the popular press's offerings afforded a constant supply of material to send up thrills and scares. The goal was to sell these stories like hotcakes, leaving readers to beg for more.

In the Argentine popular magazine *Caras y caretas*, several articles help us think more attentively about this problem. In one essay, "La voz interior," we are told of a sea captain from Brooklyn who promised to take his children to the theater. An interior voice advised him against it and the captain obeyed. That same night, the theater burned to the ground and three hundred spectators died (Meterlinck 1927). In an unsigned note from 1925, a man tells of a magical wall clock that predicted the deaths of loved ones. The strange coincidence of prediction and death was repeated several times; soon the clock became a sign of anguish that terrorized a community of readers ("Por el mundo del misterio" 1925). In a third note, "El sexto sentido," it is reported that a man, escaping worldly pleasures, saves the life of a shepherd. An elderly giant appears before him and promises, for his act of heroism, to grant the man his wish. The man then asks for the gift of sixth-sense perception. He dies a year later in the arms of a princess (Turcio 1927).

These strange stories of chance and death abounded in the popular journals of the day, but they also served as a basis for putting the senses on alert; they reminded the reading public that alerted perceptions might awaken an intuitive knowledge regarding fate and our control of the future. At the same time, and from the perspective of popular science, a new materiality simultaneously appeared describing the human body as a vehicle to transport electrical energies, facilitating a kind of communication that extended beyond language itself. While *Caras y caretas* published seductive ads about mesmerism and magic objects, the Argentine newspaper *El hogar* carried a daily column on strange events that defied the rules of logic ("Curiosidades, rarezas y extravagancias").

Beatriz Sarlo has written extensively on the technical imagination of the Argentine working classes of the 1920s and 1930s, but here I wish to redirect the discussion regarding popular science to other terrain: to explore how devices touched embodied experience and spiritualist aspirations; and to think of the ways in which new technologies linked individuals to collective desires. Electricity is often the feature that runs through these tissues of connection. In an issue of *El hogar* from February 10, 1922, for example, several articles inform us of the future of technology: the luminous telephone, the mystery of electrical sparks, and the cinematographic possibilities of the voice. In a later issue is an unsigned note in which the human body is regarded as a transmitter of electronic currents of radiophonic sound ("Experimentos que pueden hacerse con el aparato de la radio" 1928). Consistently crossing the boundaries of nature and culture, the human and the machine, material realities and ethereal yearnings, occult sciences and pragmatics, these essays install something akin to a synesthetic thinking in the minds of their readers. They seem to claim that all boundaries can be surpassed, introducing the shock of strangeness written upon what is familiar. This intertwining is crossed on the flesh of

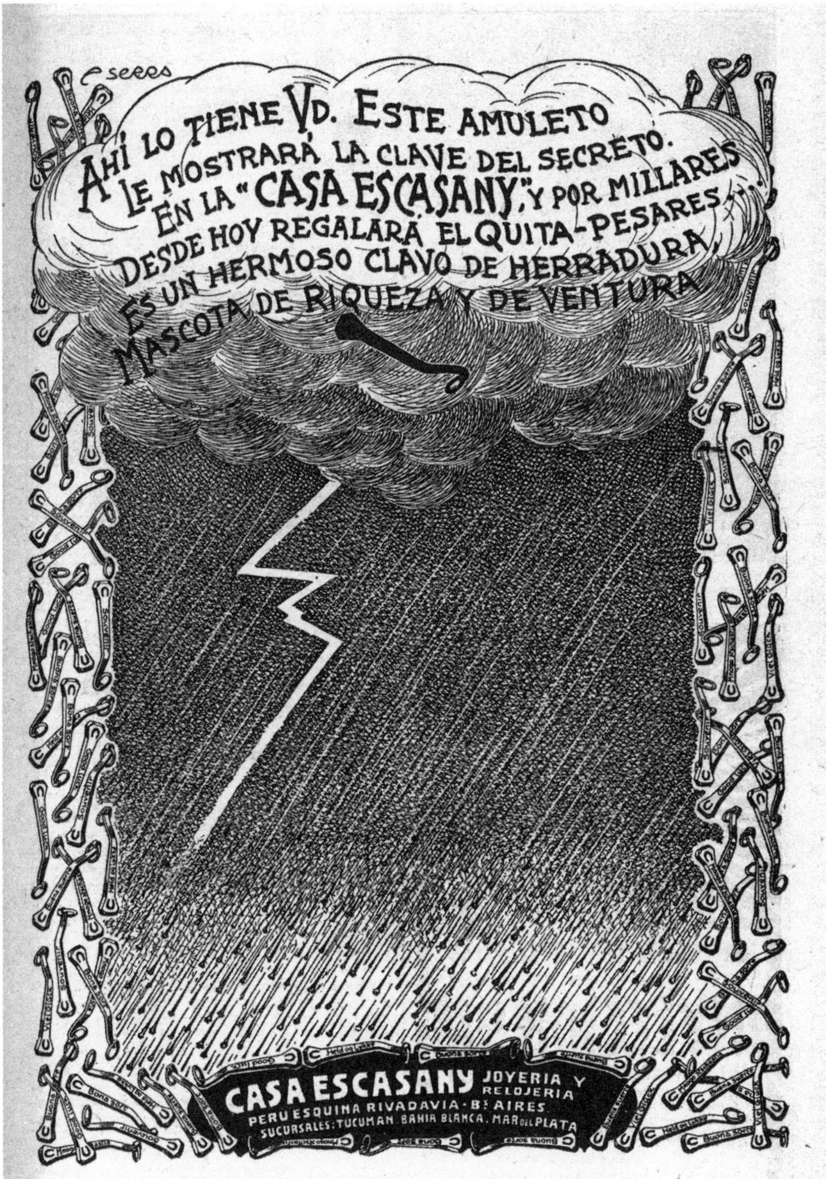
AHÍ LO TIENE VD. ESTE AMULETO
LE MOSTRARÁ LA CLAVE DEL SECRETO.
EN LA "CASA ESCASANY", Y POR MILLARES
DESDE HOY REGALARÁ EL QUITA-PESARES...
ES UN HERMOSO CLAVO DE HERRADURA,
MASCOTA DE RIQUEZA Y DE VENTURA
CASA ESCASANY JOYERIA Y RELOJERIA
PERU ESQUINA RIVADAVIA - Bs AIRES
SUCURSALES: TUCUMAN. BAHIA BLANCA. MAR DEL PLATA

Figure 3.6. Advertisement for Casa Escasany. Caras y caretas *23, no. 1118, March 6, 1920. Courtesy of University of California at Berkeley Library.*

human bodies, and indeed the body becomes the nodal point for registering the effects of one's encounters with things.

Seemingly trivial, the stories from the popular press also flooded the imaginations of creative writers, not only Horacio Quiroga and Leopoldo Lugones but also Roberto Arlt. Their fictions were supported by films like *Caligari*, and also by fantasies that sustained the self-made man and his talents for craft and invention.[33] Under the ever-present obsession with a market for sales, Arlt exploited the themes of embodied perception; shock, scandal, and the fate of the collective whole under the pressure of modernity are among his repeated motifs. He also shows the limits of what can be accomplished through synesthesia.

Trained in yellow journalism and writing for newspapers such as *El hogar*, Roberto Arlt (1900–1942) in fact published his stories on the pages of the very dailies that reported on mystic horrors and new technological inventions. He also understood the pressures that the writer felt in order to sell a story. Arlt knew that the media exercised a strange power over the shaping (and distortion) of human experience, which explains why his stories often followed a materialist approach to the narrative body, reflecting on the use of sensation and scandal as vehicles to prop up a tale. In the style of the sensational press and evoking the shock of lurid events, Arlt tells us time and again that the reader will be touched to the core, awakened from the aesthetic or political slumber into which modern man has fallen. This is made apparent in the prologue to *Los lanzallamas* (The flamethrowers), his novel of 1931. Here Arlt insists that literature embody the violence of a blow to the jaw: "Let's create our literature not by talking about literature, but by writing—in proud solitude—books that capture the violence of a 'blow to the jaw.'" (1978, 190). A wake-up call, a jolt to the body: literature was to leave a visceral effect upon the reader. Almost in the style of the Italian futurists, for whom literature was an athletic event, pushing aside the weak and defending the virility of the well-exercised reader, Arlt understood writing as a task that would attack the nerves of the reader, requiring a sensationalist strategy if anything were to be possible at all.

Arlt knew that popular-science publications, cinema, and crime sheets captured this available phenomenal world in order to shock us out of our wits; he evoked this practice in his novels to detonate bombs of rage and deception. Frustration, betrayal, or madness, even a proclivity toward crime, were woven into his unruly plots. Arlt thus moved ahead perversely, especially when he considered the linkage between sensual jolts and the awakening of the spirit. After all, his texts were neither about heightened spirituality nor even the prospects of a collective spirit that so engaged the theosophers and inventors who appeared in his novels. To the contrary, he debased those beliefs and linked them to the sales of shock and mystery that were the tabloids' pressing orders. In this environment reflecting the impact of what has been called a "neurological modernization" (Bentley 2009, 247), Arlt elaborates upon the aesthetic high that comes with acts of theft or physical assault. His oft-cited phrase "ser a través del crimen" (to become through crime) (Arlt 1978, 53) registers the euphoria of pressing one's body against the property of another and claiming it triumphantly as one's own. Here lies the shock of the new, capable of bestowing identity to the actor, thief, or inventor; it is found in a violation of the law and is expressed through physical aggression; it has the consequence of perversely awakening the self, if even for a fleeting moment. Arlt thus delivers an outburst against the avant-garde culture that I describe in this chapter; he is also poking fun at those occultists who believed they could touch the spirit.

In this respect, it comes as no surprise that Arlt in *El juguete rabioso* (The mad toy, 1926) celebrates the idea of transubstantiation *not* as a question of the reform of the human spirit (a direct challenge to Joyce's Stephen?), but as one of the everyday miracles that simple science affords. Elementary chemistry—neither art nor theosophy—is the prop for this theory of change. In a moment of automatic writing Silvio, the youthful protagonist of *El juguete rabioso*, scribbles whatever comes to mind: "limestone dissolves when you wet it" (Arlt 1969, 84). Throughout the novel, Silvio expresses wonder about the ways in which basic science enacts a transformation of matter. And although the miraculous effects of science form his backdrop, ascending into riches is Silvio's final goal; indeed, this social climbing is, in the 1920s, the most miraculous change of all. In this respect, Silvio most assuredly believes that class change is analogous to a transformation of matter that will be achieved through chemistry or crime. On the side, he makes fun of the more banal shock that is used to transform the spirit. As we observed before, this discussion flowed unremittingly in the high modernist years; mysticism, spiritualism, theosophy, desired dialogues with the dead, and the magical elixir of words engendered the metamorphosis. In Latin America, writers and artists from Lugones and Huidobro (at the start of the twentieth century) to Xul Solar, Leonora Carrington, and even Gabriela Mistral (whose work extends to the 1950s), worked under the banner of esoteric sciences in search of a common linkage between self and objects with the goal of forming a common voice. Arlt made a joke of this phenomenon in his essays and novels. At the same time, he also teased those critics and thinkers who—like de Torre, Epstein, and Ortega y Gasset—connected sensation and spirit. In other words, Arlt laughed his way through the overarching themes of his day.

Starting with his first published essay in 1920 (Arlt 1981, 9–35), he attacked the occult sciences as a fraudulent scheme to brainwash the ingenuous public and severely criticized the theosophy cults thriving in Buenos Aires. Arlt linked the spiritual experience to fanaticism and its scorn for science, but he also tied it to nostalgia for the age of miracles that people, exhausted by the tumultuous modern city, needed to express and sustain (31).[34] He also saw these cults as evidence of a colonial mentality, since after all, spiritualist cults had their roots in the United States and Europe (33). With its illusory concepts and colonial imposition of foreign beliefs, spiritualism represented for Arlt the con job of the modern age. For this reason, his characters often deliver themselves to absurd extremist beliefs ranging from theosophy and astrology to alchemy and a science of mass destruction. Perhaps Silvio and the Astrologer's team in *Los lanzallamas* sought, as Walter Benjamin did, a desired "ecstatic trance." But more important, Arlt's characters linked the dreams of premodern magic and alchemy to dreams of capitalist conquest. Synesthesia for Roberto Arlt became a summa of this experience in literature and in life.

This leads me to Arlt and his representation of the sensate world. In Arlt's mass-media inspired novels, authenticity dissolves; no one can trust to the real.[35] In this regard, Hipólita, the main female character of *Los siete locos* and *Los lanzallamas*, is an avowed consumer of mass-culture texts, insofar as they supply her with fantasies of love and perfect marriage. Although her ideal man is Tarzan, a figure from the popular press, she eventually comes to reject all romantic illusions that mass fiction supplies; instead, she turns to the idea of fake sensation, the essence of fiction itself. Mass novels have taught her to discern between *pureza* and pleasures of the flesh, between noble spirits and base passion; above all, they have taught her the wiles of deception and the know-how to put them to work. Hipólita thus takes dissimulation as her tool; she learns the value of inventing a story. As the "shock of the new" (and the shock to the body) comes under investigation, Arlt also pokes fun at the avant-garde literary experiments that exploit sensational form. Consider, for instance, his description of Hipólita's dreams, which are strikingly reminiscent of the circular movements in the early films of Marcel Duchamp:[36]

> Over her head a heavy circle spins. These are her ideas. In her head, a smaller circle also spins, wavering ever so lightly. These are her sensations. Sensations and ideas rotate in opposite directions. At times, her gums perceive the movement of her lips, pursed with impatience; she closes her eyes. The bed, which still has the bland smell of dried semen, and the slow movement of the circle of sensations drown her in an abyss. When the circle of sensations tips, she sees the top of the ellipsis, the curve of her ideas. Also spinning are the hallucinations of density, memory, and future. (Arlt 1978, 256)

For Hipólita, sensation and ideas appear in the form of circular moving shapes and piercing arrows of pain, but for Arlt's readers of a certain stripe, these images also border on a hilarious send-up of avant-garde pretensions. This is an effort to depict sensations in avant-garde visual form. From here, Hipólita goes on to think in rapid fire about the future of motherhood, revolutionary feminist cells, and the happiness she might allow herself to experience through the pores of her body (257). And if that weren't a sufficient joke on the impact of avant-garde sensation, other stimuli induce her to think about plans for extortion and murder. In this way, she rejects the awakening of nerves that might lead to any aesthetic "high," just as she turns away from the idea of moral transformation through art. Once again, the effects of the sensate world lead Arlt's characters closer to a lawless underworld than to any collective goodwill.

Arlt also engages in a secondary study of sensation when he registers on the opening page of *Los lanzallamas* the deliberately stunning effect that landscape holds on a viewer's perceptions. The novel thus begins as the Astrologer studies a blooming lemon tree on his ranch: "Lenin knew where he was going. Triangular white clouds cut though the perpendicular blue of the sky. A whirlpool of black insects bent around the vines of the roundabout. Lenin for sure knew where he was going" (191). Without making sense of nature, Arlt leaps between landscape and Lenin, provoking several questions: Is this a gap between what is seen and thought or is the Astrologer describing an unavoidable synthesis of nature and culture, a crossover of sensory perceptions that undergirds political action? Arlt will never let us know, but guides us through an environment that leaves our nerves standing on end.

Among the characters who inhabit Arlt's world, one is defined by a rhomboidal face, another has the eyes of a fish, another suffers an anguish described in geometrical form. Expressionist, grotesque, fragmented, and incoherent, the characters of *Los siete locos* and *Los lanzallamas* put realism to a test as their lame and absurdly tropistic bodies respond like primitive living forms to shards of light and darkness or stimuli that induce considerable pain. Emotion and affection are abandoned to the sidelines. In this regard, literature must be received as a "blow to the jaw." This strong physical encounter culminates in the final newspaper reports giving notice of Bizca's murder. Here we are moved to shock by the crossing of news and fiction; like readers of Dos Passos's novels, we find ourselves knocked to the floor by mass-media communiqués in fiction that sound like the kinds of alternative facts that fill our daily news feed.

Arlt also plays with the role of sensation to enact a crass reworking of the mind-body dualism dominating intellectuals of his generation. This is especially seen in the secret society, where the Astrologer presses the characters into crime and prostitution with gleeful self-affirmation. The goal, remarks the Astrologer as he thinks about putting his plans into action, is to "move . . . a mass of inert flesh" (1978, 98), to stir bodies and put them in movement. Arlt sums this up by two section headings within *Los lanzallamas*: "To exist through crime" and "To exist through pain." We can come into being by acts of crime or by painful attacks on the body; suffering, distortion, and physical discomfort awaken us to ourselves. Hence, Arlt gives us the castrated men (the Astrologer and Barsut), the prostitute with frozen feet (Hipólita), and the moribund character of Haffner. He describes the strange pain that the characters suffer and which is reflected in their faces; finally, he focuses on the inability of each to achieve felicity for the soul. Erdosain then poses the question, "When will they draw the maps of pain that run through our suffering bodies?" (220). The inability to tap that well of suffering and find an eventual epiphany is also signified by Arlt's metaphor of matter that cannot be transformed. Thus, when Remo cannot touch his soul, Arlt supplies this description: "Just as it was impossible to transform lead into gold, it was also impossible to transform the soul of man" (152). The dream of transformation expressed by Silvio Astier, and cited earlier in these pages, comes to a resounding halt.

With so much attention to the malingering body, it is not surprising to see other characters who turn around the tropes that define their corporeal bondage: "[T]hrough prostitution, one is freed of the body and . . . remains free," says Hipólita (146), reaching for a pure love that is well beyond the senses. Erdosain, about to fall asleep, is also content to lose touch with his body: "You close your eyes and it seems like your body dissolves into nothing" (78). From the sharp, piercing sensation of the flesh, which proves to Erdosain that he is alive, he also opts for sexless sex and dreams about bodies without matter. Arlt's characters thus challenge the tyranny of the body and seek incorporeal (mystical?) bliss, thereby escaping the sensational stories of the media crime sheets (153). Quite the contrast to modernists like James Joyce, who sought the body as a ground for experience and, more important, as a connection to the soul, Arlt vacillates between intense corporeality, in order to experience pain, and scenes of erased and sexless bodies that coast toward an unconventional purity with a strange theology of their own. To summarize, we might say that two contrary projects govern Arlt's fictions: on the one hand, he stirs us from slumber with incessant assaults on sensation; on the other, he frees up any adherence that characters might hold to the flesh. These divided attentions suggest a deep tear in the cultural fabric, bespeaking the effects of modernization and violence either to eradicate the body completely or to restore its capacious powers. We also have another matter at hand: Is Arlt alluding to that great paradox of literature, which takes us from words to the illusions of bodies and all the while plays with belief? Or is the "real" materiality found only in the craft of representation? These are the great moments for Arlt to reflect on the difference between shock and abstraction, between the kinetic art that Borges abjured and the still moment of ecstatic bliss that signifies aesthetic pleasure and eventual peace of the soul.

An extraordinary scene occurs in the section "Capas de oscuridad," when Erdosain, after learning of his wife's betrayal and planned separation, tries to get some sleep. Here, as he nears deep somnolence, his body is assaulted by sensory cues; he lives the simultaneous estrangement and proximity of his body in repose (Arlt 1978, 43). Because he cannot touch things close up, he turns to the intensity of physical pain, violence, or torture that might awaken his emotions. Sex has failed him; crime has failed him; communities of men have failed to redeem him.

It may here be the place to endorse Ricardo Piglia when he claims that two operations cut through Arlt's novels: a tale of inner life and anguish, on the one hand, and a study of the rules of fiction, on the other; both are seen in the ongoing narrative tensions between lies and truth (Piglia 1986, 21–22). In this vein, it is not surprising that Arlt's thoughts about this problem so often take place in the literary *bed*, the place where persons are freed from the order of the state, but where they also witness a reconfiguration of the senses and experience their alienation or pleasure. Of course, the bed is the great modernist site from which to stage the collapse or defense of the body (think of Faulkner's *As I Lay Dying* or Marcel in the first volume of *À la recherche* or the scene of Molly's final soliloquy in *Ulysses*). These writers knew that if they set a body in a fixed position, they could secure a vantage point from which to show off the novel as a treatise on sensation without the distractions of landscape or excessive external action. Too, the reposing body, much like the cadaver, locates the site that conjoins life and death in a single space. Truth and lies expose the grand fiction of life.

The second chapter of *Los lanzallamas* takes place in the hospital, where we see the slow death and decomposition of Haffner's body in bed. As his senses decline, he feels the sun bathe his face, the flies on his lips, the ponderous weight of his limbs. Thirst and sound define his experiences in this chapter:

> In vain, Haffner tries to raise his arm to shoo away the flies whose antennae tickle his lips; his limbs weigh heavily as if they had been sculpted in bronze, and with his head twisted on the pillow and a line of mist between his half-open eyelids, he lies dying.... Thirst reaches his intestines dried out like strings. The puddle of water and piss, where the horses were tied up near the forge, reappears before his eyes. (Arlt 1978, 250)

His memories come forth in faulty Italian, and, in his final moment, he even imagines a scene of sensual violence when he recalls Pibe's stabbing. In this densely corporeal scene, composed of intermittent flashbacks and streams of consciousness, Haffner also hears in present time the voices of those who would attack him: they try to get him to speak, to produce a voice that will name his assassin. Combined with his intense thirst, the sounds that Haffner is asked to utter put all attention on the mouth, as if to say that life depends on speech and voice, confession and verification, ingestion and expulsion. But Haffner cannot speak. His only reflex is a wink of the eye, though in his mind he recalls the lyrics of a Neapolitan song and a school scene drawn up from his youth. Arlt here insists on the moment in which past meets present, forcing us to adjust to different kinds of sensation and memory weaving through the pages of the chapter.

At death's door, the body is the site of meaning that predates sociability and culture. Here, Arlt draws upon a utopian fantasy that flies in the face of politics in the 1930s when he suggests (via Haffner's case) that no one can extract from the body what it will not share; no one can oblige the body to surrender to the will of the other. In other scenes, Arlt likewise tries to bring us to the point of linking nervous system and thought: "Nerves," he writes, "are the painful continuity of his thoughts, at times, mixed like water and oil, shaken by a storm; and at others, separated in dense layers, as if they had passed through a centrifugal drum" (220). Words cannot reach the depth of our anguish; instead, only through the nerve circuits can we track our consciousness and pain. The utter desperation about these irreconcilable separate spheres is repeated throughout the novel: in Hipólita's occasional streams of consciousness, in the fragmented thoughts of the agonic Rufián Melancólico (228–229), in the presleep fantasies of Erdosain (346–347) that open to the space of dreams. Certainly, they look like derivations of Joycean time and mental flow, except that Arlt always returns to scenes of utter abjection, vulgar despair, and death.[37]

Why, asks Arlt, can humans not see beyond the self-enclosed walls of their bodies? His immediate solution is to blow them up with pistols or drown them in fumes of gas. Death is an alternative for the stabbing feeling produced by contact with the world. It also signals the irreconcilable division between ailing bodies and souls. Even the separation of the novel into two halves—*Los siete locos* and *Los lanzallamas*—in itself indicates a formal duality that is like the mind/body split.

Martin Jay, suspicious of the philosophical attention to sensation, observes that the material body, placed in the physical world as a receptor of sensation, threatens to reduce the bodily experience to the "sameness of the cadaver" (qtd. in Edwards 2009, 739). But that is precisely the point: the dying or sleeping body is a transitional node that helps us reveal the Arltian project with respect to sensation. It brings us to the space where we can suture body and time, and prompts a synesthetic gesture that would collapse mental and graphic regimes, verbal and visual distinctions. There is little profane illumination here, no promise of redemption; rather, the crossover of sensation, which shocks the readers of the popular press, only allows us the chance to market a novel and perhaps earn some notice or profit.

Cultural historians depict the modernist decades as an age in which the mass public demanded sensational thrills. Even with cinema and amusement parks, electricity and radiophonic sound, the public clamored for an excess of stimulation to shock them into feeling. Describing the addictive nature of shock, Arlt placed his characters in an endless scenario of multiple sensorial assaults. His project was to expose the culture of shock as part of the insatiable culture for scandal whose fire was lit by the newspaper industry's avid hunger for sales. The problem seems to be one of surmounting distance and abbreviating urban spaces, to emphasize *direct contact* lest we forget the body. But this is only one part of the story; the modernist heyday also introduced another approach to sensate life, using the receptors of the body in order to reach a collective soul.

Blithe Spirits

In an essay of 1892, Georg Simmel acknowledged that the spiritualist mode had swept large portions of the population, and he made every attempt to denounce it. As if to anticipate Roberto Arlt's article of 1920, Simmel considered the entire realm of spiritualist pursuit best left "unexplored," reporting the experiences of believers as "childish, senseless and indifferent," a symptom of those who were unable to free themselves from the past (1997, 292–293). Although spiritualism for Simmel and Arlt was linked to nostalgia for miracles, a yearning for the past, and an inability to confront the future, in the larger Latin American context, spiritualism was often tied to liberal traditions. Even before the Spanish translation of Allan Kardec's work in 1862, the liberal elite found in spiritualist practice a way to position an anticlerical voice in Latin America; it also appealed to feminists devoted to emancipatory causes.[38] In short, intellectuals saw spiritualism less as an esoteric affair than as a transaction between science and religion, responding to the determinist nature of Roman Catholic dogma. The theosophers who emerged from this cult beginning in the 1870s attracted the attentions of important artistic and political figures throughout Latin America, all concerned with social inequities and in search of new constellations for social interconnectedness, new ways to link our sense perceptions to the spirit, and from there to propel political change. Arcadio Díaz Quiñones (2006), studying the works of the Cuban sociologist Fernando Ortiz, makes an interesting claim when he asserts that Ortiz's understanding of "transculturation" is very much connected to the spiritualist philosophies of "transmigration" of souls. The writings of Kardec entered into dialogue with Fernando Ortiz and were also essential to the projects of Francisco Madero and José Vasconcelos in Mexico. Fundamental, then, to the period in question are the links between spiritualism and materialism; even for someone like Ortiz, *mestizaje* became part of the project of transmigration, where the spirit counted more than the body (Díaz Quiñones 2006, 296). This comes to the surface with vigor among the avant-garde poets; it stands as a decided response to the culture of physical "shock." Along with writers like Amado Nervo and Leopoldo Lugones, and later Vicente Huidobro and Gabriela Mistral, visual artists like Xul Solar also discovered the importance of the spiritualist quest, less to remember the dead than to reach out to the community of the living.

The Marvelous Materiality of Xul Solar

Fresh from a long tour of Europe, Xul Solar (1887–1963) was probing alternative orders of experience that were derived from esoteric knowledge. Mysticism was to be the glue that cemented the material world together.[39] Harmony was his goal. Trained by Aleister Crowley during his years in London, Xul Solar (born Alejandro Schulz Solari) returned to Buenos Aires in 1924 as a painter and theosopher, integrating a project for spiritual renovation and social collectivity with a blending of the senses. Even the inversion in his name seems to point to an alternative way of knowing (his friends often recalled that the name Xul was an inversion of the Latin *lux*). His choice of media, watercolor, and occasionally tempera allowed him a certain fluidity to express what would be his ongoing theme—continuities and flows, synesthetic crossings, and the melding of different worlds.[40] In their most extreme dimensions, these projects signaled the mark of a painter who combined an avant-garde aesthetic with the promise of spiritual growth.

Part of the *Martín Fierro* coterie of the 1920s, Xul Solar was a reader of the mystical sciences, blending the tarot and the zodiac, the *I Ching* and the kabbalah. As astrologer, he mapped out the heavens and earth in his drawings, tracing the correspondences between color and sound, and finding the spiritual revery that was embedded in the visual image and in language itself. These synesthetic linkages were found in his paintings; in his plans to alter the structure of musical instruments, particularly his piano; in his new designs for the game of chess ("pan-chess" he called it) that demanded pieces coincide with astrological figures and particular calendar dates (whose meaning could be changed without notice!); and in his invention of a *pan-lengua*, a language that exceeded the constructs of any particular national tongue and which, like the Esperanto fad of the day, could be shared and understood by all. The goal here was to achieve what he called a *pan-conciencia* that would transcend a singularity of consciousness and individual isolation, and even point to the transhuman.

While he often conflated humans and animals in mythical inventions, he also matched men and machines as if to suggest the consequences of modernization emerging in the 1920s. Not quite the forceful statement of Chaplin in *Modern Times*, this playful melding of humans with technological novelty produced what he called *mestizo*: airplanes with the heads and feet of humans are part of this repertoire in painting. They suggest the joys of flight, an alternative to the ladders that often helped Xul, in his paintings, to reach the skies. Even spiritual heights can be achieved by mechanization. Color and sound are also presented in strange juxtapositions. Xul reorganized the musical scale in a duodecimal system taken from the kabbalah and designed a new piano whose notes corresponded to color-coded keys, with a scale corresponding to binary logic in some cases, and phonetic base in others.[41] Astrological charts of the universe and playful landscapes pointing to heaven were the staple of Xul's paintings over his long career. But most of all he insisted on the tropes of the bridge and the ladder, expressing a desire for unity and a collective harmony among men on earth. *El encuentro*, or the contact in community, was the goal of his visual proposal.

Xul's ladders in *Ruinas* (1950) offer a sturdy connection to allow individuals to scale the heights (see plate 6). Emerging from the wreck of crumbled buildings, they suggest an ongoing desire to reassemble a totality; at the summit, meanwhile, overlooking the ruins, a Christlike figure seems to beckon. Similarly, in *Puerta del este* (1935), the ladders offer an ongoing escape that helps Xul's figures reach the sky (see plate 7). And in *Zodíaco* (1949), Xul links stairways with mountains, placing twelve goddesses in the frame in order to express a unified whole (see plate 8). In these vertical orders that dominate many of Xul's later paintings, notice, too, the tiny dimensions of the few human figures; they signal our diminished importance in a world of holy symbols.

On the surface, Xul's brightly colored canvases and depictions of letters and numbers recall the paintings of Klee; Xul also represents a whimsical landscape that blends geometrical forms emerging from the soft contours of hills. His artistic practice corresponds to his unrelieved spiritualist calling. His first works, *sans signos*, were commissioned by Aleister Crowley to depict the astrological signs; his final works were a horoscope of his life's achievement and destiny. Equally important, Xul is best remembered for his ethereal paintings of worlds suspended on mountain tops, of mountain peaks as the sites for cities, of staircases leading to hilltop retreats, of the upward-lifting movement on canvas. Some might also link this to Escher, but Xul's work is clearly inscribed in a spiritual belief for collective identities in which a sense blending and a connectedness among people are his guiding forces. Geometrical forms, zodiacal signs, and kabbalistic readings provide venues for joining different levels of reality. Even his concept of *mestizaje* was designed to show physical mergers.

Vuel villa (1936) is an especially apt example (see plate 9). Here a giant airship floats over a city of pillars. The airship, however, also carries earthly structures: pagodas, guard posts, propellers, a flag, and twelve towers supporting windmills. The towers prompt us to the think of the twelve signs of the zodiac and, from theosophical thought, the number corresponding to grace and perfection. Below on earth, seven obelisks remind us of the most sacred number from the time of antiquity.[42] But let us not forget that the flying device, a city in the sky, replicates objects on earth. Land and sky mirror each other, joined in common bond. The elements of each are blended. From the division of the canvas, split by a ribbon of purple sea and by waves of wind, the different worlds merge; the fixed form of the triangle below leads to the circular balloons in the sky. Xul's cartoonlike world is, in this instance, almost spare of human subjects (a tiny human figure stands at the helm of the airship, a few stand guard at the towers), but remarkably the canvas captures human desires seen in a reach for the heavens; this is a time of waiting, with bridges that promise salvation. They all allow us to connect the pieces and remind us, as we strive toward oneness, that our desires are shaped by delivery to form, color, and rhythm. Our humanity, Xul would appear to say, is sustained by unrelieved sensorial excitement always harnessed by spiritual callings. The canvas also suggests, in a political leaning, that we might reach beyond the constraints of place if we only consent to a spiritual way.[43]

Drago (1927) captures the transnational journey to which Xul wished to subscribe (see plate 10). A dragon or serpent carrying flags of different Latin American nations traverses the whole of the canvas; upon the animal's spine stands a human figure sporting a long garment with swords at the waist and ribbons in his or her hair. In the right hand of this figure, a staff points toward the sun; at the same time, the sky's multicolored stars look down on the scene while fish look up from the sea. Meanwhile, North American and European banners are clustered in opposite corners as if to stand for spectators bearing witness to the joyous Latin American presence that fills the center of the canvas. This is a celebratory frame installed on the landscape and, for its Latin American allusion, is not far from Xul's other paintings of the period that carry such titles as *Cuatro cholas, Tlaloc, dios de la lluvia*, and *América*. The bright colors, the humanized sun and moon (both are depicted with eyes and beak-like noses), and the continuous flow of nature indicate a Pan-Americanist unity and drive home a message of dynamic harmony of intense flow and movement.[44]

The spiritual schools to which Xul belonged give an extra dimension to this frame. Some interpret the scene as a re-creation of Saint George and the Dragon in which the human figure takes the lead and brings people together;[45] others see the image as relating to syncretic African religions in which Ogún directs the people in revolt against genocide of the masses (Dinah 2007). These martial readings notwithstanding, theosophy offers a more gentle reading of the serpent, recognizing it as part of the ancient rites that lead to wisdom and hidden knowledge; carried to an extreme, the serpent is tied to the idea of life itself and is one of the principal archetypes of the soul.[46] There are also other symbols that lead us to religions, among them the adjacency of cross, crescent, and interlaced triangles of Judaism and theosophy that extend from the head of the dragon and the multiple arrows pointing to poles of electrical energy that cover the universe as we know it. Here we go beyond any nation to a reimagination of the world; everything is advancing to the harmony of waves and stars. True to the Aquarius sign that appears in all of Xul's work, the flow of water and a totalizing movement define his pictorial field. There is more, however, because the choice of colors points to forms of transcendence. Álvaro Abós reminds us that Xul studied Goethe's *Theory of Colors* under the direction of the theosopher Rudolf Steiner (Abós 2004, 100). He thus came to color in terms of refraction of light and an ongoing spectral experience that was compound and synthetic; in turn, this theory of color had its correlation in religious practice, which Xul always kept in mind. It is worth remembering in this regard that theosophical rays were represented in primary colors and stood for signs of fire; at the same time, theosophers claimed that all individuals would be contained within two color forces: neither the brightness of white nor the darkness of black would ever prevail. Instead, the harmony of colors absorbs the extremes of the world. The divine is trapped within the material world and begs for our perceptions to set it free.

Syncretic religions were not in themselves an amalgam of symbols and forms but turned to a harmonic continuum, just as they prevailed on a syncretic blending. This was at work in Xul Solar's painting in the crossing of color, sound, and movement. Perhaps participating in a *candombe* march, perhaps a military conquest, the dragon moves to the left of the scene while the waves at the top and bottom of the frame also follow in a serpentine way. The canvas thus holds together a mixture of colors and forms whose undulating movement appeals to the tactility of the viewer. But the matter of correspondence was set in the mind of Xul Solar. As he said in a published interview: "These paintings contain a description of thought, landscape and figure.... The signs are like words typed with colored keys, in which each tone corresponds to the content of words" (qtd. in Artundo 2006, 69). From this, we can derive two principles: first, an acceptance of ongoing movement as a guiding principle of Xul's art; and second, a recognition that our lives transcend categorical paths of reason. Reality here is based on correspondence and intuition; it enters the mind not simply by imprint and imposition but by an involuntary absorption and transformation of the movement and symbols set before us. In this respect, we don't passively experience the painted reality of Xul Solar; rather, he leaves enough ambiguity so that we are incited to endow the work with rhythm and formal internal properties of our own imagining. In a telling article, Xul boasted of the far-ranging extensions of his theories: "I am the creator of twelve pictorial techniques, some of surrealist origins, others that bring the sensorial, emotional world to the canvas, which produces in listening a Chopin suite, a Wagnerian prelude or a stanza sung by Beniamino Gigli" (qtd. in Artundo 2006, 76).

Xul's crossover of sensory material was also experienced in his games with language, in his efforts to override the Spanish language that he considered well out of date. He invented a series of languages, from *neo-criollo* to *pan-lengua*, systems blending different semiotic registers from romance languages, English, and classics. In his *pan-lengua*, he even tried to integrate language with astrological signs, and occasionally relied on the duodecimal system as an alphabetic base. From all these experiments, he worked with synesthetic states that necessarily linked body and spirit. Whether through architectural arrangements of words or numbers, musical notations, or pictorial pan-national leanings, Xul crossed systems of understanding in order to make us aware of failing governing orders that blocked a harmony promised between the universe and the human body. In this light, it hardly comes as a surprise that among his late-life projects was a charge to alter the human body in robotic form, making it more sensitive to matter and revelation and increasing its capacity and strength.[47] Xul had achieved the *mestizo*, or composite man, that was the object of his paintings.

A Synesthetic Ending

The essays and philosophical texts of modernism, along with literature and works of art of the early twentieth century, encircle questions of embodied knowledge. Themes of distance and closeness, the relationship between self and other, and the chance to imagine a rapprochement of the individual with the world give the trope of synesthetic blending a new horizon. It stands as the desired communal spirit that intellectuals found lacking in modern times. Arlt took this project to abject extremes (and not without some cause for laughter), while Xul Solar combined a sensual world in search of a synesthetic melding that was supposed to point to a collective, unified life of body and spirit. In their different ways, artists and writers answered the mass-media culture of sensation that was sustained for the sake of the market.

In this respect, their project was to underscore *relationality*, bringing closer contact between things and people, between events and our perceptions, and, above all, relieving the radical solitude to which modernity had consigned them. Ortega y Gasset's concluding remarks in an essay from the 1930s, "La aparición del otro," may serve us well; he writes, "[F]rom the depths of the radical solitude that is our life, we practice, again and again, a plan for interaction, to *un-lonely* ourselves by appearing before the other, wishing to give him our life and to receive his as well" (1964, 130; emphasis mine). Perhaps this is the most significant case to make for reading: sustaining the human contact.

CHAPTER 4

A Politics of Perception against the State

What happened to our bodies, our imagination, our affects?

LEÓN ROZITCHNER

The world has to be mapped with the senses and with a sense of one's body. Whoever lacks a map of his body is blind with respect to his world.

ROBERTO MATTA

In his masterpiece *Rayuela* (Hopscotch, 1963), one of the principal novels of the Latin American literary boom, Julio Cortázar's protagonist wanders aimlessly between Paris and Buenos Aires in search of the connections that will allow him fulfillment. His cultural referents are the intellectual high points of the 1950s—cool jazz, surrealist games, and the bookish culture of high modernism as it crossed through Paris. However, as the novel advances, these allusions cease to sustain him. Instead, Horacio Oliveira seeks a more concrete solution anchored in materialist perceptions. This result is made available to him in the closing chapters of the novel when he appears to discover his sentient body and the experience of physical pain. With Spanish and Latin wordplay, Cortázar, in a near final scene, turns to the human body as a way to trump verbal expression; *res non verba* he calls it—flesh for the sake of flesh, flesh overriding words. Cortázar's belated revelation—that bodily perceptions matter—comes to him after more than seven hundred pages of intellectual travels: in the end, his character admits that knowledge enters through the body. Having missed the death of baby Rocamadour while Oliveira listened to Schoenberg, having missed the magic of real-life love while he sought solace in surrealist texts, the protagonist comes to recognize the importance of embodied knowledge to place him in the world; he sets aside avant-garde culture in favor of sensate awareness. This becomes clear from a description of Oliveira's accidental fall from a window, such that the ensuing scene draws attention to the wound on his leg, to the blood and pain caused by his fall, and to the treatments that eventually cure him: in the end, Oliveira loses his energy for rambling and finally comes in touch with his body.

David Viñas (1927–2011), then a young intellectual driven by Marxist desires for social change, had little patience for Cortázar's circuitous writing and accused him of dismissing the material social conditions of Latin America in the 1950s and 1960s.[1] He tackled Cortázar for having severed the body from its social context in favor of a disinterested art; Cortázar's ongoing search for the *spirit* simply smothered the physical self. For Viñas, Cortázar suffered from unmitigated liberal thought, failing to acknowledge the material, perceptual basis of all exchanges. Cortázar's character's epiphany at the conclusion of *Rayuela* simply arrived too late. Viñas made his thesis clear in *Literatura argentina y realidad política* (1964, 1967), a book that has been hailed as the guiding text for students of Argentine literature. Here, Viñas advanced a lifelong concern: to situate the sentient body as the basis for critical thought. In the process, he opened the doors to a materialist reading of Latin American culture. Consider one of the first observations of his book: "Argentine literature is based on a towering image: rape. This blunt assault gives a defining identity to national literary evolution ... and in particular to the romantic age. "El matadero" and *Amalia*, at their base, are commentaries on the violence exercised from the outside in, from the flesh upon the spirit. From the masses against the subtle but explicit projections of heroism that the lofty Poet hoped to sustain" (Viñas 1969, 13).

This body, he goes on to argue, organizes the entire Argentine literary field from its inaugural moment and gives us a way to read politics and violence up to the present day. Not through a literary heroics or an ethereal defense of the spirit, but through the experience of flesh on flesh. Viñas's novels are no less trenchant with respect to these material claims. In *Los dueños de la tierra* (The masters of the earth, 1958), a didactic novel about the 1921–1922 military interventions against Patagonian workers, Viñas insists on keeping the body at the center of the literary text. Indians, anarchists, prostitutes, and servants wear their scars on the body in order to show the physical pain that they suffer at the hands of violent landowners and bosses. Viñas brings this into alignment through the gaze of characters as they study each other and, in turn, as each becomes an object of contemplation by others. The characters see, hear, and touch one another in a closed community of interactions. Through this circuit of perceptions, Viñas thus reminds us of the boundaries that separate one body from another, as well as their points of contact. Pungent odors, the taste of food, the texture of skin upon skin: the repetition of sensation organizes memory and moves the novel ahead. This is an economic and political experience, Viñas tells us. In fact, as prostitutes and boxers, workers and knife-wielding hoodlums cross one another in the text, they oblige us to think about political struggles emerging in present time. In the novel, the workers define themselves by tactics of encounter and contact; they stand in contrast to the bourgeois figures and government functionaries who show they lack awareness of past and future and live in a temporal vacuum. Reticent to engage in combat or love, refusing responsibility for political events, the rural bourgeoisie pretends not to know about the violence of building a nation; in the process, they expose the shortcomings of Argentine liberal thought. Vicente Vera, the protagonist and a man caught in the middle, summarizes the conflict: old-style politics is an art of contact, whereas new political exchanges are controlled by the *sociedad anónima*, or the anonymous corporation. History would soon see the emergence of new forms of biopolitical control, lacking human contact and exercised at a distance (1958, 253). Under the name of "fairness," a bewildered Vicente Vera keeps his hands clean of political debate and allows military repression to win; the army thus kills the Patagonian workers and a labor strike comes to an end. This literary scenario expressed Viñas's deep political questions. While Cortázar escaped the Peronist years by seeking refuge in Paris, where he combined his surrealist yearnings with the lure of bohemian culture, Viñas remained at home to study national crisis. He thus investigated the beleaguered face-off of state violence and liberal thought by tracking its material consequences on bodies that stood in the way. Corporeal registers were central to his approach to explain a political life. Denouncing a line of liberal thinkers who failed to take stock of the material history, Viñas pursued a desire to make sense of the body in order to define the Argentine state.

Contorno *and Material Culture: The Arrival of Merleau-Ponty*

Under his flagship journal *Contorno* (1953–1959), Viñas and other like-minded Argentine colleagues inquired about material culture and subjectivity as the basis of political readings; above all, they sought to capture the effects of political regimes on the sentient bodies of workers. Here, when the *Contorno* writers faced off with the Peronist state, they found intellectual support for their work in the writings of Sartre and Merleau-Ponty. The body-based philosophies of phenomenology—rooted in flesh and experience—provided Argentines with a materialist grounding both to register the injuries suffered under Peronist rule and to explore the historical-cultural past and anticipate change in the future. Speaking about *Contorno*'s project and its ties to French intellectual thought, Carlos Correas observed: "Phenomenology, with its insistence on the fundamental role of the body, helped us in this [national critique]. In fact, it seems evident today that phenomenology and Peronism found a match for each other in their separate proposals" (2007, 56). The matchup to which Correas alludes was built on a prevailing reality: while the *Contorno* collaborators reminded us of the slippery ways in which populism deluded the masses, phenomenology gave a stone-hard reading of experience and subject formation. It also supplied a leftist perspective that never excluded culture.[2] Embracing these critical options, Viñas found himself in good philosophical company on the *Contorno* board. In particular, León Rozitchner and Oscar Masotta, committed Marxists who linked psychoanalytical models to inquiries about philosophy and ethics, brought forward the sentient body as the first line of access to political knowledge.[3] They also expressed an unmistakable debt to Sartre and Merleau-Ponty.

It might be important to signal the ways in which Merleau-Ponty repudiated Marxist practice while he defended its philosophical positions, or to signal the split that he sustained with Sartre over political direction, but these exchanges were not necessarily central for Argentine intellectuals who, in the early 1950s, sought to mount a critique of the failures of populism under the banner of Juan Perón. Of direct importance for *Contorno*, the French philosophers reaffirmed the idea of *responsibility* among leftist intellectuals.[4] Though both were read extensively and though Sartre captivated writers for his defense of dialectical materialism,[5] Merleau-Ponty, more grounded in the body as a starting point for thought, fully sustained *Contorno*'s attention. His project was admired not so much for his search for an interior life, marked in his studies of Proust and Bergson, but for his emphasis on the concrete engagements of individuals in the world. For *Contorno*, the French philosopher's concept of experience was linked to eventual freedom and possibilities for future action.[6]

Let me briefly attend to the major disciples of Merleau-Ponty and

Sartre. Leon Rozitchner (1924–2011), a member of the *Contorno* group and later a prominent voice in modern philosophy in Argentina, first studied with Merleau-Ponty in Paris and then translated several of his books, among them *Humanism and Terror* (1947). This book would come to exercise a vast influence on Argentine thought and allowed Rozitchner to investigate terror as the basis of subject formation, alienation, and fear.[7] Terror, both Merleau-Ponty and his student Rozitchner argued, was a way to explain political man and his need to turn toward violence. In the long run, delving into the anatomy of terror was also a way to demystify liberal philosophy and its tendencies toward a defense of the spirit, an argument that Rozitchner (and Viñas) had insisted upon throughout their careers.

Early on, Rozitchner was especially interested in unfolding the tensions displayed between power and subjectivity.[8] Influenced by Merleau-Ponty's other classic, *Phenomenology of Perception* (1945), in which an ontology of the visible and the invisible cast a possibility for thinking through politics and culture, Rozitchner wrote that it was fundamentally important to redefine the nature of subjectivity in terms of experience and physical response; the individual not only produced thought but was first defined as a feeling subject, a vector for the intersection of affects, a recipient for the experiences of pleasure and pain. In this respect, the effects of terror belonging to the authoritarian state initially produced a bodily awareness in those who were the state's victims; in turn, this perceptual assault awakened original thought. In an essay published in 1986, Rozitchner offered the following observation: "It may have been that we were thinking of the coherence of the external world without asking about our interior lives: it may have offered a new way to put our bodies in the world, not in order to die, of course, but to reopen in ourselves what fear had sealed shut. Because, yes, we think with our bodies against our deepest fears" (2011, 31). Rozitchner even gives a gendered spin to these claims: before the law of the father (the state, power, civilization itself), Rozitchner turned to the maternal sphere to find contact with the body, to come in contact with the affects and pulsations that belong to nonverbal meaning. This framework allowed him a basis for his materialist reading of history, politics, and culture; a defense of the sensible self that lived surrounded by matter. In this context, the maternal was a defense of life and sensation. Following more in the line of Levinas and Kristeva than even Merleau-Ponty, Rozitchner signaled that we need to follow "Mater-iality as a point of departure" (Rozitchner 2007, 66).

Rozitchner repeatedly underscored the importance of bodies and sensation, and even in later post-*Contorno* moments, he applied theories of perception to the concept of intersecting bodies. Inspired by Merleau-Ponty's concept of "intertwining" (developed in *The Visible and the Invisible*, 1964), the gesture by which contact and interaction are sustained by social encounter (whereby no one knows who touched whom first nor where the original moment of intersection lay), Rozitchner sought forms of action without "firsts" as a main point of contention; he sought a contact among persons that would allow solidarity of the people *against* the Argentine state. These forms of transitivity thus create meaning in the present and supply a network of relational experiences, giving us identities as subjects both within and beyond strictly state-run endeavors. A paradox enters here. In Rozitchner's plan, we not only touch one another, we also (and perhaps perversely) make contact with the state; we carry it within us. Given that there is no point of origin, we can work against forms of subjection only if we can come to identify the multiple locations and points of contact that define the self; these become the *relational* dimensions of embodiment that help us overcome the brittleness of subject/object dualisms that we have learned all along.[9]

Throughout his writing career, Rozitchner was driven by questions about ways of incorporating the other in the self—whether through the symbiotic and material relationship of mother and child (in *La cosa y la cruz*) or the contact among adult bodies as agents joined in social action. For Rozitchner, the body was the basis of reading the past and our historical present. This line of inquiry was placed in evidence in his first book, where he installed the body, sensation, and affect as the prime movers for reading politics and social engagement. Based on his 1960 doctoral dissertation at the Sorbonne, Rozitchner's *Persona y comunidad: Ensayo sobre la significación de la afectividad en Max Scheler*, first published in 1962,[10] set out the major philosophical problems that would confront his generation: understanding ethics and affect by returning to the centrality of the body especially at a moment when philosophical inquiry seemed to have abandoned material readings in favor of universal abstraction.[11]

Rozitchner begins by first observing Scheler's quandary regarding the abstractions of love and spirituality. If Scheler's basic postulate is that the spirit is revealed when the senses are suppressed, Rozitchner is after something else: for him, the senses are not obstacles to the spirit but rather the interface between spirit and body:

> The senses, the sensible impulses, constitute according to Scheler the obstacle for the flowering of the spirit, which is already fully struc-

> tured. But we should ask ourselves: do we really live in the center of changing sensorial movements that are simply a spontaneous, unstable "tickling," only signaling a life form removed from its own intimate core? Or ... is what we call the spirit already an irreducible given that acquires at each moment a relationship with the world that we experience through our sense and sensibilities? If, for intellectual work, the body was the mechanism from which the impartial spirit founds its knowledge, we haven't gotten past the problem of making the body a qualitative block that the spirit would come to inhabit, from the outside. The problem isn't about signaling how the spirit descends upon a body, but in understanding the genesis of spiritual meanings that endows meaning within a material base, in understanding the passage from act to thought. (2013, 240–241)

This passage clearly argues that spirit and senses are connected, but it also signals, contrary to the great defense issued by Catholic thinkers of Scheler's abstract purity, that the starting point for this connection would be found in the body. In this regard, Rozitchner's materialism is placed in dialogue with any idealist premise belonging to a theory of the affects (which Rozitchner would later address).[12]

Rozitchner acknowledges the influence of his teacher Merleau-Ponty, who redefines carnal life, teasing out the reciprocities of body and spirit and linking them to desire and perceptions. In effect, a corporeal presence for Rozitchner (and his mentor) was seen as the medium through which humans gain access to the world. Finally, and again through Merleau-Ponty, Rozitchner insists on the affects as a buffer between spirit and body. He reaches out for embodied meanings, and finds truth first in human perceptions and later in the affects.

Persona y comunidad is foremost an entry into the not-so-obvious sensuality that guides Scheler's ethical studies of phenomenology. In particular, Rozitchner pursues Scheler's grounding in materialism and affects not without serious critique. Early in his book, Rozitchner explains: "The tragic sense of Scheler's philosophy is based upon this irreducible opposition, revealed to us as a false one: the higher stratum of the spirit and the other inferior stratum [of the flesh], the sensible set against the psychological" (2013, 52). To resolve this tension, Rozitchner goes after the totality of human experience, through which he might first link spirit, body, and matter (28); he then moves on to defend an engagement with the other through the experience of contact (55). The tropes that he uses for this encounter frequently evoke forms of contagion, but also a fusion that embraces pleasure and joy (79). This is the basis for a human community, a way to live outside the state, though it carries its own conventional sensorial burdens that are incited by state violence and shock.

Touching upon other essays by Rozitchner, Bosteels likens Rozitchner's proposal to Naomi Klein's articulation of "shock doctrine" (Bosteels 2012, 138) insofar as Rozitchner uncovers a root violence in capitalism that affects all citizens with blasts of "shock and awe" visions. But beyond this, and in another prescient anticipation, Rozitchner sees (in 1960!) the dangers of a market economy that would threaten to reduce us to "objects" (Rozitchner 2013, 244). We can only resist our identities as corporeal things when we combine bodily responses with senses and affects. Sense work, then, subsists as a break in the temporal flow established by the market's control over any sequence of events; affect, as the moment to suspend the time of labor and pay attention to our desire.

In the final sections of his book, Rozitchner devotes himself to an analysis of modesty and resentment (*pudor y resentimiento*), two affective states that constitute our resistance to the objectification of the human, two states that anticipate rage and, more important, revolution. We are about to discover the "historical character of personality" (275), Rozitchner claims, and if we insert the element of love into the mix, we can reach an art of creation that combines intimacy and communal contact. This zone of exploration is found in the hiatus (300), which might be compared to our critical focus today on the gap, the interstitial border, the in-between, or the indecipherable zone of no-man's-land that has not yet been charted on maps. Here, for Rozitchner, the desire for a communal exchange inhabits the body and straddles the divide between abstraction and concreteness. From the sensible body as a guideline, we inevitably enter the arena of social relations and the political sphere.

Contorno published some of Rozitchner's early political essays, which in turn anticipated the work of *Persona y comunidad*. Other essays in *Contorno* filled out the panorama of Rozitchner's thought by examining literary culture. In one of these, an analysis of the novelist Eduardo Mallea, Rozitchner (1955) indicts that kind of literature that fails to acknowledge the flesh. To make his case, Rozitchner reminds his readers that we cannot isolate the literary work from its social context; rather, he studies the figure of the author whose flesh-and-blood image affords us a focus on ideology and physical struggle. "To write is a way for Mallea to expose his historical situation" (1955, 28), Rozitchner says of the Argentine author, whose personality continues to be a source of mystification; Mallea prefers to delve into the invisible Argentina of the national oligarchy, while he leaves aside the visible Argentina of workers and immigrants. Stuck in a world of abstractions, Mallea shows us neither the body that suffers nor the skin that bears the blows inflicted by national history. As a result, and as Rozitchner sees it, Mallea's novels collapse and fail.

Like the other authors of the *Contorno* group, Rozitchner keeps an eye on the fleshiness of the act of writing. This kind of narrative, embodied and scarred, is the only path toward revealing history and overcoming the fate of an oppressed subject who drowns in silence and occlusion. Whether examining literature and philosophy or the political realities of the state, Rozitchner insisted on concrete realities and the responses of a sensible being. Rozitchner later writes, "What happened to our bodies, our imagination, our affects?" (2011, 33). This body, Rozitchner claims, should be linked to socially responsible action.

Rozitchner's proposal is not independent of the endeavors of David Viñas or Oscar Masotta, all participants in the *Contorno* project. Through philosophy, literature, or psychoanalysis, these three intellectuals summoned a discourse on the senses as a category for critical study. While Rozitchner and Viñas were grappling principally with the perceiving body in relation to state terror, their contemporary Oscar Masotta (1930–1979) took to mapping out theories of sensation through psychoanalytic models and, equally important for our interests here, through visual arts and literary texts.[13] Perhaps best known to the literary field for his work on Roberto Arlt, Masotta, in the decade following *Contorno*, was also a key figure in the Di Tella Institute, where he lectured on happenings and kinetic art and—their opposite—what he called "dematerialized" art, or mass-media productions that were decidedly nonauratic. His contributions represent a radical investigation of changing aesthetics in the 1960s, capturing on the one hand an art of embodiment and on the other a highly mediated and immaterial art in simulated visual spaces. Leaning on the inheritance of post-Peronist trends of the late 1950s, in which artistic experiments with new materials dominated the visual arts, Masotta took into account a corporeal experience of viewing (see Giunta 2001, 120–127) and insisted, as Merleau-Ponty did, on the ways in which bodies related to imagined space as meaningful prerational experience. Bodies, in short, contained a primary route of access to knowledge and abstraction; beyond this, Masotta was also aware of the impact of mass media that was soon to change artistic production. His studies integrated both directions.

Although Masotta is more frequently identified with Sartrean thought, he attends to Merleau-Ponty in *Conciencia y estructura* (Consciousness and structure, 1968). Written during the late 1950s and 1960s, this collection of essays exposes the ways in which Masotta's original Marxist direction had been constantly reinvented as he focused his critical lens on new objects from literature and "high-art" regimes. By the late 1960s, when Masotta turned to pop art and mass-media culture, he avidly defended an art that existed on the streets and in "life," and followed with keen concern the temporalities that governed the market. Embodied knowledge is the unifying trope that organizes the first phase of his writing.

It is significant that the opening essay of his book, dating from 1958, draws upon Merleau-Ponty as a strong basis for understanding the Italian philosopher and art critic Enzo Paci, who, through his journal *Aut Aut*, set in place a number of questions about experience, time, and perception. Like Rozitchner, Oscar Masotta wanted to defend sensible experience as a precursor to reason. History, he offered in *Conciencia y estructura*, does not reside in books, but within us; we experience and create it. With this, Masotta insisted that the body was fundamental to the structuring of thought (1968, 21). Delving further, Masotta expressed his suspicions about the fundamental ambiguities of the time gap between sense perception and understanding. Is abstract thought so distant in time from the instant of knowledge drawn in through perceptions? Answering Enzo Paci, Masotta claims that relational figures aren't simple; rather, we need to situate forms of cultural apprehension within economic and historical structures, and then to regard the sites where humans and objects cross in the consumer market. To sustain his argument, Masotta cannot let go of Merleau-Ponty, and he reminds us that moments of perception depend on situations in time: "It would be legitimate to claim, regarding the organism that Merleau-Ponty says is the body, that the organism is not just a phase, but a situation" (25). But there's more. Phenomenology, Masotta sustains, focuses not only on place but also on the thick temporal processes that support history and human evolution (22). Masotta takes these questions up on two fronts: in his literary studies and in his lectures on the visual arts.

Especially in *Sexo y traición en Roberto Arlt* (1965), Masotta took the tools of phenomenology to study the sensorial universe and its effects upon the individual in the novels of Arlt. Citing Sartre, Merleau-Ponty, and Genet in order to make his case (Masotta considers Sartre's *Saint Genet* to be the most important critical work of his time), he turns to the sensible content of fiction in order to speak of the ways in which the external world affects the internal life of the subject. The first chapter begins:

> The world creates in each of us a place where we go to receive it: we can speak of the depth of that zone.... But no amount of attack or scorn can make us forget our own particular and private way of feeling ... [and] when thoughts appear, the rhythms of hope, that place—perhaps palpable for some or invisible for others—where we feel these fleeting bolts of lightning that make objects appear and disappear, the scenes and acts that never came to fruition in our minds.... When we stand before a work, it's necessary not to forget that in it a man tells us the story of a consciousness turned toward the world by an original movement that directs him to things, to other men, or to the work itself. All literature is only the vertiginous movement of comings and goings, a life dialectic between depth and the world. (1965, 23)

Masotta devotes his study to the way in which the world interacts with the flesh of the body; from this premise, he traces how liberal society impinges upon one's freedom of being and pierces one's tissue and bone. Among his most brilliant pages are those devoted to the shiny metal of the coin that incites physical and psychic symptoms; in contact with the desiring subject, the coin creates pulsations in the individual heart and stimulates a middle-class desire to rob, to lie, and to cheat. This effectively becomes Masotta's introduction to a phenomenological reading of Roberto Arlt, starting with Arlt's first novel, *El juguete rabioso* (1926).[14] Although Masotta traces the accumulated experience of humiliation and loss found in Arlt's characters, he is not interested in defining a moral map; rather, he wants to see the ways in which objects (money, books, metals) hail the consciousness of the subject and, conversely, how material forms resist or elude our desires (Masotta 1965, 71). The larger cartography marks out instances of middle-class conflict regarding bodies and conscience.

Masotta laments the ways in which this social sector is dependent on the body yet always tries to escape it by turning to abstract thought (the characters of *Los siete locos* serve as his prime examples). This behavior, for Masotta, is the early sign of a social class that loses control over its course of progress and falls—humiliated—under the shadow of desire cast by those in power. In other words, when the middle class loses contact with its sentient self, it succumbs to outside forces, especially the forces of the state. From a minimal awareness of the body, and humiliated all the same, the members of this middle class direct their frustrations through acts of violence that in turn humiliate others (77). Perceptions are sheltered under right-wing thought and thus begin with personal frustration. To get here, Masotta, borrowing from Sartre, separates image and perception in order to show how people who begin to think about their exclusion from history also harbor a social resentment:

> We don't perceive things through a consciousness absolutely capable of fixing meanings upon them nor do we perceive things as they are dictated by our individual desires. We perceive a world in which each object is not the appropriate correlative of each person's individual will, but the crossing point at which my perspective crosses with that of the other person: and as long as this intersubjective tie is invested in things, it will find itself weighed down by tradition and by a conservative ideology that emanates from the actual structures of society; it would thus not be farfetched to say that to perceive is to perceive an almost right-wing world. (104)

Arlt tracks a history of human alienation and misery so intense that the suffering subject, deadened by pain, loses the chance for awareness and freedom:

> One can see . . . the splendor and misery of Arlt's man: the damned who go from alienation to alienation, who suppress a consciousness of their own bodies in order to force others to live out a similar corporeal misery while they, the damned, confine themselves to the anguish of pure consciousness, dreaming—as we do—of a time in which all men might find among themselves an open relationship that would be sustained between bodies, when bodies might not be an instrument of alienation between one man and the other, but the vehicle of an authentic relationship of one man with himself and of each man with all others. (111)

Masotta traces the estrangement of consciousness from the abject body and shows how this split guides individuals through politics and social life.[15]

It is not my goal to continue the debates about the influence of phenomenology on Argentine intellectual life in the 1950s and 1960s or to reach forward and insist upon its interface with Masotta's inaugural studies of the work of Lacan.[16] The point, however, is to indicate that in Masotta's world, literary texts, performances, and artistic responses were embraced in order to show the integration of politics and culture under the signs of perception and sensation. Indeed, through Viñas, Rozitchner, and Masotta and their *Contorno* colleagues, we are given a narrative about the sensible body as a product of history; a body inscribed in its environs that is always culturally bound. For them, the body is the first step in the construction of subjective life inasmuch as it offers a clear resistance to commodification and a challenge to authoritarian regimes. This even determined new forms of pop art, happenings, and art-based experience.

The Di Tella Project: Bodies of Experience

In the mid-1960s, from the sphere of philosophy and literature, writers like Rozitchner and Viñas decisively insisted that the sensate subject be in the center of debates about the political economy, while Masotta, working through the Instituto Torcuato di Tella, signaled the art events known as happenings as a way to physically experience the world.[17] In effect, he captured the transitions of Argentine artists as they moved toward those materials and experiences that perforce would awaken perception.

The art object in the 1960s was certainly in transition, reconfigured as a form to be destroyed on the spot or to be physically experienced. The goal, for some, was to locate the secret laws of matter, to find their fundamental characteristics and breaking points through art, to track the way in which inert artistic material clashed with the rush of time (Pellegrini 2004, 32). Gone were the heated debates about the values of figuration or abstraction that earlier avant-garde groups had held dear. Instead, the idea was to find new sources of beauty through new materials outside the usual artistic milieu, among them manipulable objects that required the spectator's sensory engagement. Artists and poets identified with Brazilian *concretismo* were engaged in similar pursuits. Especially concerned with the materiality of objects and the sensory responses of viewers, Hélio Oiticica and Lygia Clark, for example, redefined the parameters of the subject-object encounter through their experiences with irregular substances and forms and their renewed use of everyday objects that were to be handled by the viewers of art. In their "sensorial creations," as the works have come to be known (masks, goggles, gloves, and early virtual-reality experiments of the 1960s and 1970s), these artists took their cues from

Mário Pedrosa, the art critic responsible for introducing Merleau-Ponty to a Brazilian audience in the 1950s.[18] Oiticica, Clark, and others shaped an art of perceptions.

Working between Argentina and France, Julio Le Parc insisted, for example, that art needed to find openings for alternative sensibilities, whether though exercises of bare brutality, kinetic movements defining the art piece, or radical disruptions of light that distorted the distance between spectator and artistic form (Cámara 2014, 56; Kozak 2012, 47–50). His "Elementos a ensayar" (practice elements), for example, tested the spectator's hearing and sense of touch and altered the field of vision. Jorge Romero Brest, the first director of the Di Tella Institute and the principal art critic in Argentina of the 1960s, gave another spin to this discussion when, assessing the new challenges of contemporary art in the 1960s, he recognized the end of an aesthetic system based on quality and instead declared the importance of experience. "The key is in the *experience* . . . now that artworks are in themselves, irrefutably *experience*," wrote Romero Brest in 1963 (qtd. in Katzenstein 2004, 100). It is apparent, as many critics have noted, that Romero Brest's defense of experience was sustained by the years of course lectures he delivered in the 1950s and 1960s, during which time he insisted on a curriculum based on Sartre and Merleau-Ponty that influenced scores of artists.[19] Ever eager to sustain his idea of the experiential artwork, in 1967 Romero Brest inaugurated a gallery exhibition of "experiences"—a sensorial awareness of experience itself that released us from *thinking* about the image. In his summary of the *Experiencias* exhibition, he reminds us of the phenomenological tendency that guides the art that he set in motion:

> Proof of this fundamental activity is found in the "experiences" that began under the name of "Visual Experiences" in 1967 [and which] continued with the simpler label of "Experiences" in 1968. . . . They were realized by artists who agreed about the need to show an experiential attitude in public. . . .
>
> I should add regarding the word "experience" that we want to consider the potentiary aspect of creation, art as an instrument of knowledge and not as a mere antecedent of knowledge. . . . [A]nother way of saying this is to advance that artists don't reflect their experiences through the works that they create; rather, they present them in a virginal state, exercising an awareness of imagining instead of a consciousness of the image. . . . [W]ith these experiences, we're not looking

> at gods, ideas, sentiments, desires or mandates, in the style of creators of an earlier age.
>
> These new experiences in the imaginative field correspond to a focus on phenomenology in the intellectual field, with each artist choosing a particular phenomenon and without moving beyond this to a distant imagined reality; on the side, Husserl would have said that we're leaving alone everything that covers up the originality of phenomena and blocks access to what is immediately real. (Romero Brest 1969, 90–91)

The many happenings at the Di Tella Institute took the sensible to new extremes. Central to this project was *La menesunda*, hailed in the art world as the first Argentine happening and representing a watershed moment in national art history. Developed by Marta Minujín and Rubén Santantonín, *La menesunda* (1965) was an experiment with the minor experiences of daily life: an interactive environment that was set out so that viewers might experience the lives of others. This first version of the happening was called an environmental signal and was designed to provoke a heightened awareness of the materials with which art is constructed. In dialogue with this work, Romero Brest described *La menesunda* as "a multiexperiential project for those whom we would not call contemplative observers, but active creators of their own reality" (1992, 79). In the same vein, this art critic reminded his readers that experience was the center of a dynamic truth; basing his ideas on John Dewey, who argued art as experiential, and on an earlier Kantian concept in which perceptions determined experience that was later synthesized in consciousness, Romero Brest moved through different experiences with the modern work of art. It is not that visual images reflected experiences similar to ours, he claimed, but that art creates experience through the vehicle of perceptions.[20]

In Romero Brest's curation of the show *Experiencias*, one saw up close a display of social-political experiences that emphasized perceptions (Romero Brest 1969, 95). In Romero Brest's words, the artists were to "try to overcome dislocation by eliminating the intermediary. In other words, they tried to compress the distance between people who proposed situations and those who created them. This process has often been called the bringing together of art and life" (qtd. in Katzenstein 2004, 131). Romero Brest focused on artistic experience as active engagement and construction; whether he picked up on the multisensorial projects of avant-garde artists of the 1960s or led them deliberately on this course through his orchestration at the Di Tella is a topic up for grabs, but what is clear is that experiential art had come to claim its day throughout the Americas.

Consider these few examples. In the Di Tella exhibition of 1967 entitled *Visual Experiences*, the artist Oscar Bony designed an installation composed of chain-link fencing set on a floor, a film projector, and a required walkway for spectators to move through the exhibit. Entitled *60 metros cuadrados y su información* (60 square meters and its information, 1967), the installation invited viewers to walk on fencing material in order to experience a tactile perception (the texture, weave, and pressure of wire under the feet); at the same time, a projector showed a film of a chain-link fence. It was left to the viewer to form a mental connection between the film image and the tactile experience. Bony, like Masotta, was interested in the redundancy of experience such that material experienced in vivo alongside its filmic reproduction would be brought together as information that the viewer was supposed to unite.

A similar strategy is observable in David Lamelas's work *Office of Information about the Vietnam War on Three Levels: The Visual Image, Text and Audio* (1968). Here, Lamelas offers an office scene (desks, telephones, Olivetti typewriter, tape recorder, Telex, and microphone) situated behind a plexiglass panel: the idea is to bring the viewer's attention to the multimedia production of the newsroom along with the important communications devices that enabled sound and print in the 1960s. On the outer side of the plexiglass plate, a pair of attached headphones invites the viewer to listen to the sounds of the office. The visitor thus hears news tapes of the Vietnam War (with voices in French, Spanish, and Italian) just as they were captured by the Telex machine stationed in the office. All the while, the plexiglass shield keeps the viewer at a distance: while time, image, sound, and touch are at a remove from the viewer, the sounds heard on the headphones problematize the gap. A strange condensation of time and sensorial effect thus occurs: everything that was heard in the distant past, now of almost reliquary status, is made immediate; print is confused with voice. Through the devices of sound, moreover, the distant office scene comes within our sensorial grasp; we hear news as it once happened. Image and auditory functions are crossed; temporal lapses (from 1968 until the present) are reduced, while spatial distance (our physical distance from the office, separated from us by the plexiglass wall) is all too apparent. The distance of the newsroom from the theater of military action is also put into question, while the polyglot feast of languages heard in the audios (and presumably observed in the Telex printouts that once

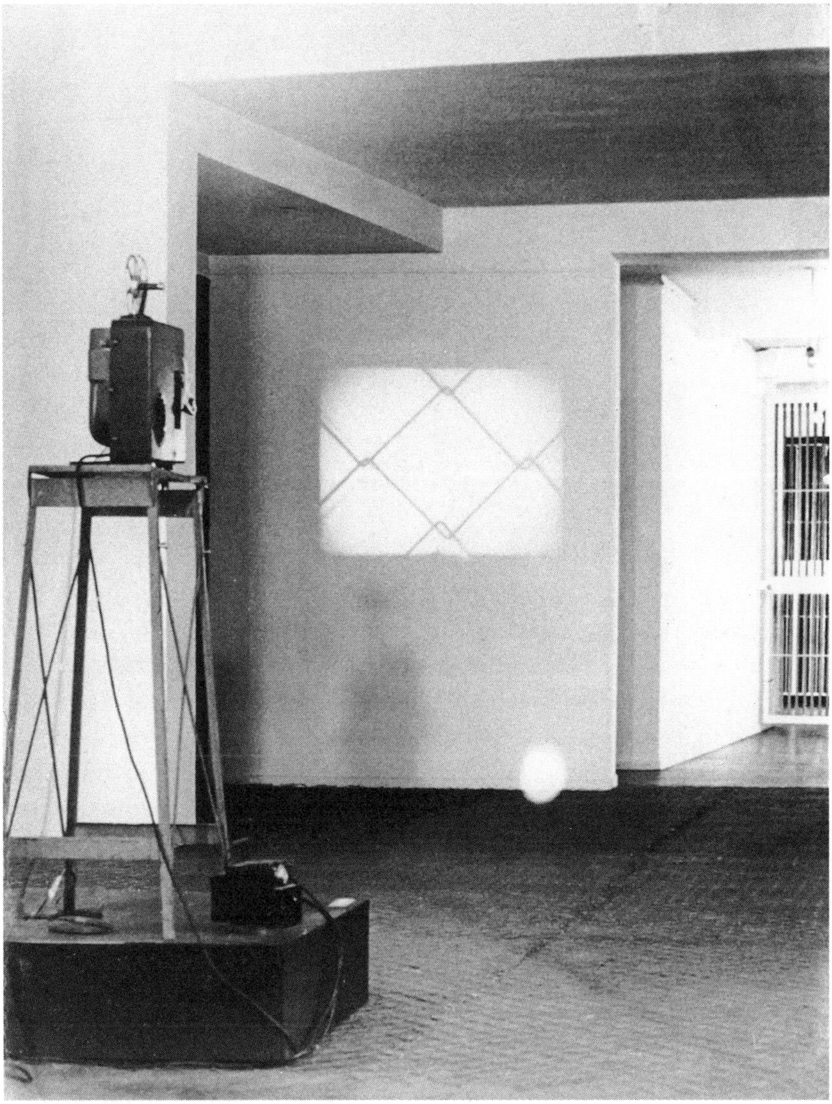

Figure 4.1. Oscar Bony, 60 Square Meters and Its Information, *1967. Courtesy of Carola Bony and the archive of the artist.*

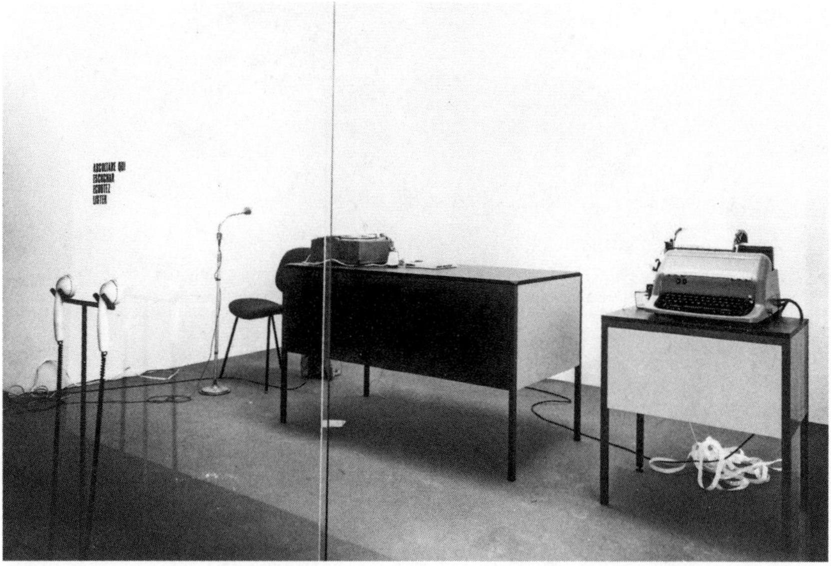

Figure 4.2. David Lamelas, Office of Information about the Vietnam War on Three Levels: The Visual Image, Text and Audio, *1968. Courtesy of the artist.*

rolled off the office machine) eradicate any sense of an "original" news feed that we might have accepted as truth. It is no wonder that the sensorial complexity of the experience obliges us to revisit our silent assumptions held about time, space, and language, not to mention the construction and reception of a political event witnessed through the media. Even in the art exhibition of 1968, these categories of distance held firm.

Marta Minujín also refocused our understanding of distance and proximity by addressing the kinds of sensorial awakening that occur in daily life. She thus insisted that her art objects needed physical experience in order to place us in the present, and tested audience consciousness of materials and one's delivery to the sensuality of the cities. Neon tunnels, television monitors lining a walkway, couples lying in bed, art workshops for the public: they all formed part of her mega-installation that shocked as it engaged. As Oscar Masotta describes it, Minujín attempted to work in the intermediary space "between the raw, animal world of the senses and the artifice of culture" (2004, 282). Her art event sustained these observable tensions, prolonging what Masotta had called the power of "environmentalist works" (*obras ambientacionales*). Masotta went on to describe these efforts as part of a project whose "goal was to envelop the audience in direct media and sensory stimulation (smells, colors, etc.). And if there is a difference between an environmentalist work and a Happening, since at least in the latter the audience can be moved from one place to another, both types of works require the quantitative determination of the audience. One could not imagine a Happening, for example, in which no viewer was called to 'participate,' just as one could not imagine a Happening without 'spectators'" (2004, 374–375).

If it is true that the goal in the new art of the sixties was, as Aldo Pellegrini put it, "a smashing of the lines between figuration and abstraction" (qtd. in Pacheco 2004, 25), it was also marked by an appeal to experience and sensation. Kinetic art, action art, a visual field that brought viewer interaction: these new forms emerging in the 1960s relied on the power of perceptions both to arouse the spectator and to rethink the dialogic function that the art object awakened. My goal here is not to homogenize the differences between these artists but to signal an overall concern with their sensorial interest in marking the gap between perception and reflection and measuring their distance from history.

Masotta found himself deeply immersed in these issues in these years, but while he cultivated a theoretical interest in kinetic art and perceptions, he was also interested in what came to be known as a dematerialized art, based in part on Soviet productivist art of the 1920s (and inspired by El Lissitzky's ideas on the future of the book) and looking forward to what we might call today a devotion to the media or virtual culture. Aware of the diminished physical materiality brought about by new technologies (and remember in this regard that Masotta's colleague Eduardo Costa was studying tape-recorded voices and making installations based on sound and other intractable forms, just as Oscar Bony and David Lamelas were experimenting with technological supplements in image and sound),[21] Masotta sought out the "liberating energy" of new forms of immaterial expression.[22] The idea here was to move attention from the values of uniqueness, origin, and permanence in order to focus on the experiences that the object or machine could engender. To work in this direction, one had to embrace materials that stood beyond the usual artistic purview: ordinary objects, austere and brutal forms, discarded waste or fragments; any common object could trigger sensation. Therein lay the emancipatory possibility of mass culture and communications.[23]

Although the Di Tella artists of the 1960s could hardly have imagined the current radical experiences of shock and awe provoked by today's visual arts, their emphasis on a new range of sensory effects left a definite mark on culture. The movement was not without its opponents. While the Di Tella experiments gave a conceptual focus for intellectuals to shape a desiring body in response to the stimuli of light and film, pain, and market promotion, others among leftist circles refused to engage with Di Tella, finding the institute too attached to movements of a global market.[24] Regardless of the polarizing debates, however, the political crisis of the late 1960s brought all conversations to a rapid ending: in 1968, the repressive forces of the Onganía regime intervened in the Di Tella and closed its artistic wing.[25]

The entire discourse on sensation represented in the Di Tella art world thus came to a slowdown and eventual halt. Although the art center was only closed for several days and, according to John King, became a "happening" in itself,[26] the military intervention nonetheless was an alert of things to come. And indeed as news of an ascendant political order using strong-arm tactics came to be heard, it demanded a different kind of art to answer oppression and violence. Withdrawing from the gallery system, then, many artists began to work in the streets; through groups like Tucumán Arde, they responded with greater political investment than ever before. From the often gratuitous sensual "experiences" fomented by the Di Tella Institute, artists now devoted themselves to the representation of physical pain.

Dictatorships of Sense and State

The years between the late 1960s and the decade of the 1980s brought two incompatible worlds into strange and unexpected contact. In effect, as the dictatorships took hold, the bodily and psychic experiences of terror took writers and artists on a different course. A different engagement with the sensorial world was budding. While avant-garde artists of the 1960s experimented with sensory effects in order to awaken their viewers, the military regimes brought new meaning to the engagement of body and state. Indeed, the dictators discovered that tools to exacerbate perceptions would produce information and exercise control of bodies and voices. By intensifying the assaults on the body with electrical instruments and other technologies, the state inflicted lasting harm on those whom it detained and surveilled. The human body, reduced to a "cell state" under conditions of martial law, was deprived of its humanity and driven by sensation alone. For more than a decade, the repellent physical acts imposed upon prisoners in their "bare life" conditions were suppressed from public knowledge; a black hole of silence and censorship surrounded the news feeds about the prison camps that cropped up throughout Latin America.

Years later, we learned of these base realities through the reports of human rights commissions on the detained and disappeared. In Argentina, the Argentine National Commission on the Disappeared (CONADEP) produced the Nunca Más (Never again) report of 1984, giving documented evidence of the abuses sustained under military rule; in Chile, with the fall of Pinochet, the Commission for Truth and Reconciliation similarly published the Rettig Report in 1991 to expose a dark world of state terror that exploited its victims through physical abuse and torture. Determined to extirpate the communist leanings of workers and student activists, and eventually pursuing any individual who appeared to oppose or even to question the legitimacy of military regimes, agents of the state resorted to sensory provocation (through deprivation or excess) and varieties of physical battery that were both sadistic and extreme; presumably to extract information from their victims (to make the body speak, as so many people have observed), the torture methods survived through the protections of secrecy and power. At times they even produced pleasure in those who administered the pain. They were acts of "ultimate brutality and absolute caprice," wrote Ronald Dworkin in his prefatory remarks to the English-language translation of *Nunca Más: Comisión Nacional sobre la Desaparición de Personas* (1986, 2). Under the general rubric of "N.N.," or disappeared, those who were detained rarely returned to speak of their torture or to account for the vast dehumanization of life staged in detention centers. Nevertheless, when their voices were heard, they filled the black hole of darkness with reports of exacerbated damage to the body and unmitigated pain. Consider, for example, this testimony reported by Nélson Eduardo Dean and included in the *Nunca Más* report:

> They tied a rope or chain to the handcuffs and pulled my arms up as high as they could without dislocating them. I was in that position, literally hanging at a distance of about 30 centimeters from the floor, for a period of time which is not possible to determine in hours, only in terms of pain. Because of the great suffering induced by … torture, one loses all track of time.

> I think it's only possible to offer a tragic caricature of what it was like. Two things might prove useful as examples and give some idea: some actual physical events and some sensation....
>
> > (a) After torture, the soles of the feet were burnt and layers of hard skin would form, which peeled off later. Obviously the skin was burnt from the electric shocks.
> > (b) During the application of electricity, one would lose all control over one's senses, such torture provoking permanent vomiting, almost constant defecation, etc.
>
> As for sensations, electricity begins to rise up the body. All the parts with wires attached to them feel as though they are being torn from the body. Thus at first, it's the feet which feel as though they are being torn off, then the legs, testicles, thorax, etc. (Comisión Nacional sobre la Desaparición de Personas 1986, 39)

Three items deserve our attention: the exacerbated work on sensation that erases any perception of time; the sadistic attacks launched by one human being upon another through what might be called technologies of pain; the vast intensities that the victim feels and that resist description. Testimony, in this instance, is the genre best used to convey the material of direct perceptions, to narrate the embodied experiences that will expose otherwise-hidden truths. As the author of this denunciation goes on to reveal: "These practices were carried out in a diabolical setting: the torturers, some drinking, others laughing, hitting, and insulting, tried to extract the name of Uruguayans living in Argentina" (1986, 40). When shielded by a state of exception and when all rule of law was lost, it was never clear if the military operands solely sought out information or if their sadistic pleasure before the pain of others was sufficient unto itself. In any event, the punishment that they launched formed part, in Foucault's terms, of an "economy of suspended right" (1995, 11).

The status of the detained and disappeared—people without voice or body—was contested from the world beyond prison with imagined depictions of pain and horror. While government forces insisted upon silence (the "nothing happened here" dictum became the official mantra), oppositional voices filled these dark and silent spaces with bodies, perceptions, and sounds. The dyad deserves exploration. On the one hand, we are at the scene of Kant's radical evil, where under guarded silence, torture tactics were used to humiliate prisoners, to extract a voice of supposed truth that might protect the interests of the state. On the other, artists and writers populated their books and canvases with violent sensory shocks, awakening viewers to the details of horror that were not reported by the state.

In Argentina the plight of the detained and disappeared has been reenacted by radical art collectives since the 1960s: Tucumán Arde, a group committed to protest art in the time of Onganía, began in 1968 to link art and social protest. Theater groups staged allegories of violence and disappearance, among them Grippo in 1980, followed by Teatro Abierto and the puppet theater of Arturo Carrera and Emeterio Cerro. Art actions by León Ferrari, Roberto Jacoby, and Marta Minujín continued from the sixties. [27] Liliana Maresca insisted on what has been called a visceral poetics in order to expose the horror of dismembered bodies and the plight of the disappeared; in photography, she even figured her own body as a victim of torture devices.

While autobiographical texts supplied testimonies of pain and stories about abjection, sound installations and public art projects reproduced sensations of horror. Elsewhere, the Chilean Catalina Parra developed a series on the *imbunches* (see plate 11), the mythical figures from Mapuche lore whose orifices were sewn shut by witches in order to suppress their hearing, sight, and touch and also prohibit them from speaking. Parra's work was an obvious reference to censorship under the military regime, to the way in which dimensions of the sensible were foreclosed by authoritarian rule. From a different corner, the Brazilian Adriana Varejão continues to work with carnal images to show the abuse of the flesh under colonialism and authoritarian rule. Abused labor and pounds of human flesh contribute to a carnal density (as Linda Williams put it) that upheld colonial law. Varejão lets these visceral bulges of organs and blood seep through colonial-era tiles, thus contrasting the beauty of artisan craft with the tissue of human meat that undergirds colonialism as a whole (see plate 12). Together, these artists remember the many abuses enacted by first-wave colonialism in America or call attention to the violence of authoritarian regimes, the dismemberment of their populations, or the abridgement or intensification of sensory perceptions.

This is not only a Latin American project, but corresponds to a heightened attention worldwide for recording experience and highlighting sensation. While Latin American artists and writers turned to body work to expose the uses of torture that had been covered up by military regimes in the 1970s and 1980s, a parallel rise in corporeal art was also traced across

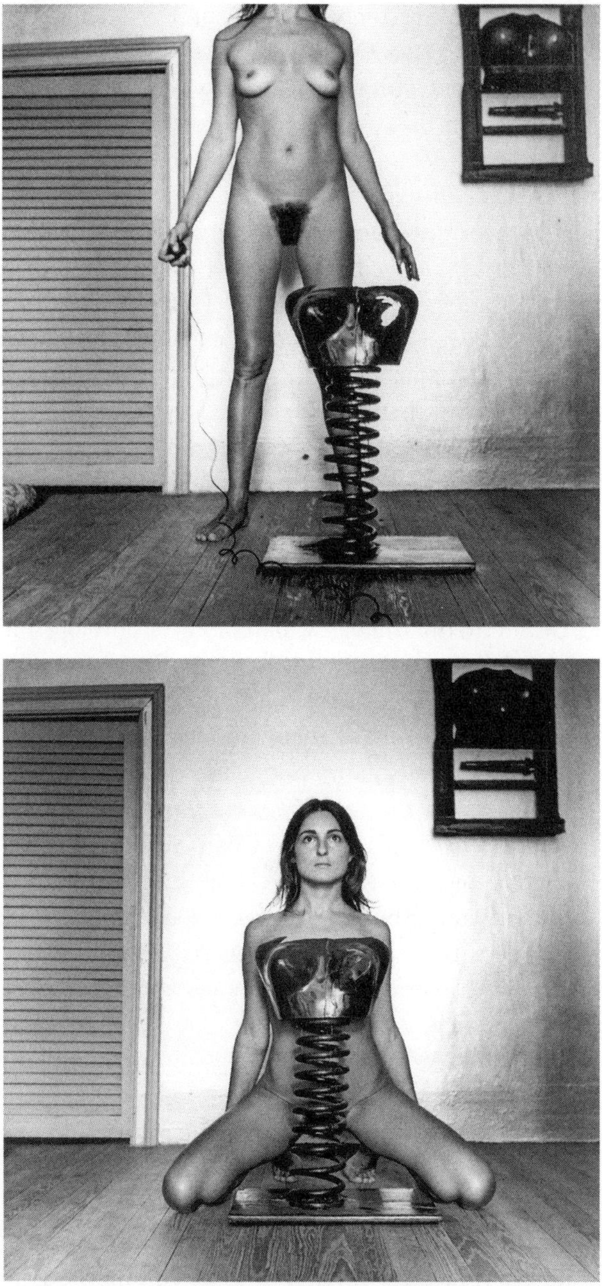

Figure 4.3. Liliana Maresca, untitled, 1983. From the series Liliana Maresca with Her Work. *Photo-performance. Photograph by Marcos López. Courtesy of Archivo Liliana Maresca and Marcos López.*

the globe. This gesture was designed to shock and entice, to call attention to the role of the individual before the neoliberal market; but it also signaled a rising aesthetic of performance, a display of the range of bodily functions that art might attach to machines in order to produce sensation (remember the multiple plastic surgeries of Orlan that changed her physical appearance; or years later, the disfigurements of Stelarc, who surgically sewed an ear into his arm and had it controlled by transistors; or the work of Marc Quinn, who in the 1990s transfused his own blood to fill translucent sculptures of human heads, emphasizing the gap between the living body and the work of art). While Latin Americans focused on the need to reveal the physical truth of pain and protest and the status of the disappeared, recreating scenes of abjection that might have occurred in prison, a global focus simultaneously turned toward the biopolitical sphere. In the mid-1970s, for example, Michel Foucault delivered the first of his seminars on this topic as he focused on the Nazi death camps and their prisoners. Following in his footsteps, Giorgio Agamben and Roberto Esposito later inquired about states of exceptions and their effects on human life. From a different angle, Elaine Scarry offered a fundamental exploration in 1985 on pain and torture and opened the path to an intense production of trauma studies in the years that followed. As a whole, these writers exposed for critical thought the abject physical experiences that had been hidden from public view.

"Nothing Is Happening Here"

We are in a tug of war between the erasure of sense (hence, the death of the subject) and a sustained engagement with the material world that, in the hands of oppositional artists, was used to denounce authoritarian regimes. "Sense work" was being put into effect on both sides of the political divide, and the body was caught in the middle, but from the position of oppositional artists, sense work also supplied a route to remembrance. The Israeli poet Yehuda Amichai prompts us in that direction: "What is not of the body will not be remembered," he claimed, situating the labor of embodiment as both an erotic and a political gesture against forgetting.[28] In the Southern Cone, where embodied perceptions in art and literature were so important to bring down the curtain of silence sustained by the authoritarian state, the artistic community found strategies to remember the body that were not commonly expected. At times, the memory of political horror was nestled within the hazy routine of everyday life; at others, it was recalled in the steaminess of erotic contact. In yet other contexts, the memory of horror came forth in anguished portraits of dismembered limbs and bodily fluids, or simply as unnamable stains on the canvas of a painting or buried allusions within the strophes of a poem. Literature and art taught us how to perceive and identify horror, and how to experience pain. Sensory recollection in several Southern Cone cases exposes the breadth of this discussion. The Argentine novelist Juan José Saer, the Chilean poet Raúl Zurita, and the Chilean visual artist Guillermo Núñez offer substantial examples of sense work that sustains the trauma of remembering through the body. Despite the different genres that undergird them, their works signal an insistence on keeping sense perceptions alive.

Saer's Nothing Never

Considered to be among the most compelling novels about the years of military rule in Argentina, Juan José Saer's *Nadie nada nunca* (Nobody nothing never, 1980) is a narrative of sensations and affects, of rhythms and attention to details that amount to a perception of time. Like many novels of Saer (1937–2005), suffused with his experience as a poet, the thematic direction is hard to define at first; instead, we are left with experiments in perception that rarely manage to suture the gaps between present and past or navigate the ethical quandary of surviving in brutal times. With indirect references to history that the characters scarcely understand, Saer's novel is about the ways in which we fail to discern how reality touches our lives. Behind this is the unmentioned dictatorship, the disappearance of human life, the torture inflicted by military police, and the endless surveillance of citizen-subjects. Saer tells us that survivors lack the tools for apprehending the degree of state interference in our daily lives. Awakened perceptions might offer a clue or an entryway to this awareness; they have the power to alert us to a hostile reality if we are willing to pay attention at all.[29]

If the dictatorships expected a "man without qualities,"[30] the compliant "hombre masa" who during those states of exception was subjected to sensorial probes in order to produce pain, and secondarily information, in Saer's novel the hero as a sentient being intrudes upon a system of silence. Saer's narrative project is to slow down time, to place attention on minute objects and actions, to bring a halt to the fragility of history, to keep us in the longue durée of an unbearably perceptual present. Through all of this, Saer shows us an astounding breadth of human experience emerging from local rural life. Through the slowness of repetitions and the seemingly boring time of small-town existence in which little of consequence happens, Saer thins out his plot to a minimalist depiction so that even the disappearance of the protagonists slips from the reader's grasp.

Occurring over three days in rural Argentina, *Nadie nada nunca* tells the story of Gato and his lover, Elisa, who languish in a village where nothing much seems to happen and where life is quite frankly dull. Food and sex, an occasional exchange with a bather who sits by the river, the perusal of a novel that Gato reads (while the bather spends time reading comics), the appearance of a journalist and a detective, the menacing sound of an automobile motor: this string of sketchy representations sustains the novel's slow pace. That said, we also come to learn that various horses around town have been shot to death and quartered, anticipating (perhaps) the murder of the detective Caballo Leyva and the (eventual) disappearance of the major characters of the story. But nothing is clear; we don't have a clue about the assassins of horses, nor do we ever understand what motivates the death of Leyva or the roles of Gato and Elisa. Instead, Saer detains us in present time in order to show how the experience of sensing might put us on track to knowing.

What is hidden beneath this flimsy plot is a slight, submerged, and almost-undetectable reference to the arrival of a dark car at night and the possible politically driven abduction of Gato and Elisa (in truth, their destiny is not declared until Saer's later novel, *Glosa*, of 1986, where we learn that they were abducted; in the posthumous novel *La grande* of 2005, Saer returns to these figures again and tells us that Gato and Elisa's tale was in fact a political allegory about the disappeared). But to get near to this understanding within the frame of the novel at hand, Saer teaches us different ways to be perceptive, to pay attention to the details picked up by the senses, to use our skills to discern what the senses tell us, and to learn—after all is said and done—to sense what is deeply wrong.

The learning curve is gentle; first, we learn from the small gestures—the bend of an elbow, a cigarette puff, the act of setting a table—how to link vision and sound, touch and taste in order to construct a character; perceptual cues on the surface replace any search for personal depth.[31] Everything, like a French *nouveau roman*, is streamlined; the same event is told from different perspectives, each time with variant details. In this respect, it is useful for Saer to situate this novel in the provinces, a nod to the rural background that he always sustains in his texts but also a way to clear the air of the perceptual overload of the city by retreating to a space where nothing is said to happen. It is as if a minimalist treatment of sense stimulation could only take place in the calm. But there's more: the sensory stimulation that inundates this text almost seems to be a compensation for what cannot be said and thought. On the one hand, Saer leaves sense work on the surface to avoid conflicts with reason; on the other, he invites the alert reader to use that sense material to awaken political thought.

The novel thus begins: "In the beginning, there is nothing" (1993, 7). This strange negation of history and events that inaugurates the fiction declares itself against analysis and interpretation; it is a phrase reiterated throughout the novel to remind us that nothing has changed. We are thus left in a present time in which characters lack the perceptual alertness to confront an authoritarian state; hence, Saer's flatness of affect signals a lack of direction or goal. But this is just the beginning; perhaps we will learn something later. Meanwhile, what won't be named is the Argentine military government or its clamp on bodies and movement.

Instead of giving name to the horror, Saer presents us with materials and objects, carcasses of beef and horses, blood draining from the slaughterhouse. These scenes and events occupy our visual field as they also recall Argentina's earliest fiction, Echeverría's "El matadero" (The slaughterhouse, 1838–1840), the grand oppositional text against Rosas, which as I argued in chapter 1 inaugurated the "civilization versus barbarism" paradigm that endures to the present day;[32] but the bloody matter of Saer's fiction also signals the ways that we talk about matter in the absence of reason. We need perceptions to touch the real, to discern the secrets of what lies before us. After all, as the narrator observes: "There are, between us, forms, volumes, colors, movement and light, transparency and wasteland" (1993, 206). The astute observer will learn to apprehend this earthbound material and give it name and meaning.

The sense work performed by bodies under dictatorial rule must here submit to a didactic process in which the human protagonists learn to discern. Discern, whose root word from Latin leads us to the idea of "secret," is here a hermeneutic approach to the surface details of the text through which we search for deeper meaning. It lets us know that beyond perceptions another layer of events emerges, altering the significance of scenes and of the context of what we hear and see. Beatriz Sarlo sees the advantages of this narrative project: "Saer eliminates the ellipsis where classical narrative evoked it, and he repeats the narrative events in order to demonstrate, against what we might assume, that repetition makes them literally unending. He can do this because, like no one else in Argentine literature, his sense of a concrete sensorial experience is applied to ephemeral matter: the reverberation of light, the moment captured as successive snapshots, the processes that affect solid bodies" (Sarlo 1993, 31).[33]

Sarlo is correct in her understanding of Saer's sensibilities and aids my thinking here. For Saer, perception is both a narrative strategy and a problem for writing. Saer explains in an essay: "The world is difficult to perceive.... Perception is difficult to communicate. The subjective is unverifiable. Description is impossible. Experience and memory are inseparable. To write is to dive deep and to gather filaments and splinters of experience and memory in order to assemble a determined image, in the same way as one can embroider with pieces of thread of different colors ... a design upon a canvas" (1986, 17). He also understands the sensual self as a resistance to the order of the state: "Nation, separated from individual experience, consists of a series of extractions that belong to the lexicon of those in power. It is the translation, on an ideological plane, of a sum of interests" (9). But oddly enough, the nation may also be defined by the affects: "Language, sensation, affect, emotions, pulsations, sexuality: the nation is built of these materials, we constantly want to go back to these things and we carry this with us wherever we go. Language gives the nation its particular taste" (10). In this deeply personal realm of the senses, one can eventually touch the solid rock reality of nation and self. Language comes in as the mediation that gives these pulsations their form. And it is all maintained in the present.

Two perspectives mark out this sensual world: a third-person narrator and the first-person voice of Gato. Both keep their senses alert to the miniscule changes of landscapes and sensations. Early on, Gato describes the objects and sensations that awaken his attention:

> I am naked. The pair of white shorts is lying in a damp heap on the floor: for a few seconds I do nothing.
>
> Now the warm rain runs, with a monotonous murmur, down my body, gradually washing away the soap. I am standing with my eyes closed, thinking of nothing, remembering nothing, in the warm rain, simply helping, with my hands, to wash the soap away with the water:

> thinking of nothing and remembering nothing, in a darkness filled only with the sound of water. (1993, 17–18)

This passage, which appears early in the book, gives an idea of how perceptions shape the narrative world of Saer. Gato's body lies at the center of the text: he first perceives the damp clothing on the floor; he later feels the warm water and hears its monotonous murmur. Hands and body are at work as the mind remains in an enduring void. This is akin to a birthing scene that features the awakening of the senses, a ground zero of perception before reason; a synesthetic beginning that is a primary grounding for future experience and thought. And the first of the in utero sensations is, of course, the pressure of touch. Why is touch so important? The experience of tactility, as we have come to learn it, is not simply and passively haptic; rather, as Fulkerson explains, it evolves to a distinction between active and passive subjects and shows a state of individual control or involuntary reception (2014, 6–7).[34] Saer's scenes of tactile perception build upon these dimensions, departing from a scene of nothingness in order to show the emergence of subjectivity, of passive or active behavior. The oft-cited phrase, "In the beginning, there is nothing," allows Saer to go forward, each time underscoring the slowly emergent body and its encounter with the palpable world; it also allows him to dive into the materiality of present time without need for analysis or historical extension. We assume that in later scenes something of import will happen.

In repose, Gato feels his surroundings: "There is not a breath of air, and not a sound reaches the porch: the entire afternoon heat is a single transparent block of mineral, hot and compact, in which everything, hollowed out inside, is at once close at hand and unreachable" (Saer 1993, 41). Here, Gato's encounter with the universe expands in small steps: though wind and sound don't reach him, he perceives the density of place. Time and nature come to a halt and distance does its work. In reality, he cannot reach the surrounding objects; they are present but out of his reach, though he nonetheless feels their pressure. Compared with the previous passage, Saer's world here begins to expand. If in the first passage Gato experienced water and warmth on his body as he stood in a kind of prebirth uterine darkness, in the second, he lies in a mineral block: the room contains his inert form, which slowly awakens to the proximity of things. This scene recalls the infant's encounter with the objects of his world; it is this moment of primary sensation that Saer wants to make clear for his readers. In what follows, the character comes in contact with smell, sound, taste, and tactility that guide him through the everyday:

> My fingertips touch, at most, the polished glass without knowing beforehand that it was there and they experience, instead of the expected roughness, a uniform, monotonous smoothness. The smell of the coffee that I am unhurriedly making, in the kitchen, gets me out, in the beginning, of the dull delirium, but it too, after a few minutes, settles down inside me and loses its strength. The calls and voices of the bathers . . . don't modify even for a moment, even once, anything about everything. . . . My eyes have nothing to look at. (44)

Notice here that the narrator now reaches out to touch the glass, to inhale the aroma of the drink, to defy the enduring silence; nevertheless, and despite his efforts, nothing is changed by this new alertness. The eyes still fail to see; the ears fail to hear. A few pages later, the narrator begins to perceive color and form. He finally begins to *see*:

> The white walls, the black doors, the red tile floor and the few articles of furniture next to the walls, the big table, surrounded by chairs with straw-bottomed seats in the living room, with the commode to one side, the beds in the three bedrooms, the little library, the refrigerator, everything, as I wander aimlessly about the house, would seem to be in the process of coming out, laboriously, from something black, formless, nameless. Finally, I see the ash tray of fired clay, on the floor, in the main room, and squat down. (48)

The field of vision is populated by objects: furniture, doors, beds, and tables appear in random order as they catch the narrator's eye. The narrator's walk through the space of the house determines their rhythm of appearance. Movement, light, and vision thus combine to produce the objects on the page; from the formlessness of the dark, objects take shape and acquire a name. Still, there is no sound ("Not a single sound is heard in the town" [59]). As the novel advances, however, noise comes within the narrator's range:

> Now, in the darkness, the sounds, the murmurs, the chorus of cicadas, the barking of a dog at the other end of town, begin, gradually, to come

> unbound from each other, to separate, building up, out of the black, compact mass of night, levels, dimensions, heights, various distances, a structure of sounds that produce, in the uniform blackness, a precarious, fragile space, whose distribution in the blackness continually changes shape, duration, and one might even say, to put it in words somehow, place. (86)

From the scenes of darkness, Saer gradually endows his characters with the qualities of vision, hapticity, and hearing. Taste will figure later at the scene of an *asado* (122). A perceiving subject is born—just in time, or so it appears, in order to make sense of the political world.

Susan Stewart supplies a formidable reading of modern poetry and the senses that enables our approach to Saer. Likening sensual arousal to the biblical creation of the world, Stewart proposes that all sense work emerges from a sky of darkness. "The darkness presses against us and yet has no boundary; without edge or end, it erases and mutes the limits of our being," she writes (2002, 1). Here the work of the senses comes to break up that unlimited void. Similarly, when Saer puts his characters through a slow sensorial awakening—the political dimensions of waking from darkness—the drama begins (Saer 1993, 122–127) and lasts until the final page when Saer returns us to "the universal nothingness" (218). This cycle of awakening and return constitutes Saer's aesthetic project of breaking the bleakness of silence and effacement; it makes an incursion into light and captures, through perceptions, a missing truth of the world. Is it the truth of a tortured or disappeared body? Or does the recursive sense work show in fact that nothing happens here? Saer's insistence on the present tense would seem to emphasize stasis, avoiding the linear flow of time that organizes history and calls for action. This is the present time to which Gumbrecht (2014) alluded, a present that denies all motive, a time that thickens with immediate experience and with the senses as open receptors. It is also a time of returning—at the novel's close—to an originary moment of darkness.

Perceptions in Saer's novel are sustained by repetition and movement, and occasionally by the sound of a voice that penetrates nocturnal darkness. In this direction, Saer steadfastly makes note of the rhythms of bodies: the couples making love, the sounds of the boatman who rows quietly through the water, the polysyndetons that give movement to a phrase and anchor the reader as well. Finally, from the void, the shrill sound of a voice emerges: "A shout comes, all of a sudden, from the beach, broken, discontinuous, emerging from its nothingness without, to all appearances, seeing a precise destination, a neutral vocal emission that someone brings forth out of the blackness not in order to say something but to see how, in violent jerks, quavering, hesitant, a shout comes into being" (Saer 1993, 71). Once again, sound is born from darkness; meaning is not the factor here as much as tone and timbre. Evoking almost a prelapsarian call that disregards the power of words, Saer situates us in the embrace of sound, the vibrations of voice that exist before language, and, just as the novel at the same moment closes in on the conflation of past and present, he lets us sink into the gaps that are, in the novel's final sentence, "inexpressible, into the universal nothingness" (218).

Does perception help us apprehend reality without depth as it is, or is it only the starting point for a symptomatic comprehension? Does the reader bask in the pleasure of the text or search deeply for the allegorical meanings that lie beneath these scenes of sensing? To answer this, Saer elaborates a picture of light, movement, and time ("it is earth, air, fire, water" [74]) and proposes, accordingly, that the earth in itself is proof of our existence. We have several choices here: to take the scene as pure description without any clue of meaning or to fill the landscape with the reason of inquiry until we reach a tightly sealed story, linking the flow of past, present, and future within a narrative project.

Theorists have returned to this difficult contrast between description and narration, though not necessarily in the context of a military regime pressing upon styles of writing. From Henry James (showing vs. telling) or Lukács (description vs. narration) to Genette (who observes that it is impossible to pull narration away from description), there is a sense that description is a secondary endeavor, subordinated to narration. It is considered a dead moment or pause in the novel in which nothing really happens; it is irrelevant to the greater aims of the story. But we can also turn this around: after all, description, despite its peripheral detail, *interrupts* the flow of narrative; its portrayal of ornamental scenes proposes another kind of thinking beyond the linearity of plot. Of course, the descriptive moments of a novel allow for reading on the surface; they cut short the hermeneutic thrust that seems crucial to our critical desires. Stephen Best and Sharon Marcus (2009) refer to a "surface reading" as a challenge to layered critique. Their proposal resists the depths of analysis or our desire to read through textual lacunae; they reject the force of domination and inequality that this reading tactic implies. They thus move against the "symptomatic" reading that looks for the repressed in writing, and instead they seek to glide on the textual surface to show how networks of perceptions work on a single plane. These readings also allow us to bathe in the rhythms and pulsations of the material that the text supplies, and in the process remind us of the freedom that attentiveness unleashes; when everything is on the surface, there is no mystification. Perhaps, as Jonathan Crary has written, attention is the major object "within the modernization of subjectivity" (1999, 17).

In an earlier chapter, I referred to Fredric Jameson; let me evoke him again. In *The Antimonies of Realism*, Jameson (2013) offers a twist on what might be considered a surface reading in order to approach the "reality" effects of the nineteenth-century realist novel. Jameson sees the training of the novel as a way not simply for the reader to mark the advance of time (by tracking the narration of past to future), but for the reader to learn to perceive the value of events from the intricacies of narrative description. This exercise prepares the emergent bourgeoisie to learn perceptual acuity, to support its call for power (and assume the observant eye of the state), but it also trains the bourgeois reader to cultivate and identify affect. We learn to respond to descriptive details and thereby learn how to feel. Jameson sees the novel as a pedagogy for the affects that prepared the nineteenth-century reader to be socialized for bourgeois culture. In that respect, reading for description—an accounting of perceptions in the literature under discussion—is more than a lesson about writing style; not only does it prepare us for the fragmented narratives that will reach their height in the high modernism of Joyce, but it also carries the weight of a political proposal. Saer trains his audience in perceptions in order to touch, feel, and hear, to visualize what cannot be seen, and to recognize in our immobility that we have no recourse to action.

Can we build an allegory for disappearance? Can we receive it in tiny measures? In a particularly humorous insertion, Saer refers to a newspaper report written by a Leopold Bloom who refers to the habits of tribal groups in Oceania that regularly murder animals of a species as a symbolic gesture meant to signify the death of the species as a whole. Bloom calls this a "ritual synecdoche" (Saer 1993, 192) and reminds us of the Joycean paradigms that also inform this novel. Like *Ulysses*, that great book that relies on the human body and its perceptions in order to explain a day of life in Ireland under colonial rule, *Nadie nada nunca* also goes in pursuit of a partial story grounded in human perceptions, but Saer paints a larger picture of one's inaction under the weight of national horror. As much as Roberto Arlt may have borrowed from Joyce in order to explain the struggles of middle-class culture in the early part of the twentieth century (as I detailed in chapter 3), here Saer leans upon the Irish writer to explain the cultural politics of silence that are subsumed under a supposed investigation of acts of listening and seeing and tasting. Like Joyce, Saer allows us to believe that an epiphany is forthcoming, although it isn't clear when a *political* awakening will occur—if it occurs at all. Certainly, there are clues that tell us events are about to change, that a consciousness will take form (perhaps as the characters prepare their meal or when they hear the sound of a running motor, something begins to stir). But Saer cuts this promise short: "When she reached the black car she had the feeling that . . . Elisa said on the porch" (130). The ellipsis belongs to Saer and is laden with content. Does Elisa have a sensation of fear? Can she intuit danger? Have we missed a significant feeling that might help us understand all events? Descriptive episodes might invite an expansion to narration, but Saer in this passage won't release his control of the scene. In fact, the ellipsis breaks off the description of a sense that has no name. We are thus stuck irremediably in the void of contemplation and stasis, in the darkness of not knowing.

Florencia Garramuño (2009, 91) argues that Saer's writing circles around the irreconcilable split between experience and narration, but what she misses is the education of the senses that follows in this elliptical break. In this interstitial zone, Saer teaches us how to assemble a story that leads to eventual critique. Through a reservoir of sensation, supplements that take place in no-man's-land—in the in-between of narration—Saer gives the reader an illusion of nearness to the real. Here, he signals a path of learning that leads to political awareness. With it, we come to value description and to discern what lies beyond it; we learn to detain the flow of time in order to learn how to feel. This, then, is an education of the senses that takes place in Argentina from the vantage of narrative culture: while the military government exacerbates the senses to get prisoners to denounce their brothers, Saer teaches us to read through the senses to uncover traces of political meaning.

What Can Poetry Do?

As we reach the point of the political impasse, we also draw close to an age-old question: what can literature do? Is it the charge of literature to study the world and make apparent what on first contact cannot be seen or perceived? To bring in for close inspection those experiences that, under a normal lens, one fails to apprehend? Or is literature for the fine-tuning of senses, to put us in touch with people, events, and things? Saer, also a poet, gives us one dimension of this literary project through the novel form; it is also sustained in poetic texts, albeit with other registers for perception.

Perhaps the novel cannot fully tell of sensation because it is pressured by the demands of narration; poetry, however, can convey the experience without contingency or emplotment. It depends more intensely upon rhythm and voice, rattling us to our very bones before we can arrive at meaning. Against instrumental reason, it is the literary genre that most allows us a physical contact with material as it resonates in our material selves. It is the face-to-face that forms the basis of this experience of reading; it not only calls up biological responses but awakens the affects as well. Poetry is, in short, an art of contact. Susan Stewart reminds us that the sense of touch, in addition to the sense of hearing, leads us to comprehend the pattern of the poem. "As touch moves and takes time, pattern becomes apparent, just as following sound, we trace a path for it: we hear and feel sound emerge, discerning its form," she writes as if to signal where to place ourselves in relation to the page (2002, 145). Density and flow, solids and lines, a text with the lightness of repeated syllabic rhyme against the sharp tones of acute accent, the silence of caesura that contrasts with the enjambment of voices: through this, we are awakened to a sense of touch that the poem sustains.

Poetry then becomes a threshold activity: it brings awareness of boundaries and difference, it allows us to plumb for the depths of rhythm that lie below the surface, it pulls us between interiority and the external world, between the thing and the way we feel it. It unsettles the world as we knew it before, it installs doubt of our bodies and minds, but it also invites an approach to intimacy, a guide to contact and regard of the other. Beginning with initial sensation, poetry allows a reflection on the power to act and the power to be affected. In this respect, poetry may put in motion the ideas of Spinoza, awakening a corporeal reason in us that in turn reaches out from the self; a way to turn the passions and affects into action, to prepare the sentient self for some kind of outward engagement. We sense first in order to advance to our agency in the world.

Because poetry has the immediacy of sensory engagement, and because it works so intensely with affects, it is a genre that allows us to speak our laments and express our deepest mourning, but it coaxes memory first with appeals to the sentient self. And because it refers us to the hapticity of language, it is also a mode for us to establish contact with the figuration of loss and remembrance. In the 1980s, poetry took up this mission through the socially committed voices of Mario Benedetti and Juan Gelman, whose sorrow for lives lost to military rule guided their lyric visions. It was also found in the metaphoric excess with which a poet like Néstor Perlongher masked his anger about the disappeared and allowed him to scream out the ironies of life under the military regime. Their project was to give voice to mourning and to expose the horror that remained unspoken. This work was inevitably corporeal, and when it turned to neobaroque extravagance, as in Perlongher's case, its thick ornamentality—based on submerged and multiple meanings—resisted all turns at translation. Its opaqueness resisted the state. This poetry represented the body's vulnerability as a tissue between personal intimacies and the vigilant eye of security forces. It provoked a scream that comes from human depths, and later—only later—anticipated thought and healing. From the first readings of these antidictatorship texts, we slipped into the space of pain; the poem let us in to the sense perceptions of contact and loss, of perverse sight and disturbing audition. Poetic inflections of this kind were set in place during the military regimes: for many, they continued in the present. The Chilean poet Raúl Zurita (1950–) is a main example.

Considering the exigencies of poetic language and structure, Zurita observes that the poetic genre requires the human body. "The body is registered, physically, in the poem," he claims (2016b). His work exposes the reader to situations that tear at the nervous system and, in the end, at the soul. Here, the purpose is to register loss and leave us vulnerable to pain. Zurita seeks that state of "unshieldedness" which for Heidegger (citing Rilke) represented the *summa* and *terminus ad quem* for all of poetry's work, helping us find our presence in what is present, helping us find a way to respond.[35] This condition exposes the rhythms of physical pain and leads to the rhythms of the social.

A poet affected by the dictatorship and, later, by the universal need to express the depths of mourning, Zurita is relentless in his pursuit of the unspoken. His poetry is a lament for the disappeared and the dead; it borders upon taboo. Zurita thus takes physical pain and repulsion and carries this in the language of the body. After all, he would seem to say, taboo is what we keep silent despite the body's need to speak it. And here the silence encircles the matter of physical and spiritual pain. His search is not akin to that of Pablo Neruda, who, as he reached the summit of Machu

Picchu, declared that he had come to speak through the dead mouths of those who went before him ("Yo vengo a hablar por vuestras bocas muertas" [I come to speak through your dead mouths]). Zurita's work is not the epic of exiled heroes as they watched their homeland uprooted, nor is it like the homage that Ercilla bestowed upon the fallen Araucanian natives who met the Spaniards in colonial wars. No, Zurita evokes the senses of a suffering, ailing man who cannot comprehend what he has known. The senses come in to give expression to the density of this loss in forms, images, and perceptions that remain unspeakable, lacking direct translation within the registers of speech. We know, we experience these words in the flesh, we hold them tightly wound up in perceptions, and we sense what they mean. All the same, they can't be conveyed in an easy register in Spanish (even less, in English translation). Touch thus becomes the medium to carry meaning when all speech fails. Identified with irrationality and a primitive state of things, touch is evoked to associate harm and injury of the body with the barbarism of the military regime. We come to touch bodies in harm.

Zurita makes a point to escort his readers to the scene of unnamable pain; touching, hearing, and seeing are thus found at the center of the poem. They are not singular and separate senses, pure physiological responses, but multiple and overlapping perceptual prompts, coincidental sensations. The tropes of tattooing, writing on the body, and slashing the fleshy surface of texts carry brute physicality and, its reverse, a desire for contact. This is driven by Zurita's confidence that tactile encounters will indeed yield eventual meaning. His poetry is thus guided by principles of movement and pressure, and perceptual misalignments. Take the case of *Purgatorio* (1979), the first of Zurita's trilogy on the horrors of civilian life under Pinochet and inspired, of course, by Dante's treacherous ascent. The text is audacious in its hybrid materials; it consists of poetry, photographs and electroencephalograms (EEGs), alterations of font and script, and occasional prose poems in lieu of stanzas. The lyric voice at times goes by the name of Raquel and self-identifies as feminine; in other cases, a masculine voice orchestrates the poem. Like the gender split, the page is divided in two. Even the structure of the book is upset: the poem comes to a close with an epilogue, and after several pages of graphic interventions, the poem continues once more. A second epilogue is followed by several more poems and continues with a printout of an EEG upon which a very few lines of verse are imposed to declare suffering and self-mutilation. The wavy lines that appear horizontally on the electrical scan remind us of both the contour of the Andean mountains that rise behind the city of Santiago and the rhythmic lines that would mark the tensions within any poem; and, of course, they signal the rhythmic breaths of life that the poem suffuses. A further unevenness follows: the strophes are labeled with Roman numerals as if to put forth a logical exposition that resembles a list of pure sensations. But these Roman numerals are decidedly out of order. We skip, for example, from poem LXXXV to poem C, and are forced to doubt along the way the efficiency of linear sequence. With hallucinatory or deranged perceptions, Zurita thus exposes a fragmented world that cannot be pieced together again. In his search for meaning, Zurita also posits the untranslatability of some of his words. Consider a few lines from the final poem ("The Desert of Atacama VII") that appears before the first of two epilogues:

> Para que desolado frente a estas fachas del paisaje
> devenga una cruz extendida sobre Chile y la soledad de mi
> facha vea entonces el redimirse de las otras fachas: mi
> propia Redención en el Desierto
>
> iii. Quién diría entonces del redimirse de mi facha
>
> iv. Quién hablaría de la soledad del desierto
>
> Para que mi facha comience a tocar tu facha y tu facha
> a esa otra facha y así hasta que todo Chile no sea sino
> una sola facha con los brazos abiertos: una larga facha
> coronada de espinas . . .
>
> vii. Entonces clavados facha con facha como una Cruz
> extendida sobre Chile habremos visto para siempre
> el Solitario Expirar del Desierto de Atacama (2009b, 50)

The irregularity of the verse forms, alternating in verse and prose, is minor compared to the fugitive word choice that anchors this particular poem. *Facha*, in common parlance in the South, is understood by speakers; nonetheless, it resists a literal definition and thus defies translation. Loosely alluding to semblance or form, to the Italian *faccia*, or face, it also refers to an attitude, to a feeling of defiance. Its meaning cannot be fixed. Anna Deeny Morales, one of Zurita's most perseverant translators, addresses the impossibility of rendering this word in English (in Zurita 2016a, 6–8). She links the enunciation of *facha* as a convergence of multiple exchanges between the speaker and his interlocutors; for her, the word offers an initial accounting, in a Levinasian way, of a communal encounter. However, her translation for *facha* is "form," not "face":

> So that desolate before these forms the landscape becomes
> a cross extended over Chile and the loneliness of my form
> then sees the redemption of the other forms: my own
> Redemption in the Desert
>
> iii. Then who would speak of the redemption of my form
>
> iv. Who would tell of the desert's loneliness
>
> So that my form begins to touch your form and your form
> that other form like that until all of Chile is nothing but
> one form with open arms: a long form crowned with thorns . . .
>
> vii. Then   nailed form to form   like a Cross
> extended over Chile   we will have seen forever
> the Final Solitary Breath of the Desert of Atacama
> (Zurita 2009b, 51)

Facha is clearly a blind spot in the poem, a place where language fails us or where popular expression holds its own and prevails without exact translation. As such, it leads to the vague sensations that the sound of the word elicits. The "ch" of *facha* is a material collision of sounds that sets off a chain reaction until, as Zurita proposes to his readers, all of Chile may be reunited under the signs of Christian agony and pain. I am concerned about this magnet word that pulls in many more meanings than it can possibly settle. It brings to mind the ways in which amorphous sensation gives rise to cognition, and signals the diffusion of pain. It also signals the ways in which popular speech manages to capture a truth that eludes standard Spanish.

In general terms, critics have recently turned their attentions to the expression of pain; perhaps more than pleasure, the topic of pain elicits a confrontation between dissidents and the state, especially in the late twentieth century. From Foucault's famous *Discipline and Punish* (1979), a text that coincides with the rise of authoritarianism in Latin America in the years that are covered here, we determined a way to install the body between power and opposition. But pain also signals a route of contact, an encounter of matter with the body, an experience that is felt and that also needs to be shared. Eve Kosofsky Sedgwick, in tandem with the critical tendency toward surface readings to which I earlier referred, acknowledges the "hermeneutics of suspicion" as a strategy for exposing the atrocities of state violence and making visible the cases of oppression that once and for all confirm our paranoia about lurking evil (2003, 140–142). In the same essay, Sedgwick asks if there may not be another way of explaining things beyond the unveiling of hidden repressions; she thus makes a case for a reparative reading that restores community rather than digging deep to destroy it.

In the world that Zurita's poetry offers, where pain more than pleasure guides him, he also leads to reparation and healing. Of course, he captures in words the pressure upon bodies exerted by air and wind during airplane drops to the sea; he tries to describe the pain experienced by incisions or blows to the flesh. In a landscape installation, he also inscribes his verses on the cliffs of Chile, overlooking the sea, as if to appeal to the eyes of the drowned and disappeared to read and partake of his lyrics (while at the same time, the landlocked lovers of poetic verse would never have a chance to see them). This is Zurita's reach of empathy extended to Pinochet's victims. But his poetry is neither univocal nor driven by a single motive. Through movement—the bodies pushed through air, the exiled travelers scaling mountains—this pain takes pleasurable form in the poetic text. It is against the pressures of an outside force that the body is touched and, even in an extreme act of violence, turns from anguished discomfort to feel the beauty of encounter. "Touch," writes Adam Gopnick, "is the unsung sense—the one that we depend on most and talk about least" (2016, 58). Zurita indeed takes the tactile art to talk about injury and harm, but he also understands the sense of hapticity that is configured when we touch the other and when we are touched in return. Equally important, Zurita's reparative measure comes from the poem itself, from the harmony of the rhythm and repetition of tone that the verse bestows. This curious juxtaposition of the horrors of war with the great poetic traditions communicates a gift of sound and feeling that shares a page with unresolved grief. It speaks to the liminal zone between beauty and pain;

it announces multiple forms of touch and contact that are based on our desire to bridge the gaps between us rather than stress our difference. This becomes a site of healing.

In Zurita's work, somatically bound, almost untranslatable utterances pick up these threads of feeling; they transmute as the volume grows louder and corroborate Zurita's claims that just as the skin can sense, so, too, language as a living thing becomes a perceptive form. "A language is an absolutely living body," he claimed in a recent lecture (2016b). Language has its own fleshiness due to its sounds, tone, timbre, and form; it changes upon the context of its use and the direction of its message. Above all, its somatic charge is guided by perceptions; how we see, hear, and touch the word inspires a breach of traditional meaning. It opens to what is new as language acquires palpable form. Even language in the pages of his work acquires palpable form. Imagine, then, in his volume *INRI*, that the disappearances whet the poet's desire to recuperate a sense of touch; they awaken his general longing to be immersed in perceptions: "Te palpo, te toco, y las yemas de mis dedos buscan / las tuyas . . . mis dedos palpan a tientas los tuyos porque si yo te / toco y tú me tocas tal vez no todo esté perdido" (2003, 82).[36] The text is followed by a page of Braille script, as if to remind us that reading invites the physical experience of touch. This occurs midway through *INRI*, declaring that at the center of the book lies a physical contact with the word. Poetry—like love, like life itself—demands tactility and sensation. We are asked to read from the body. In this respect, consider Zurita's land art,[37] where he stamps lines of poetry on the desert or sky, or his recent *Sea of Pain*, an installation at the Kochi-Muziris Biennial (2016–2017), in which he requires his viewers to walk through several inches of water in order to identify with the palpable experience of Galip Kurdi, a five-year-old Syrian refugee whose body washed ashore and whose painful death is the focus of Zurita's poem (posted on the walls of the installation). In both works, he strives to combine hapticity and language, to mark the kinetic art of contact that gives shape to sea and land, but also to touch the meaning of words that bespeak loss and emotion.

In this direction, Zurita again considers the multiply valenced words that cannot be settled by a single meaning. In *INRI* (2003), for example, we can follow the word *carnadas* (bait) as it moves through a sequence of poems bearing the title "El mar":

> Sorprendentes carnadas llueven del cielo.
> Sorprendentes carnadas sobre el mar. Abajo el

> océano, arriba las inusitadas nubes de un día
> claro. Sorprendentes carnadas llueven sobre el
> mar. Hubo un amor que llueve, hubo un día
> claro que llueve ahora sobre el mar. (2003, 17)

Like the word *facha*, open to multiple meanings, *carnadas* provokes uneasy responses. William Rowe's translation lures us with "baits," while Anna Deeny Morales goes directly to "flesh":

> Strange baits rain from the sky. Surprising bait
> Falls upon the sea. Down below the ocean, up
> Above unusual clouds on a clear day. Surprising
> Baits rain on the sea. There was a love raining,
> There was a clear day that's raining now on the sea.
> (Zurita 2009a, 7)

> Strange flesh rains from the sky. Strange flesh
> over the sea. Below the ocean, above the
> unusual clouds on a cloudless day. Strange
> flesh rains over the sea. There was a love that
> rains, there was a cloudless day that now rains
> over the sea. (Zurita 2016a, 171)

Zurita is pressing us to recognize the bodies that fall from military aircraft and find their way to the ocean floor. This resists our comprehension in whichever language we choose, just as it increases the reader's sorrow. But the destiny of flesh made bait runs parallel to another airdrop: love rains upon the sea.

Zurita's poem (and his poetry in general) works on a vertical axis, taking us from dizzying heights to deepest valleys of sea and land. The repetitive up and down ("arriba ... abajo") creates a lilting movement that, on the one hand, rocks the reader as if in a cradle, and on the other, announces death, pushing one to recall the merciless airdrops that pierced the clouds of Chile. A cycle of life and death, with past and present verb tenses crossing in the verses, thus serializes historical time. In the midst of this somatic pull, an ironic adjective, *sorprendentes* (surprising), cuts like acid through it all. How are we meant to *feel* what is never to be seen? Is it tragic or banal? Shocking in a devastating way or lightly unexpected? Unlike Saer, who only alluded to the actions that disappeared lives in the Argentina of the 1970s through cues of indirection, Zurita gives us a screen of pathos crossed with *love*, banality crossed with sadness,[38] such that both sustain the unnamable horror and scatter our sentiments widely. In each, the trail of perceptions expands in different ways. If Saer, after training us how to see, touch, and hear, leaves us in the no-man's-land of "universal nothing," Zurita begs for something more as we read his untranslatable feelings that are alternately ephemeral and rooted. It is only from perceptions, from feeling the depth of an experience from which we as readers were spared and which we don't know how to assemble, that we can try to touch a communal relationship of intersubjective range. Senses cross with affects.

Let me return briefly to Merleau-Ponty, who as we saw in earlier pages has enjoyed a definite audience among Latin Americans since the 1950s. Merleau-Ponty raises the idea of an intertwining or "chiasmus" through the point of contact with flesh, where a pivotal encounter is sustained between subjects through the experience of sight and touch (1968). In other words, from his perspective, flesh is the agent of seeing and being seen, of touching and being touched. The thickness and porosity of the flesh make possible this interconnection with the other; it is the synergetic place of contact and feeling, the entry point to cognition. Often these senses are crossed ("Vision is a palpation with the look," Merleau-Ponty [1968, 134] wrote in *The Visible and the Invisible*). But insofar as flesh contains this synesthetic reversibility, its message can also return to the sender. Everything is in movement. Merleau-Ponty thus insists on the experience of things in the making instead of things already made. He refuses to accept what is given and instead privileges lived reality as the intense discovery of truth. It is another way to formulate his defense of the "Primacy of Perception" as he insists on the ways in which bodies are entwined; consciousness here becomes a matter of merged spaces and locations. That said, Merleau-Ponty is not settled in the reformulation of the senses alone. He is also concerned with ethical responsibility: to respond to the earth and its people, both living and dead. Passion, desire, touch, and mourning are the results of this embodied perspective that emerges from intertwined subjects. To achieve this, Zurita upsets the registers of perception; he moves us from the visual dimensions of experience to the sonic and the haptic. Perhaps this strategy responds to the biographical details of the poet, who we know attempted to dash acid on his eyes as a protest against the government's denial that there were horrors left to be seen. Or perhaps the perceptual registers are decoupled from biographical threads and signal something else. The point is that Zurita is teaching his readers to experience the full dimensions of embodied perception, to feel without the restrictions of separated sensory charges.

Nelly Richard is right when she says that body art in Chile begins in response to the Pinochet coup, with Zurita (along with the artist Carlos Leppe) as initiators of this trend (Richard 1986, 65–66). While she acknowledges Zurita's literary body as a site for painful acts of sacrifice, here I hope to go further, to think of the ways in which Zurita's literary body also expands a range of perceptions. First of all, Zurita posits listening bodies that capture not only sound but also vision and touch. This synesthetic experience begins as Zurita repeats the stories of others. "El mar, *se dice* del mar. *Se dice* de carnadas que / llueven y de días claros pegados a ellas, se dice de / amores inconclusos . . ." (2003, 17; emphasis mine).[39] The reflexive voice ("*se* dice": it says) puts the responsibility upon us to listen: *we* hear these words; *we* pay attention; *we* are recipients not only of news, but also of sounds, images, and ideas. The next poem thus continues with the principal attention to sound: "*Se oyen* días enteros hundiéndose, *se oyen* extrañas mañanas soleadas, amores inconclusos, despedidas truncas que se hunden en el mar. Se oyen sorprendentes carnadas" (18; emphasis mine).[40] The dense repetition suggests the endless scenes of pain that we scarcely begin to hear. And just as the fleshy bait gives us pause, so, too, the strangeness of dawn and love cut short also reaches us through sound. This synesthetic confusion continues: the poet *hears* the sky and the sea in the following poem ("Oí un cielo y un mar alucinantes, oí soles estallados de amor cayendo como frutos, oí torbellinos de peces devorando las carnes rosa [*sic*] de sorprendentes carnadas" [19]),[41] bearing witness to such a horror that it can only disturb the senses. Seeing and hearing are confused because, in fact, we cannot endure the horrors of the fleshy bait that has been released to the water; and because, in the realm of poetry, we must also learn to hear in order to understand. It is no wonder that Zurita prevails upon synesthetic disorder; it not only expresses the overloaded perceptual registry that is the human body, but it also stands for the undoing of the rational prescriptions that guide human life. Synesthetic phrases in literary texts thus press against the calculations of military rule and neoliberal order. Zurita, in this sequence of poems, undoes the power of seeing in the metropolis (Who cannot be reminded of Simmel, who observed this phenomenon more than a century ago?) and thus proposes that we release the senses not only to express our overburdened suffering, but to more widely apprehend the hidden breakdown of history. After all, Zurita seems to tell us, experience isn't simple, and narrative cannot catch it all. In this regard, indefinite multiplicities of experience are needed to capture the real. Merleau-Ponty phrases this as a "tissue of probabilities" (1964c, 193). In Zurita's case, the tissue is discovered in the crossing of sensations where one beholds at once the landscape, the seas and sky, the vibrant colors of nature, and the water that surrounds the body; where one finds a way to see and touch, and to be touched as well; where one feels the pain of others and assumes it as one's own.

It is not surprising that the last poem of the series concludes by evoking purification through a painful oxymoron of sight and sound: "He aquí el mar quemándose," Zurita writes (2003, 26).[42] Not unlike Joyce, who depended on tropes of transubstantiation to explain the workings of literary art, the magical moment when spirit and flesh merge as one, here the synesthetic experience of sight, audition, and contact meets the power of metaphor, transforming the sea into a burning field, enacting a change in both the perceiving subject and the landscape he beholds. This is as difficult to comprehend as Zurita's image of a country that has been shipwrecked eternally in the desert (2003, 50).

Only in death, Zurita observes, will this crisscrossing of multiple experiences shut down and come to a halt. In an ode to Cesare Pavese ("El memorial del dolor"), Zurita begins: "Eres la tierra y la muerte ... eres sólo dolor, lo tienes en los ojos / y en la sangre, / pero no sientes. Vives como vive una piedra, / como la tierra dura / y te visitan sueños, movimientos, sollozos / que ignoras" (2007, 95).[43] Citing the title of Pavese's famous book, *Verrà la morte e avrà i tuoi occhi* (Death will come and it will have your eyes), Zurita observes that in death the Italian master is in pain but cannot feel it. He is a stone that leaves only ripples when it falls into the water. He is a stone that resists all encroachment of touch, for he cannot again awaken. Nonetheless, the stone in water radiates endless hope and inspires feeling in others. Here, Zurita makes a case about what poetry can do. If in life we are expected to feel, to carry out interactions with others, in death our materials, likened to earth and stone, continue to inspire life. Time and temporality, then, belong to the human spirit insofar as it still has the capacity to awaken perceptions in others; the living spirit polishes the surface that joins death with life, and poetry carries this mission.

"Language is the space of encounter where the living meet the dead," Zurita says (2016b); it is also the space to awaken the feelings that lead to reparation, for responsibility and hope, a place for permanent resurrection that reminds us that we are still alive.[44] Pain is thus brought into the writing system, not unlike the way in which César Vallejo sustained it in his poems of civil war in Spain, to show us the intensity of experience that the body registers and remembers. The worst that can happen, Zurita tells us, is not to see at all, to be blinded by our incapacity to behold and grasp the truth. "You'll see not seeing and you will weep," he admonishes at the close of his monumental volume *Zurita* (2011, 735–736).

Feeling Radical Pain

Moving forward with the representation of the senses under duress of authoritarian regimes, artists and writers continue to focus on perceptions of pain. The visual sense work of the Chilean painter Guillermo Núñez (1930–) puts this in radical perspective insofar as he seeks to depict the dimensions of pain to awaken a political awareness in viewers. Núñez has devoted his life to exposing the injustices enacted by Pinochet's regime. One of the great masters of Latin America's visual arts for over fifty years, Núñez was imprisoned in 1974 and later spent more than a decade living in exile in France. Upon his return to Chile, he continued to expose the violence of dictatorship and to represent the exacerbations of pain. Indeed, the above-cited verse of Rául Zurita, "You'll see not seeing and you will weep," aptly defines the tropes of blindness and visibility that give form to Núñez's art.

Núñez shows what cannot be seen; he exposes the bodies that slowly die in the prisons of darkness, but he also refers to a personal condition of blindness that belongs to his days in prison. Blindfolded for most of the day while in Pinochet's jails, Núñez refers to his loss of vision as a grave personal force, while it also gives him an aesthetic trope to describe our general struggle to "see." Thinking about the trope of visibility, John Berger offers an aestheticized explanation of this experience: "Painting is first an affirmation of the visible which surrounds us and which continually appears and disappears. Without the disappearing, there would perhaps be no impulse to paint" (2001, 14). Núñez takes advantage of this aesthetic tension in order to speak to ethical issues. His suffering figures are placed before the viewer's eye, quartered and dismembered. Along with this, abstract forms on canvas call out to awaken perceptions. Bright colors, contrasting hues, geometric forms that are superimposed appeal to both the visual and haptic sense, and play with the limits of form. In one example, Núñez paints two hanging figures (see plate 13). Their inverted torsos and heads with dangling tongues are imposed upon a red-stained background; a third victim faintly appears between them, etched so lightly that it seems like a ghost or simulacrum or an anticipation of what is to come. Repetition becomes the theme and reminds us of ongoing horror. At the same time, Núñez appeals through textures to the viewer's sense of touch, and through the pressures of color on canvas. Flesh comes to us in palpable, visible form in a scene of unrelieved infernal heat. We are witnessing bodies in hell.

These alarming scenes are always accompanied by tropes of blindness; the victims are shown as limbs without eyes, or in other instances appear as masked figures, blindfolded and sightless. This signals both the conditions to which prisoners were subjected and the condition of a viewing public that refuses to see. As a strategy, then, Núñez inquires about the different ways in which we come to perceive the real, with the hope of finding humanity within a collective whole. Didi-Huberman notes that the gaze is designed to recuperate the human; we need not only to see the horror, but also to restore the humanity that belongs unmistakably to the victims. In the process, we rescue what the state has hidden from the public and then bring it into view (2008, 42).

But this is just one route of entry. Núñez's work provokes other avenues of perception that exceed the visual mode: we touch the wound, we feel the heat of torture, we hear the grating teeth of the victims and their limbs as they are torn apart. At times, his art is interactive and demands the hand and body of viewers to complete the work of art. It's not enough that we simply view a body in pain: guts, bones, dismembered torsos, severed tongues that dangle from mouths. Beyond this, a haptic experience also guides our encounter with the canvas. From the boniness that protrudes from the frame or from the blood clots staining a scene, from the collage of barbed wire and photos, from the black splashes that cover wounded bodies like a cloud around our focalization, we are brought in close; we feel the witnessing close up; we feel the plight of faceless victims and sense their torturous pain.

Touch becomes central to this process, a trope to anchor the civilization-and-barbarism split, to signal a border between interior feeling and horrific assaults from beyond. It evokes liminality and pressure but also serves as a warning, a red-light alert and pulsation that courses through the viewer's body: through touch, we learn when extremes of danger are near—prodding, pushing, and roughing up bodies, treading over limbs and torsos. Through touch, we know when predators encroach upon our freedom. And while of course it brings signs of pleasure, in this instance it announces fear. Touch is thus a basic anchor for the communal experience that Núñez hopes to create, since we all know—and are united in—the feeling and knowledge of pain. The thinking might work like this: if you tell me you put your hand on a fire, I know immediately how that feels even if I've not been burned. Tactile experience, along with a sense of smell, is the most primitive or animalistic of senses. We don't need language to explain it. Paradoxically, the converse is also true; the language of politics can be unfolded by the sense of touch. War, torture, aggression, gunshot wounds, and the slashes of sabres: touch registers a political dimension that is external to our rational choices. We feel the state on our fingertips, on our torsos, in our bellies, on our teeth. Everyone reacts the same. "Let the void howl.... And let the sound leave its wound," Núñez writes regarding his paintings (2014, n.p.). He asks that we assume the bodily experience of these victims in order to understand the truth of torture.

The experience becomes a cross of palpable and visceral forms. Núñez himself explains: "Perhaps we don't have to comprehend or understand art, but live it, make it flesh within ourselves."[45] The material of painting is essential to this sensual collaboration between painter and public. Núñez goes on to write: "The most important thing is the material available; this is the immediate, tangible reality—the different papers, their thickness, their smooth or rough condition, the brushes or blades, the state of preservation.... A pencil almost without a point serves to puncture the paper, to cause it to ripple, to give it stigmata, to make it weak. My intention is to wound the paper."[46] If the materials of painting are the first line of physical encounter, a second is fielded through print discourse—the subtitles and poems that frequently accompany Núñez's paintings and drawings. In itself, this order demands multiple activities for our apprehension of an artistic work, and as a double text (poetry and drawings, prose and painting, drawings and oil-based paint), it also teaches us the many ways to feel the effects of torture on the body.

Over Núñez's more than fifty-year career, each successive canvas up to his recent retrospective, *Dibujar con sangre en el ojo* (To sketch with blood in your eye, 2015), leaves us with questions of how to feel. This is not the old sympathy ploy, but a series of works that begin with a sensorial body and lead us to a critical capacity to think. Hence in his little book on pain, *Dolor*, which was part of the *Galaxia* oscura exhibition (2000–2003), he enumerates the possible physical ills that might attack the body: from the toothache to kidney stones, even indigestion, he leads to the larger pains of discrimination and exclusion. All this begins with the body in order to give a place and name to pain. The goal here is to disconcert the viewer but also to make us see the centuries of political damage that have been done to the flesh. He looks back through history. And he does this on very large canvases and also in the "libro objeto" (book as object), where he combines image with poetry or prose.

Simon Morgan Wortham observes the great number of intellectuals who have emerged in the late twentieth century to study the topic of evil: from Joan Copjec to Susan Neiman, and before them Adorno and Arendt, they tie their inquiries to a problem for political philosophy and a test of moral certitudes (Wortham 2015, 1–20). The other side of this question draws attention to pain. Núñez, in effect, wants to inhabit the experience of dictatorial oppression, and to do this, he tries repeatedly to portray a canvas of effects in order to show the weight of military practice on the citizen-body. But how can the artist move pain on the space of the canvas? Is there a color for suffering? A brush stroke corresponding to violence? Are we expected in the end to heal, to find reparation, to arm ourselves against future attacks on the body? Núñez would situate us in the heroics of self-awareness. In his works, he communicates violence without realist figuration. Slices of color disturb order and provoke dissymmetry and chaos; they sustain uneven textures and drive the depth of experience. In this respect, Núñez shows not only pain's endurance, but also its intensity in the moment.

Núñez's work appeals to an extreme physical encounter with form; the red lines (arteries and veins?) and exposed guts of his victims cross through a black-and-white space that is geometrically ordered (see plate 14). The image arouses a sense of disruption in which color comes from the body and spills onto the visual neatness of a black-and-white canvas. One might say that Núñez invites us to toggle between abstract universality (with its clear formal lines) and the material basics of the body in pain; in the process, he asks us to stage a conceptual query: How do we measure the injustice of dictatorship? How do we expose the denial of rights? Both questions are imposed as a battle between form and formlessness on the canvas. His painting becomes a place to link ideas of justice with artistic practice.

Núñez chooses former detention centers in Chile as sites to stage his work. There, the public is invited to enter and feel the entrapment that victims once experienced during the years of the Pinochet regime. But Núñez also asks us to look at the Chilean violence as it intersects with familiar images from history, ranging from the European Shoah to human rights atrocities in other Latin American countries across the 1970s and 1980s. In this temporal collage of present imposed upon past, the materiality of the artist's work combines with art from earlier decades. He juxtaposes images of Chilean jails with photos of detention centers in Europe, for example, to cross circuit the matrix of pain. Nonetheless, he would acknowledge, global reiteration of horrors fails to guarantee healing and cure. In the *Galaxia* series, in this regard, he adds streaks of color, at times even monstrous bulges, to well-known photos of prisoners at Auschwitz (see plate 15). He then imposes a few lines of verse denouncing the cruelty that has been directed at prisoners throughout historical time. Through this juxtaposition, we are at once situated and placeless; through art, we try to cut through the familiar surface, and to break toward something new, but we are also drawn to the past. In this respect, Núñez conveys a persistent desire to *understand*. Failing this, he seems to say, we would be left like Bolaño's character Delorme, in the novel *Distant Star*, who spilled his body on the pages of books in the attempt to make physical contact with words, but who failed to make any ethical sense of the experience of that encounter.

The social theorist Davide Panagia writes that "[p]olitics is a fundamentally perceptual enterprise" (2009, 5), referring to the vigilant eye that the state casts over its citizen-subjects. With this, he signals only one dimension of political-physiological power, but we can easily stretch this to cover the complete range of sensory controls. Rancière addresses this broader range when he speaks of the "distribution of the sensible" as a tug-of-war between state and subjects, a set of a priori laws that train or condition us in what it is possible to see, feel, or hear. Rancière is also concerned with the ways in which a social world is determined by establishing different modes of apprehension and assigning value to what is felt. This sets the border of what is seen and hidden, heard and inaudible. It also implies both inclusion and exclusion of certain persons in the social milieu. Finally, it establishes the scene for a turning around of this order through creative resistance.

In this respect, Núñez takes up the perceptual enterprise first as the body's immediate response to situations of abjection, and then as an indissoluble part of a protest that runs counter to the force of the state. What the state refuses to let us see and touch is at the center of Núñez's project. Núñez begins by making apparent what is shielded from view, but he also invites us to take a step into remembrance and history. In this respect, he writes: "I can't turn my back on my dead ones, on this recalcitrant and stubborn memory. So I drew up an archaeology of pain and fear; from what is still unformed, from silence, from darkness and chaos, come unreason, nightmares, and agony. From the twilight, a brilliance, a tiny stream of light, a frozen scream. Text, body, sound, asphyxiation, mourning" (2003, n.p.). These remarks come from the catalogue for Núñez's *La quinta del sordo* (The deaf man's villa, 2003), an exhibition focusing on the multiple temporalities and pulsations coursing through the visual image. Inspired by Goya,[47] Núñez gives his viewers a broad historical canvas to comprehend the trail of abuses from the time of nineteenth-century civil wars to the regime of Pinochet. But Núñez does not expect us to behold identical forms of pain, nor to respond with monochromatic feeling. Rather, he moves us through unequal fields of experience, forcing us to recombine our memories and expand the possible permutations of horror, weaving them into a weblike composition. Material encounters and distant memory are intertwined to reach a degree of understanding. In this way we might say that he scrambles any fixed distribution of the sensible, in the terms that Rancière set forth.

For this reason, Núñez's major work is usually supplemented by minor prints and essays, small handcrafted artisanal books, brief citations of poems, instruction kits for the viewer, and lyric reflections on the function of art. These are not part of any exhibition catalogue, Núñez explains, but rather a sign of pressure to keep telling and awakening the senses of the viewing public. Even the order of these supplements is random; they are assembled arbitrarily in cardboard boxes without a preordained order. Sometimes they accompany an exhibition; sometimes they appear years later. Thus an extra book of drawings, a surplus of explanations, add-ons to image and text tell us that history will not come to an end with a single linear story. It's as if there is no peace or finitude for the artist who pursues reparation. At the same time, this open work invites the viewer to assemble and interpret. The choice is ours to continue perceiving, to continue to make sense of the whole, or simply to walk away from the work of art.

But while Núñez asks us to become fully engaged, he asks for comprehension, never banal shock. In *Minima Moralia,* Adorno set up the parameters of this problem when he reminded us of how the Third Reich used sensual stimuli to incite the weakened affects of the masses; sensationalism, he argued, weakened one's capacity for judgment (1974, 237–238). In a similar way, Núñez rejects exalted perceptions of shock since they only lead to disorder. Instead, he insists on reflection. Auschwitz, Buchenwald, Vietnam, and Villa Grimaldi are of course sites of terror recorded in history, but they also require comprehension once our senses have been awakened. At the risk of a facile didacticism, Núñez reminds us that in the history of art the body is always the point of departure to enter a critique of politics and art. Here, I could again evoke Terry Eagleton, who takes us back to classical antiquity in order to claim that art begins with the body (1990, 13), or Adorno, who referred to this bodily experience as the "somatic moment" of cognition, that piercing instant of consciousness that is felt first in the body but is never fully sustained by the body alone (Eagleton 1990, 344). Núñez works through this frame just as he engages the tensions between figuration and abstraction as different routes to comprehend pain. In the second half of the twentieth century, intellectuals like Núñez circled around the somatic body as the basis for understanding politics and art. While this focus allowed them to critique the perversions of the authoritarian state and give vent to their unrelieved mourning, they were not yet ready to move to another dimension that captures the present day: I refer here to the drive for an unending present that even leads to a posthuman power. This next step, the ultimate and most contemporary instance of sense work, intersects with the free market's sway and will be the focus of the final chapter of this book.

CHAPTER 5

By Way of a Conclusion

A Sense of the "Now"

My task: to give matter to the voice, to give a voice to matter.

NUNO RAMOS

The Brazilian artist and writer Nuno Ramos sets up a problem for contemporary culture: how to define the human body with regard to a life of "things." Considered the material center of perceptions, the source of gestures and modes of contact, the human body in the work of Ramos is the starting point from which to explore the physicality of self in relation to palpable objects: to test sights and sounds, to feel the density of stone or the lightness of grasses, to sense the pressures of wind and rain. Often beginning as a natural occurrence, unmediated and unplanned, the body/object encounter is the basis of Ramos's creative writing as well as his visual art. What he calls a "tactile anxiety" (2014, 35) gives rise to these chance meetings: he rubs his fingers over metal and cloth, over cubes of cement or dampened clay; he touches the oily water on the surface of Brazil's polluted rivers. He considers the texture of nylon, the roughness of grain, the silk petals of flowers. He figures the materiality of letters as an imposition of paints and oils on the surface of a canvas. We are indeed speaking of an art of contact in which touch, temperature, and pressure are central to Ramos's descriptions. But the perceptual encounters that define Nuno Ramos's art also expand to another arena: to the presence of sound, utterance, and voice. Ramos thus refers in amazement to the human capacity for producing ephemeral, immaterial sound, all the while seeking phenomenological evidence of the voice's capacity to sustain routes of memory and the illusion of physical contact. Often new technologies reorganize these intentions.

In *O* (2014), a hybrid text consisting of chronicle and autofiction,

Ramos moves close to these questions when he reflects on body and sound in relationship to their material form. The slim volume consists of twenty-five chapters that begin with a reflection on his physical presence in the world and end with the narrator observing his face in a mirror as he slowly washes his hands. Minor details—scars and spots, freckles and fat—give him a particular identity and lead him to think of the materialities that mark the temporal process of aging.[1] At uneven intervals, seven interspersed chapters carry the title of "O" and show the problematics of voice and sound as they take physical form from his body. In Portuguese, "O" is also a way to hail the other—"Look," "Pay attention," "Wake up." Moreover, "O" refers not just to the mouth, but also to the anus, a site for the production of pleasure and the expulsion of solid matter. But "O" also elicits *ohlo*: eye joins anus and mouth as modes of sensible contact. Through these figures, Ramos's book becomes an essay about the body's alertness to material, whether it embraces the grittiness of food and waste, the decay and rebirth of forms, or, in quite a Barthesian way, when it locates in the human voice a solid physical core. Ramos thus delves into the place of subjectivity, both "inside" and "outside" the body. His concern is first directed toward the materiality of the orifice that controls voice and communication; in the process, he studies the political and somatic role of the human mouth. If we follow Davide Panagia, the mouth is a site for political incitement; it is either a conduit for thought (expressed in speech) or an orifice that enables consumption (2009, 123). By extension, taste links politics and eating; the mouth links taste and sound; the mouth, to continue, is the start of a tunnel that facilitates movement of matter from one place to another.

This guiding trope brings us to our final reflections about the senses. Indeed, in the tracing of modern experience as a somatic affair, we move close to a desired connection between individuals and their world, and we learn to balance ideas and matter, even life and death. But as human experience is redefined, our expectation for a narrative about the senses also suffers disturbance. We traditionally expect narrative to normativize change, to plot advances in the name of progress; but twenty-first-century narrative style turns to unpredictability, and often forsakes what seems like any overarching governing precept that is under human control. In some cases, the contingency of perceptions dislodges human life from a philosophical center; in others, the autonomous machine reroutes any originary perception to extend beyond the reach of human desire. Regardless, we are faced with a set of stimuli and scenes that we fail to fully embrace; matter drifts through space and time, and, in its most extreme examples, sometimes loses its human anchor.

In *O*, Nuno Ramos guides us through the construction of the body as if he were observing a detachable object. Ramos speaks of his desire to touch the bit of tissue that he imagines protrudes from his tooth; he follows his flesh as it folds on his belly; he studies the flab that has so much excess that it appears to be separate from his person. He uses the skin to think of surface and depth, inside and out combined, or what Lacan might have referred to as the strangeness of *extimacy* that cancels the distinction between borders of self and other and joins them on one single plane. It is the flesh that connects them. Ramos then writes, toward the end of his book, that all knowledge comes from the body (2014, 172). Here, as readers, we find ourselves in the comfort of a phenomenological truth that I have sustained throughout these pages. The body, animallike in its sensory apprehension, gives proof of presence. Experience is above all somatic. Ramos reports the sound of clocks without informing us of the passing of time; he attends to odors, he feels the pain of his limbs, he suffers an inflamed throat. Life finds a way to breathe on its own, overcoming the abstractions of reason. As such, Ramos acknowledges the body as an instrument to register weights and measures, and also a vehicle for contact, visuality, and audition. But this perceiving body is far from perfect. It fails to surpass the inadequacies of language, to overcome cliché; it lacks an ethos with which to describe the encounter of body and things. Life here is led by contingencies rather than scripted direction. This is the new condition of personhood, left alone to the immediacy of the flesh:

> We're sinking into our flesh, with few windows of connection. All language, all science, all poetry wants to expand the transparency of that fragile glass but winds up increasing its darkness—instead of letting the epiphanies last, these discourses introduce new layers of alienation. As if we were in a kind of progressive irreversible asthma, we distance ourselves from the fresh air that helps our breathing, and we block our paths with the very artifacts that we have invented. We can't perceive the wind, or the cold, or the leaves that brush past our bodies. (174–175)

Ramos notes an unnatural process in which our perceptions fall out of sync. Not only that, but we are in the process of losing our capacity to reach others. We are in the moment of sense experience, but alienation disables us and keeps us far from any potential beauty that we might behold. In this respect, Ramos takes a daring leap and tries to rehabilitate vocal sound in its material form. Hence, Ramos's phrase that serves as an epigraph to this chapter: "My task: to give matter to the voice, to give a voice to matter" (105). Without this pact, writing is impossible; we cannot grasp the living, pulsating sounds that reach the ears of others. Without matter and voice connected, we are flattened by the winds of happenstance and left alone in the world. We have no way to explain the sounds that rumble within us or to link our voices to nature, to plants and animals or minerals and stone. Who or what will hear us?

> Without deciding whether life is a blessing or dumb material, let's examine with patience the stones and fossils, the patterns we see in the clouds, the markings, the letters inscribed in smoke, the rhyme that is made of detritus, the immense landscape imprisoned by walls, the ringing in an ear, the glow of a micro-organism, the heartbeats of animals, the components that belong to inert matter; and we should absorb the whole horizon as one who wants to choose and then fails: "Is this matter or language?" (11–12)

Matter or language: the one embraces the other. For this reason, Ramos studies the relationship between bodies and preverbal sound; he listens for patterns of breathing, the utterance of noise, and the tie between animals and humans who share a similar practice of vocalization. Thinkers from the time of Plato have insisted on the voice as a challenge to logos insofar as its preverbal sounds might resist the calls of reason. Adriana Cavarero also understands the voice as a presemantic expression that escapes the discipline of codes; it works as a register of an economy of drives that cannot be charted precisely (2005, 11–15). In this respect, Cavarero helps us to think about *O* as Ramos seeks to trace the vibrant materiality that belongs to a sea of sounds.

He is driven by a set of questions: Can we get beyond language to sound alone? Can we reach the synesthetic scene where color and image coincide with noise? Where water rubbing on stone produces a sound as well as a visual trace of time? And where human intervention is not necessarily the founding gesture to inaugurate a trail of voices? For this reason, in Ramos's writings, the animal voice becomes the collective wisdom of beings on earth (Ramos 2014, 102). It is a voice unfettered by the complexities of representation that so obsess the human species. Our task, among others, is to absorb the animal voice and give it a place next to human speech. Or to listen to the animal voice and learn its expressive contours. To trace a history of sound.

A brief video by Nuno Ramos, with Eduardo Climachauska, underscores this experimental direction. *Luz negra* (Black light, 2002) is a sound citation of the Pereira dos Santos film *Vidas secas* (Barren lives, 1963), a monumental exploration of poverty and displacement in the Brazilian sertão. Ramos's film begins and ends with a screeching noise of the wheel of a wooden oxcart; here, we are obliged to sense the friction of matter on matter that belonged to the earlier film and which, as Pereira dos Santos tell us, vitally shows impoverished lives that lack for other modes of travel (Pereira dos Santos 2007, 334). We are thus introduced to a historical memory whose figuration derives from sensual recall of a particular *sound* and from the *visual* experience of a barren land. Borrowing from Pereira dos Santos, Nuno Ramos in his video manages to capture both. No language is needed to establish this connection nor to explain the plight of the poor. In *Luz negra*, Ramos begins by showing the movement of silent workers who drag a large box over the arid sertão. As they laboriously carry that heavy and oversized object, we only hear their footsteps, the sound of the wind, and the occasional bark of a nearby dog (a clear citation of the dog Baleia, who defined the opening segment of both the Pereira dos Santos film and before that, Graciliano Ramos's novel); in any event, no one seems to be talking. When the men reach their destination, a close-up reveals that the giant box is in fact a stereo speaker[2] that is lowered—like a coffin—deep into an excavation resembling a grave (see plate 16). The exercise is repeated several times, and with each interment, the workers remove wires from the sunken speaker and carry them to some electrical connection that is beyond the camera's eye; they then seal the speakers in earth, much like a burial of humans. At this point, Ramos becomes defiant. As the last shovelfuls of soil cover the buried boxes, a song comes seemingly from below the land—we hear the famous "Final Judgment" samba that was written by Nelson Cavaquinho. The workers retreat and disappear; only the dog and the song remain. In the final scenes of the video we hear the full samba played, while from an aerial view capturing brilliant sunlight, we see the parched earth that harbors numerous excavations resembling graves. The film ends with the incessant grating of the oxcart wheels with which the film began. Noise thus abounds, but, as

Cavaquinho's famous samba tells us, a black light surrounds this heartless age whose meaning we cannot discern.[3]

This minimalist experience recalls the "resonant tomb" that Jonathan Sterne (2003) evoked in order to describe the early gramophones that captured the voices of the nearly dead. Sound appears to acquire physicality as it emanates from the soil, enacting a breach in experience: we appear to reach the core of voice, but only a voice machine is speaking; meanwhile, the humans in the film remain in total silence. How can we read this? Most obviously, one can surmise a political history of Brazilian workers, who in the film are clearly voiceless; meanwhile, interventions of technology—the wire, the speakers, the sound system—absorb all human intention.[4] *Luz negra*, in this regard, is an appeal to a sensorial dehumanized present. An allegory for the sertão as a site for the past production of meaning, the film enacts a sound transmission only through technological devices; its artificial transmission haunts us with a trace of the past. The film thus becomes an archive of human and nonhuman sounds, and however much we may wish to interpret the film as an exposure of social injustice, Ramos obliges us to focus first on the "thingness" that constitutes sound. Through this, its materiality reorganizes our history of connection to bodies.

Giuliana Bruno has spoken of the ways in which material relations are activated in order to "refashion our sense of space and contact" (2014, 8). Similarly, the works of artists from the traditional avant-garde to our contemporary wave have addressed the power of nonverbal speech as a material force; these range from Hugo Ball's Dada experiments and the last canto of Huidobro's *Altazor* to the "uncreative writing" of the contemporary performance poet Kenneth Goldsmith in New York and the "polipoesía" of the Italian Enzo Minarelli that was carried to Barcelona and Buenos Aires. More recently, the Argentine Nicolás Varchausky devotes himself to compositions for 3-D sound to explore the resonance of phonemes as objects that unfold in space. He thus asks for a total immersion in soundscapes, in his words "the smallest sonic units capable of conveying a distinction in meaning" such that "the series becomes a search for language's ultimate acoustic matter and meaning" (Varchausky n.d.). Nuno Ramos also continues his quest for the materiality of sound and words when he explores the *durée* of alphabetic letters in an installation. Here, the letters are designed from petroleum jelly, but as time advances, the letters melt away, leaving only stains on the canvas (see plate 17). Language becomes only a greasy residue whose original semantic order can no longer be found. This experiment brings our perceptions in focus in order to reach for the thickness of matter, to apprehend words in their material form; finally, it refuses the traditional routes of meaning that once informed the historical past.

On the listening end, the utterances of voice once again raise the matter of attention. I take my cue from James MacDonald, who wrote regarding John Cage that "the difference between silence and sound is not so much acoustic as a matter of attention" (qtd. in Jiménez, loc. 91). In this respect, attention serves as a link, a red thread between the voice and the ear, a first step of a phenomenological analysis, but also a first step that reminds us that we are alive and in tune with the world. Attention, then, is a way of confirming our own acoustic presence with respect to resonating objects and animals as they are given to sound. Finally, attention is a way to note the start of community, which in this case, begins by *listening*. Jean-Luc Nancy writes on this topic in a way that very much seems to coincide with Ramos's texts: "To be listening is to be at the same time inside and outside. To be open from without and from within, hence from one to the other and from one in the other. Listening thus forms the aesthetic condition as such: the sharing of an inside/outside, division and participation, de-connection and contagion" (2007, 12–13).

Unlike Juan José Saer, who invested himself in the perceptual turn in order to break the wall of silenced knowledge surrounding the horrors of military rule; unlike Guillermo Núñez, who makes us aware of the interface between images of tortured bodies so that we come close to feelings of pain; and finally, unlike Raúl Zurita, who dwelled—and continues to dwell—on despair as he struggles to find a language that might connect the living with the dead, Nuno Ramos focuses on the sensorial present in order to create a real-time performance in the *now*. His revelation is that the materiality of the voice has a beauty all in the moment and is thereby worthy of capture; he arrests its sound and tone, its rhythms and breathing, and its pulsations, and pries it free from the body. This is a voice defined by a grain of matter that gives it density and substance; a tiny speck or material form that survives regardless of the body that it normally inhabits. It is the voice as object, just like a stone, that gives us material for our fixation. And in what has to be a tenuous paradox, both the elusive evaporation of the voice after its moment of sounding *and* the stone's inertness remind us of duration in time. Some may see this as the birthing of a misaligned synesthesia that crosses the sensorial archive;

its unexpected combinations surprise or shock the system. Others will go in a different direction, and find through contact of voice and stone that we awaken the human within us. In this latter extreme, we find a way to use our voices in order to form a story, and thus to sustain a life. But in Nuno Ramos's proposal, the voice neither sets demands for coherence nor carries expectations for the future. It is utterance in the instant, in the here and now.

The question this opens is far from simple. While artists like Nuno Ramos find a point of materiality that can reach the ear or eye, other artists would press these elements to move decidedly to a posthuman connection. Sensations are there for artistic study, but not to be used as proof of any human achievement or endeavor. This is a far stretch from the essays of Derrida, where he proposed that the phenomenological voice—to its degree of fleshiness and embodiment—was a link between consciousness and signs. By contrast, Ramos brings us closer to a material center preceding logos, instantiating pleasure in the ear of the listener, sounding the friction between matter and music, floating syllables untied from meaning, allowing us to feel the substance of letters.

Sense Work without Bodies?

As the millennium begins, we face an artistic culture that draws persistent reference to sensations, often by setting human life in competition with technologies of the virtual. This is perhaps the artistic equivalent of neoliberal discourse, indulging surface readings that are swift and quick, surpassing all regard for reason. Mabel Moraña describes the rise of a perceptual-affective climate in art and literature as a tool to answer a globalized world in a postideological age; it opens to modes of sociability that Marxist analysis had formerly eschewed (2012, 314–315). Dierdra Reber regards our present moment as an age of "feeling soma"—a headless body that "thinks by feeling" (2016, xviii); this is a collective (and mindless) response to numbing global logic, a time of affective and physical intensities that supplant sequential order. In a different direction, Martin Jay (2003) observes the rise of kinesthetic formations in art—what he calls "somaesthetics"—as an answer to contemplative slowness. At a time when no utopia is possible and we face universal violence, the work of sensation in the *now* supplies a ready answer; it pays homage to the agonistic moment of democratic practice that "is always in front of us, never fully achieved" (Jay 2003, 174). Jacques Rancière situates this crisis as a matter of state control. His phrase "the partition of the sensible" refers to the state's organization and control of perceptions and affects; this model alerts us to the policing of the senses through which the state determines the "delimitation of spaces and times, of the visible and the invisible, speech and noise" (2004, 12–13). He also claims that the turn toward perceptions might open, in a best-case scenario, the chance for a forceful response to injuries caused by the state. In these instances, new forms of subjectivity emerge under pressure from the neoliberal market and state directives. Often, from the perspective of culture, the senses are reconfigured to stand apart from market dictates; in the furthest extreme, disembodied senses are enmeshed with nonhuman forms.

What is this all about? Sense work without bodies? In some cases, this articulation speaks to the artist's anxiety regarding the loss of liberal humanism as we knew it in earlier times; in others, it speaks to the loss of value engendered at a moment when the machine appears to surpass human control. In mass culture, the zombie phenomenon endorses the idea that we are the "living undead," threatening to contaminate others. This goes far beyond the projections anticipated by Deleuze and Guattari in their landmark *A Thousand Plateaus* and brings us closer to what has often been defined as the realm of the posthuman, an "anthropological exodus," as Hardt and Negri choose to call it (2000, 176). Katherine Hayles (1999) maps this out when she traces a late-twentieth-century evolutionary curve from the years in which homeostasis informed much of critical theory to our current moment dominated by a culture of the virtually real. Technological advances have thus reconstructed our idea of the human subject, reaching our present time in which the domain of the senses is enmeshed with posthuman machines. Rejecting the kind of liberal thought that insisted on the centrality of the body and, in more pedestrian terms, the ownership of oneself, Hayles proposes in this posthuman condition in which we live that perhaps embodiment is not essential to our being. Following her lead, Paula Sibilia observes, in the fusion of humans with technology, that the human body is becoming obsolete (2009, 12). Worse, argues David Le Breton, technoscience leads us to disdain what belongs to the body. Le Breton, who in general argues for a humanistic version of body art insofar as he sees sensation as the guiding pathway to social practices, a first step in pedagogy for life and in learning, laments that the body is now subordinated to the machine (2010, 10–11).

Literature and art take up these mediations in countless ways, allowing us to participate in a scenario of "technowriting" and endless prostheses that often border on the fantastic. A few examples: In Carmen Boullosa's *La novela perfecta* (2006), a frustrated Mexican writer in Brooklyn allows a sensor to be attached to his tongue in order that ideas be produced by signals carried directly from brain to computer. The character's novel is an unprocessed absorption of sensory impulses without the intervention of logos. There is no ordering of events, no slow narration of plot or themes. Rather, the sensor announces the interface of synaptic awakenings and virtual events, just as it conflates creativity and science and, in the end, proclaims the crossing of North and South via Mexico and Brooklyn: they all merge in a hapless effort designed to make sense of the whole. In the high-tech age, it appears that crossing vectors of information will supplement human performance and diminish human authority and style. Neuroscience, at least in Boullosa's novel, points a path to chaotic futures. Pedro Cabiya's *La cabeza* (2007) also entertains the power of science to reformulate bodily senses and our idea of eros. On the edge of a new grotesque in twenty-first-century writing, the Puerto Rican novelist brings under inspection the posthuman conditions that are sustained by technological intervention. This is about the mind/body split, the severance of the mind from perceptions, a machine that can awaken deadened senses without the need for a body. Some may read *La cabeza* for a story about sadistic love in the modern age since, after all, the protagonist's wife is surgically reduced to a head and kept alive through tubes and wires; others will see this as a ludic charge of the posthuman moment that, despite its flashy irreverence, shows us that we still need a narrative logos in order to produce a sensual pleasure—not just to save the character's head, but to save the head of the reader. Mario Bellatin's entire corpus sustains a meditation on prosthesis, evoking his real-life condition as a man lacking an arm, but also revealing a way to mark the construction of classical narrative fiction from the space of absence. When he asks how to feel sensation in an arm that has long ceased to exist, Bellatin gives us a formula for the art of representation and notes the gap between word and experience, between a long-lost original form and its copy. In *Los fantasmas del masajista* (2009), he tells the story of a therapeutic masseur who palpates the missing limbs of his patients in order to stimulate their lost sensation. But this is also a trope for the invisibility of a literary style that the reader brings into existence, a play on imagination that is reified through the word and then felt in the body. Consider, too, the science-fiction narratives that are the purview of Marcelo Cohen as he bridges the human and the cyborg. The pairings of machine and human beings, real and imagined cities, real bodies and their prosthetic replacements course through all his fictions, but the Argentine writer Cohen combats the details of human deterioration by insisting on the pulsations and rhythmic chains that transcend the boundaries of these binary worlds. Life is sustained in a novel like *Balada* (2011) by a cadence of repetitions that we feel in our lungs and breathing, in the material engagement of the body that we invest in the literary texts. Here, we return however obliquely to the realm of the human; it is found in the reader's commitment to intuitions of rhythm and sound, contact and human value. This is the art of literature that Cohen refuses to surrender to the cyborg or the transhuman.

We have come a long way since the early episodes of this book in which Rivadavia and Jefferson brought the philosophy of French sensationalist theory to American shores. A follow-up to this close focus on perceptions led to the famous staging of the "civilization versus barbarism" trope in the cultural imagination of Southern Cone intellectuals, while in the North, where the enslavement of bodies was intensely embraced in discussion, a writer like Melville constructed embodied protests and an art of black and white contact only in those literary fictions that he could safely set offshore. We are far from this today. Now, nearly two centuries later, we work in the light of disembodied perceptions, surrendering to an affective world in which *things* have an agency that human-centered discourses seem to lack. A response to neoliberal market conditions that have diminished human potential? An exaltation of objects and matter that seem endowed with a life of their own? A route of political expedience to press for equality among animals, matter, and people? Perhaps.

To be sure, we witness a new materiality in our culture, with its emphasis on bodies and things. Jane Bennett refers to this as "vibrant matter," and (following Bruno Latour) she praises the encounter of materialities that gain identities as actants, those sources of action that can be human or nonhuman, alive or inert, and that produce effects and events and have the capacity to trigger sensation (Bennett 2010, viii). The goal is to surpass the binary opposite of life and matter, or the distinctions between human and animal, in order to find political resonance in effects, perceptions, and senses. We are all activated, human and animal alike, to trace force fields that will not necessarily end in human subjectivity alone. Indeed, as Deleuze once put it, these force fields are found in the reciprocal exchange of bodies that affect one another (1992, 93). Or at times, while inanimate materials act onstage, we stand on the sidelines and only hope that they might carry traces of something that once was human. Here, I am reminded of the Argentine artist Liliana Porter, whose photographs and paintings of celebrity bobbleheads stand next to plastic models of saints, and whose busts of dead political figures sit in close range of ceramic martyrs (see plates 18 and 19). Left alone, the little images are no more than simulacra sculpted in plaster or metal molds, examples of global kitsch to be sure; but when we bring our arsenal of affective and sensorial alerts in order to observe them, we endow them with lifelike forces. By the work of our imagination, set in motion by Liliana Porter, we give these figurines and tiny dolls the capacity to see, hear, and listen, to come in contact with one another; we allow them to speak their discomforts or pleasures, just as we hear their voices in conversation. Porter calls attention to the humanistic defense with which we put our senses to work, our need to sense on multiple levels and to project this onto others. Space, size, the distribution of objects on canvas, the height and depth of figurines aligned on a board all contribute to our imagining; they build us up as subjects. In the process, we embrace a world of inert objects to sustain our own metaphors and dreams. Through sensual proximity and familiar contact facilitated in her paintings by banal souvenirs, Porter pushes us to witness a plastic, posthuman world to which our human condition lays claim, taking us at several removes in time and place from what we used to believe was "real."

Art and literature of our times bring us within the realm of multisensory experience, and they often press for a synesthesia designed to confuse the senses by joining form and movement, fluid and cold, color and taste, sound and audition, and a sense of touch that in its depth is responsive to multiple pressures and to a barrage of assaults on the body. These are all part of a contemporary aesthetic attention that is increasingly interactive, joining humans to the artwork or to nonhuman matter while at the same time relying on intermedial strategies (mixing media, multiple languages, varying perspectives), all of which tend to upend expected sequential order. But the new materialism that this aesthetic assumes also responds to technological advances, to the overwhelming physical attacks on our intimate selves by virtual images or the digital web; in the process, it also answers the power of globalization and the biopolitical order.

Frequently, artists meet the challenge through different kinds of biological responses. Claudia Kozak, in a valuable guide to Argentine technopoetics, signals the details of contemporary bio art as a guiding force to handle nature and artifice and also to sustain an interface among living and inert things (2012, 22–30). A product of this way of thinking, the

Argentine Biolab project, which has worked since 2008 on the merger of living organisms of different species, has used biological materials to grow genetically altered tissue as the basis of art. The sensorial life of plants or the perceptions of robots enters into this project whose goal, as Eduardo Kac explains, is to create not just new objects but also new feeling subjects (2007, 8).[5] The Neuroartes group, a trans-American collective devoted to neuroscience and arts, not only studies human perception and the senses but also seeks to recover the biological impulses behind works of art (Delannoy 2015, 15–49).

I want to focus on two examples of recent materialist art that put human sensations to the test using the interface of computer technology and other mechanical supports. Eduardo Kac and Demian Schopf, visual artists from Brazil and Chile, respectively, take questions of materiality and sensation to a powerful critical dimension. Eduardo Kac, a conceptual artist whose work has been widely studied, focuses on the robotic interactions that produce sensation; he also attends to the ways in which human bodies learn sensation from mechanical form. In particular, he is interested in creating in robotic form some range of human experience that can be reproduced and sustained. This idea is not to replace the body, but to expand sensation and perception. In an early manifesto on what he calls "transgenic art," Kac outlined his major concerns: "New technologies culturally mutate our perception of the human body from a naturally self-regulated system to an artificially controlled and electronically transformed object" (1998, 4). The human is under siege. Bodies are reformulated by machines; identities are reconstructed; in the process, the uniqueness of human memory is refashioned by the computer. This technological sweep comes through virtual reality, through avatars and robots, and through medical advances that cover everything from plastic surgery to prosthesis. Biotechnology, from genetic engineering to electronic implants, controls us and changes our lives. Here, Kac thinks of the resistances of art that might preserve the body by exploiting technological control; he envisions a moment in which the body reclaims its rights to sensation and perception or situations in which we take control of the new forms of life.

> Transgenic art, I propose, is a new art form based on the use of genetic engineering techniques to transfer synthetic genes to an organism or to transfer natural genetic material from one species into another, to create unique living beings. Molecular genetics allows the artist to

> engineer the plant and animal genome and create new life forms. The nature of this new art is defined not only by the birth and growth of a new plant or animal but above all by the nature of the relationship between artist, public, and transgenic organism. (1998, 4)

This is the body's refusal to surrender. Kac wants to rethink embodiment such that the body subsumes technology and tames it for its own purpose or use—in this case, to continue a memory of sensation. Kac thus passes human sensation through computers and robots; a telepresence spreads his experiment over several geographical locations at once. His works remark on the rootlessness that belongs to our times, but also test displaced sensation. Finally, Kac's celebration of electronic work, insofar as it builds upon body art of the 1980s, also relativizes the experience of sensation as a unique encounter; no longer can we speak of a singular sensorial event in a fixed location.[6]

It is interesting that while Kac's earlier work of the 1990s emphasized the role of the robot and reproducible sensory perceptions, his more recent work is devoted to capturing sensation in order to keep it in place. Kac's *Holopoetry* of 2007 speaks to the infinite varieties of perception that are opened by this kind of art, stimulating multiple ways of reading, and human kinetic interactions with words that float, move, and disappear, or interact with color.[7] *Aromapoetry* (2011) is Kac's attempt to unlock scents from the pages of a book. The poet writes with scents, he explains; through chemical intervention and nanotechnology, the poem becomes an active olfactory experience. The goal is to release stimuli within reach of the human body and, with this, to invigorate modes of perception that might not be normally available through vehicles such as the traditional book.

Demian Schopf supplies a second case of sensorial experience. A philosopher and an art critic, Schopf is most importantly a multimedia artist who studies the relationship between the body and materiality while entertaining conceptual problems that traverse the axis of traditional and modern cultures in the Andean region. History is conveyed through the senses. Almost to echo Karl Marx, who saw the evolution of world labor as a history of sensory deployment, Schopf traces a history of Latin America since the Conquest as a permutation and recombination of ornament, textures, touch, and tones colliding in different times and spaces. Through this, Schopf enters the deep layers of materials that put pressure against our bodies over time, starting with the arrival of the conquerors in the Andes. This was first conveyed when Schopf staged a New World baroque (*La revolución silenciosa*, 2001), reconstructing paintings of the eighteenth-century angel-soldiers (*ángeles arcabuceros*) in his photorealist treatments (see plates 20 and 21). Schopf thus transforms the viceroyalty images by using manikins dressed as soldiers who carry, along with lances and muskets, diverse weapons of defense, from pitchforks to machine guns; in addition, taxidermied animals and fake tropical plants surround the angel-soldiers, reminding us that we are unmistakably in the realm of simulacra. The doubling of images, surely a nod to Deleuze's "fold," contributes to the artificiality of the scene and shouts out the ornamentality of the Spanish baroque in America. Furthermore, Schopf crosses these new syncretic extremes with various temporalities and climates (note the modern shoes, the tropical African beasts, the guns), appealing to the affective and sensorial multiplicity that the baroque still evokes today.

This continues more recently in Schopf's photo series *The Minor Choirs* (*Los coros menores*, 2011), focusing on the native poor in the north of Chile and Bolivia who celebrate in costume at the festival of La Tirana. Many Chilean poets and artists have addressed this hallucinatory fete where identities are transgressed and confused, but Schopf removes his subjects from the famous carnival and positions them instead in a nearby waste dump where they pose in costume for the camera (see plate 22). Clothed in distinctive apparel drawn from mass-market imaging (some are dressed as action figures from comic-book fame; others stand in dragon costumes associated with the Chinese New Year), the subjects remind us that we fall squarely before a mixture of borrowed cultures where no cultural inflection is "pure." Local and foreign imaginaries shape the colonial horizon, while, with the garbage field in plain view, human lives intersect with litter. The idea of recycling is both a matter of aesthetic choice and a tactic of waste management. Yet there's something else: the excesses of color and fabric belonging to the carnival subjects (we feel the texture of animal hairs on the wearer's costume; we embrace the metallic adornments of the Chinese ceremonial figure) are muted by a memento mori of the gray-white litter behind them. Schopf appears to tell us that the fate of the poor in Latin America cannot be sustained by the senses alone. Eventually, they will fuse with rubble. And in this reminder, the strategy of the seventeenth-century baroque remains with us still.

Schopf's eye on the Andean baroque brings attention to a multilayering of physical presence as a step toward comprehending the politics of present and past. History becomes tactile and draws the eye, while a performance of excessive dress and design appeals to the haptic; together, they let us negotiate conceptual abstractions alongside physical presence. In this regard, the fleetingness of time that so concerned poets like Góngora or Quevedo here becomes a materialized force entangled with pagan and religious appeal, ornamentality and waste. Note, too, that Schopf has no shyness about figural representation; in this respect, he makes a formal decision about the aesthetic and political potential of popular and foreign material that, when draped upon his human subjects (as live models in *Los tíos del diablo* or as manikins in his earlier work), brings forward reminders of the original baroque of seventeenth-century Spain and the oppositional neobaroque of Latin America in the 1980s and 1990s. Both question the role of the state with respect to its marginal subjects, just as they interrogate the durability of the senses and our perceptions of time.

In what appears at first to be an extreme shift in aesthetic direction, but in fact continues his long concern for the modality and materials of perception, Schopf's more recent work, *Máquina Cóndor* (2006–2016), abandons human figuration completely and goes to the interface between language and computation (see plate 23). Here, Schopf develops a writing machine that at first recalls Alan Turing's algorithmic code breaking during World War II and would seem to anticipate the artificial-intelligence work prevailing in our culture today. Schopf, however, is not breaking a code; rather, he seeks the rules of interchangeability among letters and words that are the basis of poetic expression. He thus works with the materiality of words, as we saw in the case of Nuno Ramos, just as he posits an inquiry about borders and the efficacy of containment. Schopf's work is therefore limited neither to a single space nor to a single time. Rather, he expands the unpredictable supplements that put the singular word to the test; he calls attention to the aleatory factors that shape all composition, and he has them sprout up on multiple monitors and screens that he stations in different places. Here, the new poem is born. More than anything else, the materiality of the word and its permutations are the center of Schopf's work; the letters occupy the computer screens as if by autonomous gesture. Beneath it all, we find an undeniable political component pushing the experiment along.

If Schopf's interest in computation brings Alan Turing to mind, other references to war and espionage are also evident in his work. After all, *Máquina Cóndor* reminds us of the Cold War spy program first used by the Soviet Union and later adopted by Southern Cone dictators during the "Dirty Wars" of the 1970s and 1980s. Under Operation Condor, death squads from the Southern Cone countries crossed over national boundaries in order to kidnap political opponents who had sought refuge in other lands. Schopf uses the sinister nature of the Condor plan—policing beyond all frontiers—for another purpose: borderless, like its military antecedent (and akin to the decodings of Turing), *Máquina Cóndor* is an apparatus capable of producing infinite permutations in its viral-like spread. In that way, if it resists policing that belonged to the years of state terror, its algorithms swing between determinism and escape; the recombination of words in new contexts proposes an aleatory feature that in the long run flees all control, leading to a sensory and creative release that, on the monitors, looks like a poem.

Schopf toggles back and forth in this play of freedom and intricate planning. In this respect, the machines yield words by combinations guided by chance and expand our idea of agency, time, and space. Obliquely, they evoke the body. In some cases, for example, a seismometer attached to the computers registers the footsteps of passersby; the pressure of nearby human weight and the sound of human voices awaken a spin-off of words in the poem. Human movement, in this case, is at the center of the machine's production. In other instances, however, the computer acts alone in the production of words, supplementing and ultimately displacing the human role as actant. Spread over different sites, the computer screens challenge the matter of space, while time becomes a variable of permutations and combinations.

Máquina Cóndor consists of many television monitors and obsolete computers from the 1980s and 1990s; as such, the installation refuses to participate in technology of the latest moment (perhaps a comment about the Latin American time lag with regard to innovation). At the same time, the words that appear on the screens are drawn from different lexical values. For instance, words from the poetry of Góngora and Gabriela Mistral are in turn combined with a database of vocabulary of war and economy taken from foreign press publications. An experiment in "media archaeology," as Schopf likes to describe it, the various computers of the Condor Machine spew words belonging to different eras; and while modernists might hope for an original voice from all that is read on the screens, in fact we might only be asked to reflect on the deterministic nature of the algorithm that runs against its ephemeral product. A third distortion of temporal dimension is added by the rhythm of word production: every several minutes, at carefully staged intervals, a stanza appears on the screens. This is a way to grasp the thickness of time not restricted to singular linear flow, but as clusters or chunks of historical precision where words carry the weight of the past. Schopf thus manipulates the time of history, the time of production of output, and the times that are signified by the different technologies and voices in use. And because the programs can be shown on multiple monitors and not in any specific location, space is also unmoored. Schopf would have us ask the following questions: How do our perceptions of time and space interact with the apparently infinite modalities of the many machines at work? And how do we employ our sentient selves to master the course of poetry and history? The encounter of the machine and the human sets its weight upon conflicting perceptions; it forces us to think of material traces and ephemeral forms. Underlying this is a political question about autonomy and integration.

Sensing the End

The early twenty-first century brings us to a confrontation of humans with the machine. At times, the sensory effects of technology excite the human imagination; at times, the experience is numbing. If in the first instance, the virtual produces a sequence of *effects* in the viewer, in the second, we shut ourselves down to the overload in order to protect us from future shock. The virtual keeps everything on the surface, as Brian Massumi (2002, 135) tells us; it works from the immediacy of effects in order to keep us engaged. Attention is both visceral and tactile; it shakes us to the core, as contemporary critics from Hayles to Hansen have recently claimed. At the same time, the unreserved power of the virtual even transforms the shapes of the book, announcing in its most recent rebirth its condition of "thingness." Can the "thing" that is the literary text compete with the machine? Can the machine and the book interact so that the technologies of each set new expectations for the perceiving body? Craig Epplin has made us aware again of the book as an "experimental object" for interaction, a medium rather than a transcendent vehicle of knowledge (2014, 5). In this respect, the sense work that emerges from our contact with the book becomes much more than a vehicle for abstract knowledge; it requires that we first encounter the book as a field of materialities, ranging from the paper content of the pages to its codes for digital writing; it then demands that we assess the book for its sensual appeal, ranging from texture and color to tactility and scent. Underneath it all, this encounter occupies a place on the political horizon. Of course, in the Southern Cone, in the aftermath of dictatorships, the persistent attention to remembrance guides many aspects of creative exploration, but often this discourse turns to a postfoundationalist proposal: sensory material, the figurative treatments of shock and torture, the status of the subject whose interiority is diminished while its body functions as a pure receptor of assaults from a field of "things" all redefine the way we might recall events of a distant past. Combined with this, the prominence of the neoliberal market makes us alert to velocity and speed, movement and transnational time. The art of perception and sense work responds to these callings. The book in the contemporary age grasps for these material questions. Within this framework, human interaction with digital technologies brings forth the tensions of the global and the local. If the human sensorium is the vehicle that registers the effects of the machine (and remember that the machine is not just the video game and the construction of virtual worlds, but also the apparatus of war and repression sustained by electronic devices), technology puts a steady pressure on embodied knowledge. Remembering through the body, sensing the power of the state. Not unexpectedly, literary texts may have the last word on these modern dilemmas.

Let me close with a brief reflection on the work of the Chilean Diamela Eltit, who, in her usual brilliance, helps me set this story straight. Since the 1980s, Eltit has been known for her novels about politics and bodies; her early work addressed the effects of Pinochet's repression upon the female body, while her later novels addressed the somatic effects of neoliberalism under the transition to democracy. In recent years, however, Eltit's work has gained an accelerated urgency in defending the damaged self, in speaking of the ways in which contemporary history deposits its sediments of violence upon the flesh of the poor and diminishes the value of human agency while altering the paths of affect and eros. If in earlier centuries, in Foucauldian terms, we witnessed the "birth of man," when the dominance of external and abstract reason gave way to organic experience and perceptions as a path to knowledge, today's fabric of interaction between the human and its others (organic or electronic) gives evidence that the model is once again in the process of change. Replacing the self-made man is a kind of *Homo bacteria* (the term belongs to Ficino)—that is, a pulsating subject that responds to sense stimuli but claims no agency of its own. This new version of the human responds to light and heat, food and sustenance; it flees pounding violence, it seeks escape from harm. It responds to sound, gesture, and the proximity of others' bodies; it perceives movement and velocity, pressure and cold; it pulsates with life forms while often lacking the force of logos. This sensate subject is frequently situated in the space of the posthuman, either linked to the animal world or confronted with the machine. For many this figure signals a crisis in humanist thought, the eclipse of an age of reason. It also invites further speculation about politics in our times.

Eltit's new work intersects with these currents in philosophical thought as she also supplies an ongoing critique of the global age in which we happen to live. In the process, her novels unfold upon human bodies and upon the materialities that cross these figures, especially the bodies of women. Her recent novels, however, reach far new explorations and in fact run in tandem with the kind of sense work that guides this final chapter. In one novel, she takes up the life in cell state, to which humans have been reduced (*Jamás el fuego nunca*, 2007); in a later text, she focuses on the biopolitical control exercised by the state over its female subjects (*Impuesto a la carne*, 2010). In *Fuerzas especiales* (2013), Eltit goes one step further by addressing global culture and its impact on the poor. Here, cyber forces and the interaction of humans and machines stand front and center. Because Eltit echoes the trajectory that I have been trying to establish in this chapter regarding sense work in the present, I want to linger on her proposals.

Eltit's tenth novel, *Fuerzas especiales* (Special forces), brings us to our current state of affairs, registering human sensory interaction with a global system that controls taste, desire, and knowledge. This system offers as a primary attraction a vast array of novel consumer products, along with the overarching fantasy that one day we all might possess them. In particular, the technological interface allows this fantasy to persist, stimulating an appetite for new levels of velocity and sound and new engagements with foreign objects insofar as they are brought into a local context through the World Wide Web. The stimulus passes through perceptions, so that light, velocity, color, and sound awaken the viewer's attention. What is not so evident from the start, however, is the way we reach this global compact through our human exchange with machines. "Embodying technesis," Mark Hansen (2000) calls it, outlining the ways in which the computer reshapes human perceptions and intervenes in our minds and bodies; the materiality of images on the screen delivers (in Benjaminian terms) a shock to the physical body; it also appeals to a presubjective realm of pure addiction that requires no language at all. Nevertheless, in this instance, a new kind of cognition emerges, leading to new desires and needs that fail to be directed by standard reason: "reception as embodiment," Hansen writes, working up to what he describes as the nonrepresentational experience of embodied sensation (2000, 261).

Eltit in *Fuerzas especiales* embarks upon a similar adventure, trying to build a narrative about human interactions with the machine. She situates her global story in the poor outlying neighborhoods around Santiago de Chile, enacting the drama both in a single place and, because of the cyberspace feature, in a space that is remarkably placeless. Between these two extremes—the local and the global—Eltit first installs a story of abject and aimless people, hungry and unemployed, to show the violent disruptions of their psycho-affective world. Their lives find no autonomous pleasure, no joy of communication, no seeds of social protest; instead, like entropic subjects, Eltit's protagonists move as mere pulsations. They dodge the danger of violence by police and the aggressions they enact on each other; they sell their bodies through prostitution in order to barely scrape by. Above all, physiology defines them: broken ribs, a painful tooth, and the palpitations of rough and decadent bodies that lie within reach of each other. In this condition, pleasure and dreams of progress are absent. The second violent disruption occurs with their encounter with electronic technology in the cybercafe.

A first-person female narrator alternates between passive and active voices; she toggles between the reported speech contained by indirect discourse and her direct expression of the physical pain that she feels. It would appear that the senses perform all the work, that human agency is lacking. After all, the narrator's only affirmations engage bodily perceptions: "The noisy din gives me nausea, and pushes me toward a strange and prolonged hunger. I am a parasitic creature of myself. I know that my sister trembles as she lies in our bed" (Eltit 2013, 11). From the very start, the narrator is pushed around and loses contact with her own desire. Her friends Omar and Lucho share a similar experience of inertia. Meanwhile, the neighbors are also passive: an incontinent woman languishes in bed, a mother talks to herself, others are deafened by various measures of sound without logos. Only cyberspace offers a marvelous distraction from so much urban blight. It is here that Eltit seizes the occasion to introduce a posthuman subject that is attached increasingly to an electronic machine.

The encounter with cyberspace is physical and urgent, though it speaks at first of a diminished agency that the narrator admits and assumes: "I go to the cybercafe like a woman who between the screens seeks out her food. Everyone eats everyone else. They eat me too. They pull down my underpants in front of the screens" (11). One might say that the character lives in bare-life extremes, as Agamben might have described it. Eltit describes this as a "larva state" (103) that presses upon human life; through cyber enticement, we enter a global war as seen from the margin of the margin. The poor lack control over their bodies; they lose their human dimensions.

Let's look at this cyborg expression. The larva-like stimulation of characters depends on their interface with media ecology; chat rooms and internet ads sustain their fragile imagination and shape their language as well. The computer gives them keys to touch, sounds to hear, images to see. Light and color guide their eyes; movement and velocity bombard them; synesthetic intensities attract their attention and create hunger for more of the same. Laura Marks has called the film screen a "portable sensorium" (2000, 243), a site that triggers sensory response and awakens audience perceptions. Eltit's computer monitors act in similar ways, dragging characters from their barrio lives and stirring their sensations. Memory here is diminished as the text moves in an endless present, but cyber life also creates a reflux language that vomits out new images, traveling from the computer back into the characters' daily routines. This is the start of the posthuman environment for the senses that gradually will be exposed in the novel.

Characters think in metaphors that the World Wide Web supplies. Hungarian bric-a-brac, Korean games, a trip to a Viennese circus, Italian and Japanese bridal gowns, French window displays: these images are drawn from cyberspace ads and flood the minds of the characters, who in turn use these images as metaphors to refer to their lives at home. Parallel to this parade of "things" is a review of military weapons at steady intervals throughout the book. The novel thus opens with the observations, "There were two thousand Webley Green .455. There were one thousand three hundred Bareta [*sic*] Target 90" (11); in the last line of the novel, we read, "There were four billion XM82 Excalibur artillery projectiles tele-directed at long range" (165). Ciphers and weapons abound; violence shapes the imagination. They mobilize the basic wants of characters who feel compelled to spend and consume in an environment of massive destruction. They also set a poetic rhythm in the novel in an age in which poetry is lacking.

The title *Fuerzas especiales* works from a triple meaning: Most notably, it evokes the Chilean security police (set in place by Pinochet) whose task it was to root out delinquency from marginal neighborhoods; it also refers to the special forces that poor people still need in order to survive the travails of the day-to-day; and then the title alludes to the special forces controlled by the Web, taking hold of its global subscribers and never letting them go. There is also a fourth and final meaning that emerges in the conclusion of the book and refers to the special forces of creativity that the characters ultimately claim. Together, these are the "special forces" that drag the poor out of their barrio homes into the global flow; they allude to the sentient body that is pulled in by the machine. Eltit does not circle around any moral precept as she builds this story; rather, she shows how sense work moves through the global Web and sets the tone and imaginings of all who fall into its clutches.

David Howes speaks of the hyperesthesia of late capitalism, by extension in its global phase, which is remarkably different from the actions of earlier times, when we were driven by the fantasy of accumulation and savings. Now we squander investments in order to indulge new habits of consumption; sensation in the present moment is the guiding stimulus for the circulation of images and our appetite for "things." Consumer capitalism, he argues, emerges inextricably from the demands of sensory stimulation (Howes 2005, 284). But these matters are never simple. While the economy offers substantial sensual enticement in order to trigger consumption, often the mediation of cyberspace recalibrates human responses. Cyber technology certainly whets a hunger for new sensation, and it also awakens a desire to cross over to a new transhuman engagement. On these terms, novel forms of creativity—along with sense work in its fullest expression—demand that men and women merge with cyborg life.

Two parallel and unsettling events govern the direction of Eltit's novel. On the one hand, a police invasion destroys neighborhoods and families; on the other, a cyber presence rewires the characters' desires such that they become engaged with the appeal of distant global products offered for sale (the already-noted guns and bric-a-brac, foreign food and fashion), which alter their sense of where they live and confuse the machine/life borders. In other words, this new and seductive disposition of modern globalization requires that individuals on the margins finally forget who they are. Eltit sustains this landscape of issues as her novel advances, frequently turning to the structure of indirect discourse to remind us that characters are no longer capable of managing their own stories and instead tell the stories of others; they thus pass their authority to the voice of someone else. "Dice que . . ." (They say that . . .) is this common phrasing; it is a way to tell the stories of others, to create a doubling of information, a repetition and shadow of former events that announce our loss of ambition to tell the story in terms uniquely our own. At the same time, the characters are acted upon and rarely initiate actions. This begins with the narrator's surrender to the violence of the Chilean police:

> It's more than a year since the [violent] images of the children flooded the papers and news shows, and broke into the social media. . . . This time they managed to condense my body and at the same time, break it up into infinite fragments of sensation because the children, yes, they were born again before me. (Eltit 2013, 17)

> They oblige us to behave like twisted technological toys. . . . Like that, like beacons, we have turned into untethered sounds screaming before an imminent arrest. (47)

Notice the Kafka-like changes as the characters are transformed by the powers of police harassment. As the novel advances, however, the cyber world takes over and takes claim of the characters' lives. The narrator synthetically notes this transition: "I have to forget the neighborhood building, the kids, the teeth, the helmets. I have to forget who I am in order to surrender in body and soul to the transparency of the radiant screen" (39). In this context, and despite the police bullets, hunger, and drugs, a social change is enacted; the machine is now the constitutive basis for the birth of the posthuman body. Access to the electronic screen becomes the characters' air and lungs. It alone can awaken the senses; it alone can keep people alive. The primacy of the body was the ontological access to the self, as Merleau-Ponty once taught us; now it is bridged by a computer world and an uncharted digital life. Indeed, we've come a long way since phenomenologists gave priority to the perceiving body as a linking between mind and world. Now we are in a technoculture that absorbs its human subjects, bringing the human into the digital realm, where it forms part of the evolving code.

In Eltit's novel, the first effect of the cyber world is experienced through one's distortion of time: "The hardheaded Lucho can't understand numbers in the cybercafe because he confuses himself with time and isn't able to tell a half hour from a fifteen-minute segment" (47). Digital time affects perceptions and sets interior clocks; it creates an urgent hunger for recycling and repetition. Moreover, as the narrator observes, it signals the edge of radical change: "Time is the element that flies over the human surface to show its powerful apocalyptic angle" (85). The pressure of time is experienced by characters as an addictive thirst for cyberspace programs that would leave all other obligations of city life on hold; temporality is gauged by the time of online access or by the repetitions of virtual wars and on-screen bombings and explosions.

The cyber world concedes a life-giving force through the "special forces" that come from perception: tactile, visual, and sonic prompts uphold the new version of the human that emerges in *Fuerzas especiales*. Human life is powered by one's interactions with machines, with the power of action and movement; it is sustained by the insatiable craving to always ask for more. More important, cyber life relieves the daily discomfort of the poor people of Santiago, their humiliation by the police, and their limited survival options; they seek "an image, a memory, a smell that would be capable of admitting new sensations to cancel out the malaise" (Eltit 2013, 101). Clearly, the global/local split needs a resolution.

As the novel advances, the electronic environment becomes increasingly life sustaining; it stands for technogenesis of all new sensation. And while Eltit defines the intersection of technological power with biological form as a testing ground for the senses, she also exposes the political force fields that are crossed by global hegemony and strong local resistance. This is focused on the characters' choices. "We're cyber, not the street, no" (156), the narrator avidly proclaims. For this reason, when the electricity is cut, when the lines of communication die, when cell phones cease to function and the radio connection fails (141–142), the characters begin to panic. Are they at the end of the human line, so pressed by the need for a sensory fix that they put aside the life of the mind? Or have characters accepted this routine of self-annihilation to save themselves from neighborhood violence? Eltit points to a confusing yet ingenious narrative solution.

Following a dramatic penultimate chapter in which the cyber connections are severed and no one has online access, a closing episode yields a remarkable end that brings us to the questions that I have raised in this chapter. The characters, no longer passive, become stars of a video game; they cross the barriers between machine and life and emerge as something new. "We are parapeted into cyberspace. Now we digitalize ourselves. . . . We navigate through the cubicle to test out the first Chilean video. A rapid game of defense designed by Lucho, set to music by Omar, and perfected by me. . . . And then we appear on-screen with the title that we invented: Fuckin' Cops" (165). Eltit offers two ways to read this dramatic ending: either the machine has absorbed us, locking us up in a relentless chamber of horrors, or, in a genuinely creative leap, we have become one with the computer game, its inventors and creators but also its actors and stars. The characters—in an almost Pirandellian move—have seized the chance to write a script of their own and install themselves as characters in the global cyberspace context. They have invented the first Chilean video game; they are celebrities of art and life. They thus return us to an auratic ending that we might have assumed to be forever lost. Directed toward a creative lens, sense work here reaches new advances; under the sign of the cyborg, the characters—through their exalted perceptions—celebrate their newfound freedom. And here in the final pages, Eltit explains her cryptic epigraph, which she has taken from Severo Sarduy: "I am an electronic Joan of Arc, right now." Auratic or oppressive? Creative movement or a sign of containment, a kind of death at the stake? The role of the artist in *Fuerzas especiales* is certainly up for grabs. To be sure, the utopian dream of the poor is tied to electronic awakening; their final answer clings to the potential auratic illusion. We are left here with the power of creativity as it comes from the South, the "special forces" that continue to hold out a promise of a local Latin American future. If sense work cannot lead to this situated identity and basic root, then we will not find the human within us; we'll await, instead, the death of our species, with no route for reading ourselves. Or maybe, in the end, it's all about reading for senses that matter.

Notes

Introduction

1. Though nearly lost to Anglo-American readers, Hudson's work still retains considerable interest in Latin America today. See, for example, the recent homages to Hudson that include contributions by significant critics in the Latin American field (Gómez and Castro-Klarén 2012; Vegh and Barnabé 2005).

Chapter 1: Sensing the Early Republic

1. All translations from Spanish are mine unless otherwise noted.

2. For a summary of the backwardness of the Spanish administration in America in part as an effect of scholastic thinking, see Alejandro Korn, who points to its dogmatic intolerance and absolutist objectives (1949, 47), a critique typical among Argentine historians (see also Chiabra in Chorroarín 1911; Torchia Estrada 1961; and Chiaramonte 2007a). Note, however, that the effect of scholasticism in Latin America is not the same throughout. For example, while scholastic thought all but collapsed in the early postindependence years in Argentina, it lingered until the 1840s in countries like Mexico. For a brief and general history of scholasticism in Latin America, see Lanning (1940). On the Mexican case, see Coronado (2014).

3. In Sarmiento's words, Funes understood that there was no need "to defer to the barbarism of gothic times, to which the precepts of ecclesiastical ministry subjected students" (Sarmiento 2005, 96).

4. Chiabra notes, and with reason, that Chorroarín never fully separated from scholastic thought, although he was certainly willing to entertain new philosophies, as his course notes show (see Chiabra's foreword in Chorroarín 1911, xvi–xvii). And indeed, Chorroarín's course notes reveal a constant interest in integrating sense theory with Christian doctrine. In one case, he explains: "The testimony of the senses, subjected to certain conditions, is the rule and criterion of many truths. This proposition goes against academics and Cartesians. In effect: 1, all of our knowledge that we acquire through induction and experiments cannot be proven by means other than through sense testimony; 2. Christ, affirming faith in resurrection, used the testimony of the senses. Touch, he said, and see, because the spirit has flesh and bones" (Chorroarín 1911, 98).

5. On the scandal of Lafinur's teaching, see the Franciscan priest Francisco de Paula

Castañeda, who vilified "the noble yet failed" Lafinur for his sensualist lessons (Groussac 1918, 137). Castañeda declared war against "Philosophism," and in various issues of the cultural journal *El Argos*, he attacked all philosophies that failed to respect Catholic doctrine (see Gallo 2006, 49–52). Manuel Belgrano and Diego de Alcorta were present as students in Lafinur's course.

6. See Halperin Donghi (1988, 50) and Palti (2007, 106–114) for the contradictions inherent in the neoscholastic pact insofar as it defined the role of the pueblo within the political order. The deep dilemma of sovereignty that scholasticism never resolved was brought into crisis with the fall of the Spanish monarchy in 1808. From there, the colonies took a cue that led to a call for independence.

7. For a convincing view of the general backlash against scholasticism not only in Argentina but elsewhere in Latin America, see Castro Gómez (2004).

8. This is unlike the evolution of French philosophy in Chile, where the strongly religious concerns of Juan Egaña, rector and founder in 1813 of the Instituto Nacional, were replaced by modern topics only when the French scholar Charles Lozier was appointed rector in 1826; Lozier then promoted Condillac as a major figure in philosophy. Among the students of Lozier was the future Chilean president Manuel Montt (Jaksic 1989, 17).

9. Destutt's *Lecciones elementales de ideología* (Spanish translation unsigned) also appeared as an appendix to the course notes of José Joaquín de Mora, who was teaching in Chile. Mora, in the notes to Destutt's book, is critical of the emphasis on sensation. He writes: "If the author wants to say that thinking is only having sensations, memories, judgments, and desires, we have to challenge him. Beasts also have sensations, memories, judgments, and desires, but they'll have to go a far way until we can claim that they have the same intellectual faculties as man" (1849, n4, n.p.).

10. Richard Herr notes the degree to which Condillac left a definite mark on the Spanish Enlightenment (1958, 69). A Spanish translation of Condillac's *Logique* appeared in 1784 in Madrid, followed by a translation of his *Cours d'études* two years later. Condillac in Spain was considered an heir to Descartes and Locke rather than as a friend of the encyclopedists. He was cited amply, and was the source of various plagiarisms. See also Alejandro E. Parada, who refers to the authors whose books were sold through routine advertisements in the Gaceta mercantil of the 1820s. Among the philosophers, Rousseau and Bentham sold most, followed by Voltaire, Condillac, and Destutt de Tracy. In addition to Bentham, Scottish philosophers also circulated in Buenos Aires, among them Bacon and Thomas Reid (Parada 1998, 58–62). As these sensationalists and common sense philosophers appeared in the Argentine book market in the decades following independence, Parada notes a simultaneous decline in the number of religious titles (59). See Korn, who claims that when Mariano Moreno founded the first public library in Buenos Aires in the preindependence years, the collection held only one philosophy text, Condillac's *Logique*, and his treatise on political economy (Korn 1949, 113).

11. For access to these documents, see their reproductions in Chiaramonte (2007b) as "Documento 1: Manuel Belgrano, 'Educación'" (2–5), and "Documento 2: Manuel Belgrano, 'Metafísica'" (6–8).

12. See Halperin Donghi (2014, 81–83), who refers to Belgrano's translation from French (in 1794) of François Quesnay's *General Maxims*, a physiocratic plan for the development of agricultural economy.

13. On the period of the *feliz experiencia*, or happy experience, see Halperin Donghi (2002, 393–424).

14. On Destutt and the Idéologues in relation to sensationalist philosophy, see O'Neal (1996, 225–244).

15. I should also note that his stay in France was complicated by a vexed conspiratorial scheme, which Rivadavia initially supported: to impose a French monarch upon the new Argentine nation and thereby resolve uncertainties at home (on this episode, see Gallo 2006, 3).

16. It is not the place here to examine the kinds of philosophy that emplotted a future for capital advancement in the new republic, but it is certain that Rivadavia's turn to the Idéologues helped him open a path for economic and managerial order. On capital cultivation of this kind in the years of transition to independence, see Halperin Donghi (2014) and Hirschman (1997).

17. In the law courses at the University of Buenos Aires, Juan María Gutiérrez taught Bentham, but in the philosophy courses, Alcorta featured the works of Condillac and Destutt de Tracy. Lafinur had also taught this course at the Colegio de la Unión del Sud, but, according to Groussac, he confused the philosophical strands of Descartes and Condillac, just as Fernández de Agüero, who taught *Principles of Ideology* at the University of Buenos Aires, also engendered conflicting ideas (Groussac 1918, 142n1). For a contrasting view of these paths of influence in England, see Catherine Gallagher (2006), *The Body Economic*, on sensation in the Victorian novel, where she points to the importance of Bentham for English writers.

18. We have access to Alcorta's course notes through a transcription by one of his students that was later recuperated by Paul Groussac. Recently, Santiago Kovadloff edited both Alcorta's lectures and the Groussac essay (Alcorta 2001).

19. See also Destutt de Tracy when, at the beginning of his *Treatise on Political Economy* (a supplement to his *Elements of Ideology*), he writes: "I have reduced the whole science of logic to observation of two facts, which result manifestly from the scrupulous examination of our intellectual operation. The first is, that our perceptions begin everything for us, we are perfectly, completely and necessarily sure of all that we actually feel. The second, which is but a consequence of that, is that none of our judgments, taken separately, can be erroneous, since, for the very reason that we see one idea in another, it must be actually there" (Destutt de Tracy 1817, 2–3).

20. The power of Condillac has returned to exercise considerable weight on today's thinkers and creative writers. See, for example, the writing of Michel Serres (2008), an homage of sorts to Condillac, and the poetry of Arturo Carrera (2004), who devotes a volume to the possibilities that Condillac's thought affords.

21. Alcorta—via Condillac—presses to link the soul and body to justify the material basis of moral inclination.

22. In this section of his lectures, Alcorta abandons Condillac's metaphor of the statue in order to consider the living body as a whole. He is especially concerned with connecting experience and feeling in what he describes as a sense impression. This is where the soul comes in, awakened by attention, reason, and will; in other words, the soul brings consciousness to experience itself (Alcorta 2001, 42).

23. Or, as a nineteenth-century Colombian thinker put it: "Without these faculties, there would be no happiness, disgrace, good and evil, moral or immoral, just and unjust, etc.... [T]hrough sensualist doctrine—and not dogma—one can articulate the public good" (qtd. in Castro Gómez 2004, 113n21). Sensualism, then, is the basis of order and even the law.

24. Jefferson was especially interested in getting to the root of the relationship between

rights of property and personality, which occupied a significant section of the *Éléments d'idéologie* (Destutt de Tracy 1817, v).

25. On Scottish common sense philosophy as an influence in the US academy and in literary formation, see Martin (1961) and Charvat (1936).

26. Tucker required Thomas Brown's *Lectures on the Philosophy of the Human Mind*, published in Philadelphia in 1824 as three volumes, as the single textbook for his course.

27. On the break with scholasticism at Harvard in the last decades of the seventeenth century, see Fiering (1981), especially chapter 6.

28. On Jefferson's late-life rejection of the sensationalists, see Kaplan (1967, 109).

29. Well into the century, Alcorta's students expressed admiration for their teacher: Mármol praised him in his novel *Amalia* (1851); Alberdi confessed to Vicente Fidel López his enduring respect for his teacher (see the comments of Vicente Fidel López in Alcorta 2001, 199n7), although toward the end of his life he sought a philosophical discourse that would greater sustain the logic of confraternity and political association that he believed Argentina needed (see his autobiography, "Mi vida privada," in Alberdi 1900, 294–295, 309). By century's end, Paul Groussac recalled the towering influence of Alcorta and his lessons upon the romantic generation (Groussac 1918, 258–259).

30. See, for example, "Del discurso al Dr. Carta" (1827).

31. See also "Ciencias" (1822).

32. See, for example, "Nuevas literarias: Fenómenos del galvanismo" (1822, 149–150).

33. *La abeja argentina* carried a monthly column on illnesses and plagues; obsessed with remedies to cure the infirm, contributors also sought places to bury the dead. Recalling Foucault's essay on heterotopia, the authors acknowledge the advantages of La Recoleta (established as a burial ground in 1822) as a choice location.

34. See Acree (2011, 7, 29) on the *fiestas mayas*; Seibel (2002, 55–81) on patriotic celebrations and theatrical spectacles in the postindependence years; Batticuore, Gallo, and Myers (2005) on public cultural expression of the 1820s in Buenos Aires; Marino and Munilla Lacasa (2017) on visual culture under Rosas; and Hallstead and Root (2017) on nineteenth-century visuality and fashion.

35. Elías Palti (2007, 105) roots the political and ideological conflicts and breaks of the independence years as a "history of effects," a term he takes from Hans Blumenberg.

36. Alberdi in this text rejects the sensualist tradition tout court, finding a replacement for Condillac in the interpretations of Cousin.

37. See Sarlo and Altamirano on this idea of incompatibility between the two aesthetic modes (1991, xxvii).

38. On the hunting trope in nineteenth-century literature, see Traisnel (2012).

39. Sarmiento in the *Viajes* wrote, "Poor Echeverría. Sick of spirit and body" (1993, 54).

40. In an annotation to "Avellaneda," Echeverría wrote: "The sensualist philosophy of Condillac and De Tracy, the utilitarian Bentham, the materialism at the time and the ignorance of duty influenced elite society in Buenos Aires and carried over into practical life" (1870–1874, 1:437–438).

41. See also Juan María Gutiérrez's defense of Echeverría's university teachings and the wide shadow of influence that Alcorta cast on his student (in Echeverría 1870–1874, xxiv). Zamudio Silva exposes the debate that followed the publication of Echeverría's poem and shows rebuttals by José Ingenieros and others (Zamudio Silva 1940, 87–89).

42. See Halperin Donghi (1951, 45–46) where he writes about the contradictory and

cloudy experiences of Echeverría's religious sentiment following his return from France. He concludes that Echeverría was led by pragmatic motives appealing to the masses.

43. Remember that taste was a widespread topic of inquiry owing to the publication of Brillat-Savarin's *Physiology of Taste* (1825).

44. On this, Hugo wrote: "[P]oetry will take a great step, a decisive step, a step which, like the upheaval of an earthquake, will change the whole face of the intellectual world. It will set about doing as nature does, mingling in its creations—but without confounding them—darkness and light, the grotesque and the sublime; in other words, the body and the soul, the beast and the intellect, for the starting-point of religion is always the starting-point of poetry. All things are connected" (Hugo 1909, 363). Noé Jitrik also refers to Hugo's famous essay in order to argue for the necessity of mixing the genres and challenging the Aristotelian unities of form; see his *El fuego de la especie* (Jitrik 1971, 65). I think, however, the mixture refers more to the epistemological uncertainties of the "material-ideal" binary that perplexed romantics like Echeverría.

45. Echeverría pretends to resist a literature of the senses, although his writings inevitably seem to move in that direction. In the prologue to his poems (1870–1874, 5:143–149), Echeverría protests sensuality of the romantic mode. Referring to himself in the third person and commenting on *La cautiva*, he writes: "He tries to use vulgar locutions and call things by their name, because he believes that poetry consists principally of ideas and circumlocutions that don't always put the object before one's eyes. If this is shocking to those who are accustomed to the high sounding and pompous speech that poetry uses, it's their fault since they are seeking what pleases them without regard for what is part of the author's vision" (5:144–146).

46. In his "Cartas a un amigo," a recollection of the death of his mother along with meditations on the countryside as he prepares to take leave of his country, nature is the site of intense sensation, and although Echeverría describes unrestrained beauty, he also names those aspects of nature that reinforce death and decay. In this respect, some of the scenes described resemble those of *La cautiva*. See, for example, the following passage: "Today, tired of the gallop and also thirsty, I reined in my horse by the side of a lagoon where plants and sparrows live. The flaming sun of midday burned the earth, and the humid steam coming off the lagoon formed a smoky cloud on the surface, reflecting luminous rays and turning the steam into a thousand sparkling irises that astonished the eyes. Quenching my thirst and exhaustion, I took a sip of water; but then I saw with surprise a multitude of fish floating dead on the swampy surface of the lagoon. A putrid odor wounded my sense of smell, and it was no longer possible to cool my inflamed body or to moisten my arid throat" (1870–1874, 5:39–40).

47. All English citations of *Facundo* are from the 2003 edition unless otherwise noted.

48. Leroux's significance in the history of ideas lies in his attempt to resuscitate community in France in the wake of the revolutionary decades of the 1790s and the Napoleonic era. As was the case with many of his romantic socialist contemporaries, Leroux sought a basis on which to establish a human community that did not rely on the pillars of the old regime, with its sense of authority, hierarchy, and respect for the Catholic Church.

49. See especially Ricardo Piglia (1980, 15–18).

50. Sarmiento is clearly obsessed with the keen sense of audition of the natives. In the section of his *Viajes* devoted to Brazil, he writes: "[I]n nature, there are tropical melodies that are imperceptible to our ear, but which move the fibers of aboriginal peoples. They hear the whispering of vegetation as it opens up, and in the palms where we hear only the waves of wind, they hear melodic African songs, rhythms that are similar to their own" (1993, 60).

51. Doris Sommer rightly called attention to the Argentine interest in Cooper's trailblazers in her comparison of Cooper and Sarmiento (Sommer 1991, 52–83).

52. See a similar comment by Josefina Ludmer (1988), who addressed tonality in gauchesca poetry. Contreras, reading Sarmiento's intonations, sees them as a time of fruitful expectation, anticipating future events (Contreras 2012, 82–83).

53. It's not just any sound that Sarmiento defends. He thus rejects the racket, or *bulla* (2003, 116), that belongs to a civil society that fails to find harmony in form.

54. Perhaps Sarmiento here engages Rousseau, who in Roberto Darnton's terms was trying to redefine the notion of reading so that it "would become not a substitute for experience but a primary emotional experience itself, a constituent of identity, a way of understanding and making one's self" (Darnton qtd. in Fliegelman 1993, 58).

55. On Sarmiento's use of optical cabinets and other devices that tricked the eye, see Lanctot (2014, 114–118).

56. Halperin Donghi observes that these reflections belong to the English theologian William Paley, whose *Natural Theology* is in fact a forebear of natural design (in Sarmiento 1998, 237).

57. While Sarmiento denounces Rosas for his perceptual errors and clumsy military maneuvers, it is only ironic to read that Sarmiento lugs an unwieldy printing press (that he purchased in Montevideo) through the battlefields of war; he carries the machine from place to place in the name of freedom of thought.

58. Sarmiento understood that he was living in a war economy, but he also knew that the war machine could best defeat barbarism not by violence but by attention to new machines and rationalized systems of exchange. He was thus attracted to trains and waterways and taken with velocity and movement; he was enthralled by visions of the countryside that a moving train or carriage might afford. This is the basis of *Campaña*—quick as the blink of an eye, an almost filmic experience of the nation. So while Sarmiento was pressing the experience of speed upon the flesh of his readers, he also announced the emergence of a new subjectivity that would not be erased by Rosas's retrograde laws. On market logic in Sarmiento, see F. A. Rodríguez (2012, 630).

59. On the design of Monticello and the importance of optics in Jefferson's design, see Breitweiser (2007).

60. Among recent critics who have drawn attention to the sensuality that informs Melville's aesthetics, see especially Samuel Otter and Geoffrey Sanborn (2011). See also Sharon Cameron (1981).

61. Similarly, Andrew Delbanco, one of Melville's recent biographers, sees the sentences of *Moby Dick* emerging from associative impulse and the art of improvisation (2005, 143).

Chapter 2: Troubled by Gender

1. See cuaderno 5 in Bacle (1947), devoted to images of the *peinetón*. Among recent scholars who have studied the historical importance of the *peinetón*, see especially Root (2010). For an overview of Bacle's political engagement with Rosas, see Acree (2011, 47–59).

2. For a history of ocularcentric discourse in the nineteenth century, see Jay (1993).

3. Lithography was invented by the German Alois Senefelder in 1796, but by the 1830s, artists practiced with multicolor lithographic printing, as in the case of Bacle's studio engravers.

4. See Tomás Buch and Carlos E. Solivérez, who refer to the arrival of the steamships with the blockade of Buenos Aires in 1838–1840 (2011, 189).

5. Clorinda Matto de Turner's journal, which she began publishing a year after her arrival in Buenos Aires, ran for eight years (1896–1901, 1905–1908) and comprised thirty-one issues. It covered a wide range of topics pertinent to women and included demands for female education and reflections on the role of science and technologies in the lives of female readers. On this and other journals by women of the late nineteenth century, see Masiello (1992, 83–109; 1994); on Matto de Turner, see Ferreira (2005).

6. "I was born to be a man!" she wrote in a letter to her son in 1852 (Sánchez de Thompson 2003, 259). She also wrote in a letter to Alberdi of 1852: "My life more resembles that of a philosophical man than that of any woman, but for the fact that I have a woman's heart and a volcanic temper, and lack the frivolity of sexual conquest that would keep me entertained" (342).

7. See the important discussion by Florian Nelle (1993) with respect to Sarmiento's admiration for the new technologies of his time.

8. See also the work of Skinner, who speaks of the effects of the telephone for the female workforce (2016, 156).

9. On the female fantastic in the late nineteenth century, see Carlos Abraham (2014) and Masiello (1992) on Gorriti.

10. See Nicolás Bolet Peraza in *Búcaro americano*, who expresses invidious comparisons between a backward Argentina and a modern United States where science, he claims, bestows an elevated place to its women: "Science did not repudiate women; rather, civilization recognized her as an ally and worthy worker and, taking her by the hand, with her brow enlightened by divine light, civilization raised her to a place of honor ... in these last, decisive battles of the century" (Bolet Peraza 1896, 141).

11. "The Mashorquero's Daughter" was published in Lima in 1863 and later appeared in Gorriti's now-celebrated book, *Sueños y realidades* (1865). All citations are from Gorriti (2003).

12. On the spectacle of the Rosas regime, see Brendan Lanctot (2014).

13. See, for example, Barker-Benfield (1992), as well the groundbreaking work of Douglas (1976) and Cohen (1999).

14. See the 1783 dictionary of Dr. Samuel Johnson in which "sensible" is "perceived by the mind or senses having the quality of being affected by moral good or ill."

15. This goes against the observations offered by Margaret Cohen with respect to the sentimental writers, whom she claims avoid description and details about material culture in favor of a pursuit of the moral truths and interior depths of the characters. The material world, for Cohen, is thus secondary to the quest for a moral certainty (1999, 49).

16. For nineteenth-century sentimental romance in Latin America, see Masiello (1992) and Sommer (1991).

17. See Pratt (1992) for a fundamental reading on visual discourses pertinent to exploration and conquest in Latin America. For a history of light and vision in nineteenth-century Britain, see Christopher Otter (2008).

18. Cited in Andrew Delbanco (2012, 44).

19. See especially James Baldwin's (1955) vitriolic critique of Stowe as an example of this perspective.

20. See Gates (2007, xxi).

21. On the idea of "sentimental men," see Chapman and Hendler (1999).

22. Years later, in collaboration with her sister Catherine, Stowe published *The American Woman's Home* (1869), a scientific design for the spatial dispositions of the kitchen and for the use of new technologies that would become the standard for daily living of the modern US family. The sisters' emphasis on order picks up on some of the detail that Harriet had supplied in her novel, but the later text also highlights the striking emphasis that continued to be attached to domestic sensorial pleasures. The home, if it is to guarantee happiness, needs not only design and order; it must also supply a place of human contact where the gaze is nourished, and also the ear and the palate. The 1869 edition represented amplification and revision of Catherine Beecher's *A Treatise on Domestic Economy* (1841) and was largely Catherine's work.

23. On the railroad in *Torn from the Nest* and in other Latin American texts, see Skinner (2016, 148–153).

24. See Matto de Turner (1896, 30): "The basis of domestic economy can be reduced to this one rule: always spend less than you earn and make sure to spend it well."

25. See Gorriti's protests in a letter of January 25, 1888, addressed to Ricardo Palma, where she writes about a strike of cooks in Buenos Aires: "We are in the middle of a horrible strike of cooks who refuse to be part of the domestic staff and declare themselves 'culinary artists.' The restaurants have closed and the pensioners have to eat at the homes of friends, where the women, tied to their aprons, are cooking over the fire. As for me, as soon as the cook joined the strike, I wasn't bothered because I lost my appetite quite a while ago. My diet is beef blood, milk, fruit, and ice cream" (2004, 42).

26. Remember that Matto de Turner had devoted herself to the genre of *costumbrismo* from the time of her *Tradiciones cuzqueñas* (1884). In the prologue to *Torn from the Nest*, she continued to insist on the merits of the sketch, claiming that literature was needed to correct the bad habits of a people.

27. Marx also wrote in the same text: "Sense perception (see Feuerbach) must be the basis of all science. Only when it proceeds from sense perception in the two-fold form of sensuous consciousness and sensuous need—that is, only when science proceeds from nature—is it true science. All history is the preparation for 'man' to become the object of sensuous consciousness and for the needs of 'man as man' to become [natural, sensuous] needs. History itself is a real part of natural history and of nature developing into man. Natural science will in time incorporate into itself the science of man, just as the science of man will incorporate into itself natural science: these will be one science" (1964, 143).

Chapter 3: Collective Synesthesia

1. William Nestrick observes that the film's scriptwriters, Hans Janowitz and Carl Mayer, responding to the manipulations by the German government over individual autonomy during World War I, designed the figure of Caligari and his subjects with German realities in mind. For Mayer, in particular, military psychiatrists embodied state control (Nestrick 1976, 7–8). Anton Kaes takes this a step further and sees the horror genre under Weimar rule as a response to the trauma of war, such that cinema staged the shock of battle without even referring to military combat; instead, it referred to domestic enactments of terror and crime far from the theater of war. Subsumed under the rubric of "shell shock cinema," *Caligari* is a principal case of the ways in which trauma was treated and alludes to the gen-

eral paranoia that was triggered by published images of mental hospitals and reported errors of psychoanalytic treatment rendered to veterans of war (Kaes 2009). See also Siegfried Kracauer's fundamental analysis of the film, in which Dr. Caligari is read as an embodiment of the authoritarian state that controls the puppet Cesare and thus anticipates the rise of Nazi rule (1990, 245).

2. Kracauer notes that Francis and his friend Alan are the signifiers of mass-culture audiences attracted to glossy sensation (1990, 208); other critics have also noted the sensationalist ways in which the film was marketed to audiences worldwide. Motion Picture News, for example, observed that a theater manager in St. Louis sold Caligari as a "film sensation that is not a sex picture," and building upon this, announced that no children would be admitted to the theater under any circumstances and advised nervous women to keep away (qtd. in Thompson 1990, 147). In another case, Motion Picture News reviewed the film: "It is like a page from Poe—a fantastic, uncanny piece of imaginative fiction—a page of diabolical scheming by a distorted, insane mind" (qtd. in Thompson 1990, 148).

3. Think only of Jung getting his start in psychoanalysis by attending a séance salon; his dissertation on the psychogenesis of spiritualist phenomena then set him on course to study the intrapsychic material that was so attractive to the avant-garde. As he expressed in a letter to Freud, "I have been dabbling in spookery again," inspiring Freud's displeasure (Jung 1977, viii).

4. On spiritualism and literature in the 1920s, see Banga (2016).

5. On Lehmann Nitsche's sound experiments, see the dissertation of Diego Ballesteros (2013).

6. Miriam Bratu Hansen also sees the ambivalence of Benjamin regarding sensational pleasures. She observes that Benjamin was afraid that theosophists would lay claim to the concept of "aura" (and only with respect to specific objects); writing against them, Benjamin wanted to see the possibility of auratic experience in all things. "In such formulations, the term shock acquires a valence quite different from, though no less in tension with, its more familiar sense of effecting, in its relentless proliferation in industrialist-capitalist labor and living, a defensive numbing of human sense perception. This alternative sense of shock also differs from the deliberate, avant-gardist staging of countershock, designed to enhance the demolition of aura (as in the artwork essay's section on Dada). Rather, it relates to the idea of an involuntary confrontation of the subject with an external, alien image of the self" (Bratu Hansen 2008, 347).

7. See especially, in *The Varieties of Religious Experience* (1902), the chapters on "The Divided Self" and "Mysticism" (James 1985).

8. For a detailed look at Ortega's engagement with phenomenology, see Philip A. Silver, who insists that Ortega's training at Marburg led to a psychological phenomenology as the defining first moment of Ortega's career, and that this early period was not part of a gradual "coming to maturity" approach with which one might see Ortega in the years 1911–1914 sowing the seeds for his later work (1978, 4).

9. See in this regard his "Ensayo de estética a manera de prólogo" (1914), where he refers to "[e]l yo como lo ejecutivo" (the I as executor) (Ortega y Gasset 2004, 667). In this essay, Ortega signals the role of bodily action (especially sense perception) that precedes one's consciousness of things. In the same line, we learn to assess performativity only after the fact; consciousness is always a posteriori, as is our sense of history.

10. Borges even carries this analysis to his focus on time: if we were to use the "I" as a

way to measure time, he claims, then this would "translate the I into a mere logical necessity, without any qualities of its own or distinctions that would separate one individual from the other" (1925, 95).

11. For his idea of "profane illumination," Benjamin took advantage of the experiments of surrealist writers (André Breton in *Nadja* and Louis Aragon in *Le paysan de Paris*), who allowed him to think of the magical experience of words with which it would be possible to transform the spirit. See especially his celebrated essay of 1929, "Surrealism: The Last Snapshot of the European Intelligentsia" (1979, 225–239). Though it would be erroneous to suggest that Benjamin was attracted to the occult in the way that Yeats or Rilke found it appealing, Benjamin was in fact open to all dimensions of the spirit: he was especially interested in the phantasmagoria that came to haunt us daily and on occasion he drew from fantastic events, from studies of graphology, and from hallucinations and hashish to introduce his reflections. Like his confreres of the decade, he believed that these alternative engagements with reality could help one reach a redemptive understanding of history, overcoming what one might otherwise experience as a facile stimulation of the senses (on this, see especially his essay of 1933, "Experience and Poverty" [2005, 732]). Elsewhere he referred admiringly to the way in which the ancients interacted with the cosmos, defining it as the "ecstatic trance" and claiming that "it is in this experience alone that we gain certain knowledge of what is nearest to us and what is remotest to us, and never of one without the other. This means, however, that man can be in ecstatic contact with the cosmos only communally" (1979, 103).

12. See Adorno's study of Wagner, especially the chapter "Music Drama," in which Adorno takes Wagner to task for his desire to link the senses as one in order to issue a challenge to the institutionalized division of labor: "The universe of perceptions at his disposal offers itself as a coherent totality of meaning, as the fullness of life; hence the fictive nature of the Wagnerian style. For in the contingent experience of individual bourgeois existence, the separate senses do not unite to create a totality, a unified and guaranteed world of essences. It is questionable, indeed, whether such a unity of sense experience has ever existed, dependent on it as Wagner's disillusioned mind may be. On the contrary, the senses, which all have a different history, end up poles apart from each other, as a consequence of the growing reification of reality as well as of the division of labour. For this not only separates men from each other but also divides each man with himself. It is for this reason that the music drama proves unable to assign meaningful functions to the different arts" (2005, 91).

13. James acknowledged the tendency toward synesthetic fusion as a rule rather than the exception of infant perception: "any number of impressions, from any number of sensory sources, falling simultaneously on a mind which has not yet experienced them separately, will fuse into a single undivided object for that mind. The law is that all things fuse that can fuse, and nothing separates except what must" (1918, 488).

14. For a history of synesthesia with emphasis on antiquity through the Renaissance, see Schrader (1975).

15. On this, see Ina Blom (2001, 209–216) and Jacques Donguy (2001, 217–220).

16. See also Henríquez Ureña (1926) on this essay.

17. It is worth reading Sanín Cano's early comments as a harbinger of the writings of Richard Sennett, who in his discussion of the value of craft devotes a chapter to the hand (Sennett 2008, 149–178).

18. For an extensive discussion of futurist noises, see Douglas Kahn (1999), esp. 56–67. Kahn makes the observation that sound is discerned through three figures—vibration, inscription, transmission—all central to the procedures of the avant-garde (16).

19. In this respect, Russolo wrote: "In modern warfare, mechanical and metallic, the element of sight is almost zero. The sense, the significance, and the expressiveness of noises, however, are infinite. And since traditional poetry lacks suitable means for rendering the reality and the values of noises, modern war cannot be expressed lyrically without the noise instrumentation of futurist free words" (1986, 49).

20. Hannah Chapelle Wojciehowski and Vittorio Gallese (2016) refer to this phenomenon as "neurohumanism." See, as an example, Jonathan Lehrer's (2007) recent popularization of the melding of neuroscience and literary fields.

21. This is the verse line that many critics have defined as an orgasmic expression; others see it as a hiccup. The point is that we apprehend a moment in which a bodily experience is expressed synesthetically and cannot be reduced. Sound becomes visual, silence is voiced, and pleasure is crossed with disruption: all are decidedly beyond language and resistant to the habitual modes of understanding that might be parsed by scholars.

22. Michelle Clayton reads the construction of the body as central to Vallejo's book of poems. Her thesis is that Vallejo in his poetry shifts from an emphasis on sight toward the other senses, and in this regard, she finds Vallejo notably different from other participants of the Latin American and international avant-gardes who in her words "seize hold of vision" (2011, 54). Throughout the course of this chapter, I have aimed to show that sense work and especially the melding of the senses have been the defining characteristics of the avant-garde in general without belonging to any one poet.

23. Taking discussion in a different direction, Beatriz Sarlo also comments on this text (1992, 39–42).

24. For a brilliant exposition of this thinking with respect to the visual arts, see Merleau-Ponty, "Cezanne's Doubt" (1964b, 9–25).

25. This may be akin to Simmel's idea about the individual's blasé attitude to the difference among things. Simmel spoke of this defining characteristic of metropolitan life as a way for a person to protect herself from the ongoing assault on the senses. Indifference, then, was a way to insulate the individual from the outside world (1950, 414).

26. On coenaesthesis, see Heller-Roazan, who explains this in terms of a sensory phenomenon that is irreducible to particular regions of the body. Cojoining all sensations, coenaesthesis can be registered as a "common feeling" or as the Aristotelian "inner touch," the "touch" that apprehends the vital force of the sensing body without locating the specificity of experience. Coenaesthetics in these terms goes beyond a single response to a single external agent; it is a super-sensual hypersensibility that makes us very aware of our bodies (2007, 247).

27. Chaplin is the model of the fatigued, overwrought hero who works off sensations and allows the audience to sense this as well. In a later essay on the senses, Epstein writes of Chaplin: "His entire performance consists of the reflex actions of a nervous, tired person. A bell or an automobile horn makes him jump, forces him to stand anxiously, his hand on his chest, because of the nervous palpitations of his heart. This isn't so much an example, but rather a synopsis of his photogenic neurasthenia" (1988, 238). I should note that Epstein enters into contradiction with the premises of his own book when he insists in the later essay that cinema is a "cyclopean art, a unisensual art.... All life and attention are in the eye.... One cannot listen and look at the same time. Truly, the cinema creates a particular system of consciousness limited to a single sense" (1988, 239–240). Here, by stressing cinema's appeal to a single sensation, he cancels his claims to the value of coenaesthesia as an aggregate of impressions generating a novel art (239).

28. The 1965 edition, under the title of *Historia de las literaturas de vanguardia*, bears little resemblance to the original text. In this edition, de Torre claims to have included the prologue to the 1925 book, but even this document has changed. To be sure, the 1965 book was edited for another clime: the youthful excesses and emotive plea for community, which I explore in chapter 3, were not to be found in the later edition, which Guillermo de Torre transformed into a proper manual for international avant-garde readings. Fortunately for current readers, a recent edition by José Luis Calvo Carilla restores the 1925 contents (see de Torre 2002). My translations of the text are based on the 1925 edition.

29. De Torre refers to Epstein's book as a path-breaking study of poetry, "the first essay to codify the psychological characteristics of the new tendencies in art" (de Torre 1925, 272–273).

30. Braque also helps his argument, "the senses deform, but the spirit forms" (de Torre 1925, 277).

31. See "The Metropolis and Mental Life," where Simmel explained: "To the extent that the metropolis creates these psychological conditions—with every crossing of the street, with the tempo and multiplicity of economic, occupational, and social life—it creates in the sensory foundations of mental life, and in the degree of awareness necessitated by our organization as creatures dependent on differences, a deep contrast with the slower, more habitual, more smoothly flowing rhythm of the sensory-mental phase of small town and rural existence" (1950, 404–405).

32. Ivan Goll, Joyce's German translator, occupies a section of de Torre's study. He was persuaded by the occult, translated occult poets, and also wrote a book on literature and its relation to the occult; at the same time, he advanced a theory of the unspoken connections among artists of the world above and beyond national borders, which was placed in evidence in his anthology of poets, *Les cinq continents* (Goll 1922).

33. Richard Sennett addresses the crisis of the craftsman in light of the industrial machine: "[T]he most radical way to contest machinery seemed, to some, to turn one's back to modernity itself. This Romantic gesture had the virtue of heroism, but it doomed the artisan, who could not work out how he or she might escape becoming the machine's victim" (2008, 145).

34. Many have called attention to this essay as an urtext for Arlt's future novels, but it should also be noted as a foundational text in which Arlt studies the sensational triggers that awaken physiological responses in the perceiver. Here he considers radiophonic sound, magnetism, and electricity as basic types of stimulation that deserve further attention (see esp. 26–27).

35. It's not surprising that John Dos Passos in his famous *USA* trilogy was also preoccupied with the ways in which modernity played with illusion; reality was a construct that was altered by the world of advertising, news reports, and radio. Often the disguise of the voice misrepresented the American people, which, he claimed, he sought to portray.

36. See in particular Marcel Duchamp's "Anémic Cinéma" (1926).

37. On the literary interactions between Arlt and Joyce, see Masiello (2004).

38. See Vicuña (2006, 37) on Kardec in America. Vicuña also notes that the Chilean hero Francisco Bilbao, a liberal Mason, was often called the "first apostle of Spiritualism in South America" (129).

39. Borges was also decidedly interested in the community of readers and writers. See, for example, p. 3 of the prologue of the 1923 edition of *Fervor de Buenos Aires*: "We are all a few; our nothingnesses hardly differ." This prologue was largely suppressed in subsequent

editions; only the final paragraph in which this sentence appeared remained, although it was also rewritten.

40. Barnitz notes that Xul's turn against naturalism and materialism determined his rejection of oil as a medium (2001, 68).

41. Other theosopher-musicians of the time were also experimenting with synesthetic possibilities for the musical scale, as did, for example, the Russian pianist Alexander Scriabin, who strung chords together in consonance with intensities of light (it should be noted in this instance that Scriabin was diagnosed with "clinical" synesthesia and that his compositions were often seen less as experiments than as signs of mental confusion).

42. See H. P. Blavatsky (n.d.), "The Number Seven."

43. By 1959, Xul gave a second thought to his city in the sky. In an essay entitled "Vuel villa" (in Artundo 2006, 188–194), Xul lamented that space travel, a fantasy in earlier decades, had now become a commercial reality. Xul, however, hoped to retain the dreams of mobility by recourse to the giant helium balloons used in the late nineteenth century, and by floating spongy platforms that could serve as walkways in the sky. All the heavy materials of construction would have to remain on land. The *vuel villa*, or *villa volante*, was in 1959 on its way to becoming a reality, driven by publicity and market needs that Xul abhorred.

44. Álvaro Abós advises us not to see the flag as a sign of nationalist pride but, following the Taoist tradition, as a sign of spirituality and protection (2004, 214–215).

45. This reading is possibly influenced by another canvas by Xul, also from 1923, entitled *Drago San Jorge*.

46. For a detailed treatment of the serpent in Xul's work, see Gradowczyk (1988, 12).

47. See "Propuestas para más vida futura. Algo semitécnico sobre mejoras anatómicas y entes nuevos" (Artundo 2006, 146–151).

Chapter 4: A Politics of Perception against the State

1. A considerable bibliography on Viñas is available. See especially Astutti and Contreras (1989); Croce (2005); Rinesi et al. (2011); Roca (2007); Valverde (1989).

2. The French philosophers were similarly interested in the work of the Argentine thinkers. Sartre, in this regard, invited the *Contorno* board to edit an issue of *Les temps modernes* about literature in Argentina in which Viñas and his colleagues presented their critical work.

3. A few years later, in socialist Cuba, where the moral insistence on the "hombre masa," or the anonymous citizen-public prevailed, dissident intellectuals produced a similarly strong reaction. The censorial actions of the state against the excesses of art, the dogmatism contained in Castro's famous phrase of 1961, "within the revolution everything, beyond the revolution nothing," and Che's moralizing definition in 1965 of the socialist New Man—an ideal worker, an ideal soldier, an ideal citizen of the state, severed from individualist desires—triggered a strong reaction among Cuba's most noted writers, who then subjected the literary body to sensual hyperindulgence. From Edmundo Desnoes's *Memorias del subdesarrollo* (Memories of underdevelopment, 1967) and the neobaroque excesses of Severo Sarduy, to the later "dirty realism" that established Pedro Juan Gutiérrez as a major dissident writer in the 1990s, a sentient man lay at the center of oppositional writing. These authors tried to correct the facelessness of the Cuban citizen as defined and controlled by the state. Desnoes was the first to expose the flattened affects that anesthetized Cuban bodies. He

responded with a voice of protest: early in *Memorias del subdesarrollo*, the narrator states, "I never felt that anything might exist outside of my body" (Desnoes 1967, 30). It is notable in the filmed version of this novel (dir. Tomás Gutiérrez Alea, 1968) that David Viñas appears in a famous roundtable scene and that a book by León Rozitchner (*Moral burguesa y revolución*, 1963) finds its way into the protagonist's hands. Perhaps with these visual cues, Gutiérrez Alea supplied a key for reading the perceptual strategies of a generation that was insistent on embodied knowledge.

4. On the influence of Merleau-Ponty and Sartre in Argentina, see Eiff (2011).

5. See Oscar Masotta (1968, 33), "La fenomenología de Sartre: Un trabajo de Daniel Lagache," in *Conciencia y estructura.*

6. See especially Merleau-Ponty's *Phenomenology of Perception* (1945), translated into Spanish in 1957; his *Elogio de la filosofía* appeared in Buenos Aires in 1957, published by Galatea-Nueva Visión.

7. See Bruno Bosteels (2012) for a discussion of Rozitchner's efforts to utilize phenomenology as a way to explain the excesses of the authoritarian state (esp. chapter 5).

8. See his doctoral dissertation on Max Scheler from 1960; it was recently republished by the Argentine Biblioteca Nacional, with a useful introduction by Cristián Sucksdorf and Diego Sztulwark (Rozitchner 2013, 9–13).

9. Judith Butler (2015) recently takes this topic up in *Senses of the Subject.*

10. It is clear that Rozitchner began working on this project in the 1950s; *Contorno* advertised the future appearance of this book in its tenth issue of 1956.

11. Emilio de Ípola notes that Rozitchner's choice of Scheler for his thesis and first book was considerably influenced by Francisco Romero, a Scheler scholar and chair of the Institute of Philosophy at the University of Buenos Aires, where Rozitchner was employed at the time. From the author's personal correspondence with de Ípola, September 2015.

12. For a similar view of the issues that Rozitchner raises, see Bosteels (2012, 142–144).

13. A handsome bibliography on Masotta exists: see especially Correas (2007); Scholten (2001); Giordano (2005).

14. See Hernán Scholten (2001) regarding the Sartrean influence in Masotta's study of Arlt. See also Nora Avaro and Analía Capdevila (1989), and Nicolás Rosa (1989) for more on this topic.

15. Nicolás Rosa expands on Masotta's reading of Arlt: "Between the reality of the world and consciousness, Arlt's characters place their own bodies, separated at once from the world and consciousness; in other words, they are inert. No one accepts that body as an immediate reality; rather, these characters watch ... over the life that the body lives. They measure it, they weigh it (there are constant references to weight in Arlt's novels), they observe it as it lives outside of consciousness, like a separate entity, as if biological life were to be contaminated by metaphysics.... The body 'is' the limit" (1989, 40). Carlos Correas writes also, "With Masotta, we tried to invent a new type of intellectual: materialists ideologically open to their own materialism" (2007, 58). Correas adds that this materialist focus served, on the one hand, to combat the abstractions of spirit of the kind that Victoria Ocampo had defended in the pages of *Sur* and, on the other, to challenge the effects of Perón's reforms for anonymous masses. It is no surprise, then, that Arlt would capture Masotta's attention.

16. On Lacan, see Masotta's (1980) posthumous *El modelo pulsional.*

17. For essential discussions of the Di Tella Institute, see Andrea Giunta (2001); Inés Katzenstein (2004); John King (1985); Jorge Romero Brest (1992); and the essays and lec-

tures by Oscar Masotta (2004) on pop art and happenings, many of these focusing on the Di Tella.

18. On this see Mario Cámara (2014, 52–55).

19. See Giunta (2001, 176n32).

20. Praising the reach of Minujín's project, Masotta was beginning to compare the direct experience of the happening to new mediatic proposals that were on the horizon: "[T]he 'material' of the Happening, the very stuff of which a Happening is made, would be closer to the sensible while the 'material' of works produced on the level of the mass media would be more immaterial ... though no less concrete" (2004, 201–202).

21. On Costa's sound tapes, see McEnaney (2016). Consider also the immaterial art proposed by Roberto Jacoby as part of his long-term defense of medial art and new technology. Against the physicality of the happening, for example, Jacoby planned staged events at which there was absolutely nothing to be seen. Sensorial contact for Jacoby was experienced in the art of networks, inviting viewers to think of mergers and flows, and effacing boundaries between feelings and form (on this see Jacoby 2011).

22. See especially Masotta's essay "Después del Pop: Nosotros desmaterializamos" (After pop we dematerialize) (2004, 218–440).

23. See Vindel (2010) for a reflection on the intersection of politics and avant-garde art in Argentina of the 1960s.

24. See Beatriz Sarlo in *King* (1985, 304).

25. The Di Tella's exhibition *Experiencias* (1967–1968), and in particular the installation by Roberto Plate on public urinals, inspired the anger of military officials and led to an intervention in 1968. Many artists subsequently retreated into exile. The Di Tella theatrical programs lasted until a final closure in 1970, although it should be noted that the social science and research branch of the institute remained open and later became the University Di Tella, which is still active today.

26. From author's personal correspondence with John King, March 8, 2017.

27. See the exhibition catalogue edited by Gabriela Rangel (2007).

28. From "Farewell." Amichai quoted from translation by Chana Kronfeld (2016, 5).

29. Luigi Vallebona (2013) makes a case for Merleau-Ponty's influence on Saer, especially in his novel *Glosa*.

30. I allude to the title of one of Saer's (1997) more famous essays, "Una literatura sin atributos," whose title plays on one from Robert Musil.

31. In an interview with Gerard de Cortanze, Saer reflects on the relationship between writing and bodies: "Writing, in the graphological sense, perfectly individualized, carries the marks of the body. And that body, whose countless signs can be carried in the traces of writing, [is] deposited little by little, across the years, in the work that is, in terms of the old Latin name that we use, a corpus. To write is thus a translation of what happens, through time, from one body to another" (Saer 1997, 298).

32. On the importance of Echeverría's story for Saer's novel, see Isabel Quintana (2001, 123).

33. Beatriz Sarlo is arguably the first critic who noted the importance of perceptions at the center of Saer's literary fictions; on this, see her "Narrar la percepción" (1980). Following her lead, others have paid attention, more generally, to the role of experience in the novels of Saer (see Garramuño 2009; Premat 2002; Quintana 2001). For a new reading of Saer, see Sarlo (2016).

34. The recent attention to touch is in part a way to dismantle the authority of the visual, in part to reinstall the full body as a perceptual organ. See Classen (2012); Connor (2004b); Deleuze and Guattari (1987); Heller-Roazen (2007); Maurette (2015); Nancy (2008); and Serres (2008).

35. See Martin Heidegger, "What Are Poets For?" (1975, 91–142).

36. "I feel you, I touch you, and the tips of my fingers seek / yours ... my fingers feel their way around to reach yours because if I / touch you and you touch me perhaps then not all is lost" (my translation).

37. On the materiality of Zurita's land art, see Juan Soros (2011).

38. The choice of the word *sorprendentes*—surprising—takes us to a quotidian level that is incommensurate with the horror observed. Though in their respective translations, Rowe uses both "surprising" and "strange," and Deeny Morales sticks with the option of "strange" (and thereby alludes to the song, made famous by Billie Holliday, about the "strange fruit" of lynchings), Zurita's use of *sorprendentes* introduces a level of irony that gives the poem a purposeful banality, playing off the public's frequent blindness and ignorance of Pinochet's terror.

39. "The sea, it says the sea. It says baits with clear / days stuck to them, with loves that were never / said. / The sea, it says the sea. It says baits that rain and / clear days stuck to them, it says unfinished / loves" (Zurita 2009a, 7).

40. "[Y]ou can hear whole days sinking, strange sunny / mornings, unfinished loves, goodbyes cut short / that sink into the sea" (Zurita 2009a, 8).

41. "I heard a sea and a sky hallucinated, I heard suns / exploding with love fall like fruits, I heard / whirlwinds of fish devouring the pink flesh of surprising baits" (2009a, 9).

42. "There is the sea in flames" (Zurita 2009a, 15).

43. "You are earth and death ... you are only pain, you carry it in your eyes / and blood, but you don't feel it. You live like a stone, like the hardened earth and dreams, movements, and sighs approach you that you ignore" (my translation).

44. "Language is the site of permanent resurrection," Zurita claims (2016b).

45. Guillermo Núñez, "Don't ask me to paint flowers," in *La quinta del sordo* (2003, n.p.).

46. Quoted in Gaspar Galaz's prologue to Núñez (2003, n.p.).

47. Legend has it that Goya lost his hearing when he went to paint at his country house, or *quinta*, outside of Madrid; there, he executed his "Black Paintings," the most notable of which is probably *Saturn Devouring His Son*, a canvas that surely inspired Núñez in expressing the darkness of Pinochet's regime.

Chapter 5: By Way of a Conclusion

1. See Florencia Garramuño, who addresses the work of Nuno Ramos at length and signals the fluidity of materials that tend to efface all borders (2015, 160–161).

2. We learn from the artist's notes on his website that these objects that resemble stereo speakers are in fact made of compressed sand, glass, and welded metal.

3. Cavaquinho's lyrics begin: "A luz negra de um destino cruel / Ilumina o teatro sem cor" (The black light of cruel destiny / Illuminates a heartless theater).

4. From a different perspective, Natalia Brizuela attends to the awakening of the sensible body as a route to political readings when she writes about Nuno Ramos's installation

"111" (2014, 197). The awakening in *Luz negra*, however, takes us in a different direction, paradoxically going beyond an actively sensible body and leaving only sound.

5. See also the online journal *Leonardo Electronic Almanac* for further interventions about recent bio art.

6. See Eduardo Kac's *Ornitorrinco*, a series of telepresence events that began in 1990 (Kac 1996).

7. Kac writes of his genre: "Holopoetry defines a new domain of poetic exploration where the text is written with the malleable medium of light, where the word is free from surface constraints, where textuality is signifiers in motion. In a holopoem, the verbal phenomenon cannot be dissociated from the spatiotemporal environment of the optical and synthetic hologram" (Kac n.d.).

Works Cited

Abós, Álvaro. 2004. *Xul Solar: Pintor del misterio*. Buenos Aires: Sudamericana.

Abraham, Carlos. 2014. "Raimunda Torres y Quiroga: Una desconocida autora de literatura fantástica en el siglo XIX." *Brumal* 2, no. 3: 127–147.

Acree, William Garrett. 2011. *Everyday Reading: Print Culture and Collective Identity in the Río de la Plata, 1780–1910*. Nashville, TN: Vanderbilt University Press.

———. 2013. "Divisas and Deberes: Women and the Symbolic Economy of War Rhetoric in the Río de la Plata, 1810–1910." *Journal of Latin American Cultural Studies: Travesía* 22, no. 2: 213–237.

Adorno, Theodor. 1974. *Minima Moralia: Reflections from Damaged Life*. Translated by E. F. N. Jephcott. London: Verso.

———. 2005. *In Search of Wagner*. Translated by Rodney Livingstone. London: Verso.

Alberdi, Juan Bautista. 1876. *La vida y los trabajos industriales de William Wheelwright en la América del Sud*. Paris: Garnier.

———. 1886. "Fragmento preliminar al estudio del derecho." In *Obras completas de Juan Bautista Alberdi*, 1:99–256. Buenos Aires: La Tribuna. First published 1837.

———. 1900. *Escritos póstumos de J. B. Alberdi: Memorias y documentos*. Vol. 15. Edited by Francisco Cruz. Buenos Aires: J. B. Alberdi.

Alcorta, Diego. 2001. *Lecciones de filosofía*. Foreword by Paul Groussac. Edited and with notes by Santiago Kovadloff. Buenos Aires: Fondo Nacional de las Artes.

Alemán, Jesse, and Shelley Streeby, eds. 2007. *Empire and the Literature of Sensation*. New Brunswick, NJ: Rutgers University Press.

Alexander, Abel, ed. 2005. *La fotografía en la historia argentina*. Buenos Aires: Clarín.

"A los que se oponen a la instrucción de las mujeres." 1830. *La aljaba*, no. 4 (Nov. 26): 1.

Amante, Adriana, ed. 2012. *Historia crítica de la literatura argentina*, vol. 4, *Sarmiento*. Buenos Aires: Emecé.

Andermann, Jens. 2007. *The Optic of the State: Visuality and Power in Argentina and Brazil*. Pittsburgh, PA: University of Pittsburgh Press.

Anderson, Benedict. 1983. *Imagined Communities: Reflections on the Origin and Spread of Nationalism*. London: Verso.

Arlt, Roberto. 1969. *El juguete rabioso*. Edited by Mirta Arlt. Buenos Aires: Mirasol.

———. 1978. *Los siete locos; Los lanzallamas*. Edited by Adolfo Prieto. Caracas: Ayacucho.

———. 1981. "Las ciencias ocultas en la ciudad de Buenos Aires." In *Obra completa*, 2:9–35. Buenos Aires: Carlos Lohlé. First published 1920.

Artundo, Patricia M., ed. 2006. *Alejandro Xul Solar: Entrevistas, artículos y textos inéditos.* Buenos Aires: Corregidor.

Astutti, Adriana, and Sandra Contreras. 1989. "Entregarse a la literatura: David Viñas." In Rosa et al. 1989, 3–21.

Aulicino, Jorge. 2011. *Libro del engaño y del desengaño.* Buenos Aires: Ediciones en Danza.

Avaro, Nora, and Analía Capdevila. 1989. "Un Ensayo Político (A propósito de *Sexo y traición en Roberto Arlt*)." In Rosa ct al. 1989, 22–30.

Bacle, César Hipólito. 1947. "Extravagancias de 1834." In *Trages y costumbres de la provincia de Buenos Aires; 36 litografías coloreadas*, cuaderno 5, nos. 1, 5. Facsimile edition. Foreword by Alejo González Garaño. Buenos Aires: Viau. First published 1833.

Badiou, Alain. 2007. *The Century*. Translated by Alberto Toscano. Cambridge, UK: Polity.

Baldwin, James. 1955. "Everybody's Protest Novel." In *Notes of a Native Son*. Boston: Beacon. First published 1949.

Ballesteros, Diego. 2013. *Los espacios de la antropología en la obra de Robert Lehmann-Nitsche, 1894–1938*. PhD diss., University of Buenos Aires.

Banga, Fabián. 2016. *Brujos, espiritistas y vanguardistas: Arlt, Huidobro y Valle Inclán.* Foreword by Francine Masiello. Buenos Aires: Leviatán.

Barker-Benfield, G. J. 1992. *The Culture of Sensibility: Sex and Society in Eighteenth-Century Britain.* Chicago: University of Chicago Press.

Barnitz, Jacqueline. 2001. *Twentieth-Century Art of Latin America.* Austin: University of Texas Press.

Barrán, José Pedro. 1990. *Historia de la sensibilidad en el Uruguay.* 2 vols. Montevideo: Ediciones de la Banda Oriental.

Barthes, Roland. 1978. "The Grain of the Voice." In *Image, Music, Text*, 172–189. Translated by Stephen Heath. New York: Hill and Wang. First published 1972.

———. 1989. "The Reality Effect." In *The Rustle of Language*, 141–148. Translated by Richard Howard. Berkeley: University of California Press. First published 1968.

Bates, David. 2012. *States of War: Enlightenment Origins of the Political.* New York: Columbia University Press.

Batticuore, Graciela, Klaus Gallo, and Jorge Myers, eds. 2005. *Resonancias románticas: Ensayos sobre historia de la cultura argentina (1820–1890).* Buenos Aires: Eudeba.

Baudelaire, Charles. 1995. "The Painter of Modern Life." In *The Painter of Modern Life and Other Essays*, 1–41. Translated by Jonathan Mayne. New York: Phaidon.

Beecher, Catherine. 1831. *Elements of Mental and Moral Philosophy Founded upon Experience, Reason, and the Bible.* Hartford, CT: Peter B. Gleason.

Beecher, Catherine, and Harriet Beecher Stowe. 1987. *The American Home; or, Principles of Domestic Science.* Introduction by Joseph Van Why. Hartford, CT: Stowe-Day Foundation. First published 1869.

Belgrano, Manuel. 2007. "Metafísica." In Chiaramonte 2007b, 6–8.

Benjamin, Walter. 1979. *One-Way Street and Other Writings.* Translated by Edmund Jephcott and Kingsley Shorter. London: New Left Books. First published 1928.

———. 2005. "Experience and Poverty." In *Walter Benjamin: Selected Writings, Volume 2: Part 2, 1931–1934*, edited by Michael W. Jennings, Howard Eiland, and Gary Smith, 731–736. Cambridge, MA: Harvard University Press. First published 1933.

———. 2006. "On Some Motifs in Baudelaire." In *The Writer of Modern Life*, edited by Michael W. Jennings and translated by Howard Eiland, Edmund Jephcott, Rodney Livingstone, and Harry Zohn, 170–210. Cambridge, MA: Harvard University Press. First published 1939.

Bennett, Jane. 2010. *Vibrant Matter: A Political Ecology of Things*. Durham, NC: Duke University Press.

Bentley, Nancy. 2009. *Frantic Panoramas: American Literature and Mass Culture, 1870–1920*. Philadelphia: University of Pennsylvania Press.

Berger, John. 2001. *The Shape of a Pocket*. New York: Vintage.

Bergmann, Emilie, Janet Greenberg, Gwen Kirkpatrick, Francine Masiello, Francesca Miller, Marta Morello-Frosch, Kathleen Newman, and Mary Louise Pratt. 1990. *Women, Culture, and Politics in Latin America*. Seminar on Feminism and Culture. Berkeley: University of California Press.

Bergson, Henri. 2008. *Materiality and Memory*. Translated by N. M. Paul and W. S. Palmer. Cambridge, MA: MIT Press. First published 1896.

Berlant, Lauren, ed. 2004. *Compassion: The Culture and Politics of an Emotion*. New York: Routledge.

Best, Stephen, and Sharon Marcus. 2009. "Surface Reading: An Introduction." *Representations* 108, no. 1 (Fall): 1–21.

Blavatsky, H. P. n.d. "The Number Seven." http://www.blavatsky.net/index.php/17-hpblavatsky/hpb-articles/175-number-seven. First published 1880.

Blom, Ina. 2011. "Raoul Hausmann, Nam June Paik, and the Transmission of New Technologies of the Avant-Garde." *Leonardo Electronic Almanac* 34, no. 3: 209–216.

Bolet Peraza, Nicolás. 1896. "La mujer en los Estados Unidos." *Búcaro americano* 1, no. 7 (June 1): 140–143.

Borges, Jorge Luis. 1923. *Fervor de Buenos Aires*. Buenos Aires: Serrantes.

———. 1925. "La nadería de la personalidad." In *Inquisiciones*, 84–95. Buenos Aires: El Inca.

Bosteels, Bruno. 2012. *Marx and Freud in Latin America: Politics, Psychoanalysis, and Religion in Times of Terror*. New York: Verso.

Bratu Hansen, Miriam. 2008. "Benjamin's Aura." *Critical Inquiry* 34 (Winter): 336–375.

Breitweiser, Mitchell. 2007. *National Melancholy: Mourning and Opportunity in Classic American Literature*. Stanford, CA: Stanford University Press.

Brizuela, Natalia. 2014. *Depois da fotografia: Uma literatura fora de si*. Rio de Janeiro: Rocca.

Brown, Bill. 2003. *A Sense of Things: The Object Matter of American Literature*. Chicago: University of Chicago Press.

Bruno, Giuliana. 2002. *The Atlas of Emotion: Journeys in Art, Architecture, and Film*. New York: Verso.

———. 2014. *Surface: Matters of Aesthetics, Materiality, and Media*. Chicago: University of Chicago Press.

Buch, Tomás, and Carlos E. Solivérez. 2011. *De los quipus a los satélites: Historia de la tecnología en la Argentina*. Buenos Aires: Universidad Nacional de Quilmes.

Budd, Mike, ed. 1990. *The Cabinet of Dr. Caligari: Texts, Contexts, Histories*. New Brunswick, NJ: Rutgers University Press.

Budgen, Frank. 1960. *James Joyce and the Making of "Ulysses."* Bloomington: Indiana University Press. First published 1934.

Burstein, Andrew. 1999. *Sentimental Democracy: The Evolution of America's Romantic Self-Image*. New York: Hill and Wang.

Butler, Judith. 2015. *Senses of the Subject*. New York: Fordham University Press.

Cabello de Carbonera, Mercedes. 1896. "Párrafos sueltos." *Búcaro americano* 1, no. 3 (March): 54–56.

Cámara, Mario. 2014. *Corpos pagãos: Usos e figuracões na cultura brasileira (1960–1980)*. Belo Horizonte: Editora UFMG.

Cameron, Sharon. 1981. *The Corporeal Self: Allegories of the Body in Melville and Hawthorne*. Baltimore, MD: Johns Hopkins University Press.

Carrera, Arturo. 2004. *Tratado de sensaciones*. Valencia: Pre-Textos.

Castro Gómez, Santiago, ed. 2004. *Pensar el siglo XIX: Cultura, biopolítica y modernidad en Colombia*. Pittsburgh, PA: Biblioteca de América.

Catanzaro, Gisela. 2011. *La nación entre naturaleza e historia; Sobre los modos de la crítica*. Buenos Aires: Fondo de Cultura Económica.

Cavarero, Adriana. 2005. *For More Than One Voice: Toward a Philosophy of Vocal Expression*. Stanford, CA: Stanford University Press.

Chapelle Wojciehowski, Hannah, and Vittorio Gallese. 2011. "How Stories Make Us Feel: Toward an Embodied Narratology." *California Italian Studies* 2, no. 1: 12–35.

Chapman, Mary, and Glenn Hendler, eds. 1999. *Sentimental Men: Masculinity and the Politics of Affect in American Culture*. Berkeley: University of California Press.

Charvat, William. 1936. "The Origins of American Critical Thought, 1810–1835." PhD diss., University of Pennsylvania.

Chiaramonte, José Carlos. 2007a. *La ilustración en el Río de la Plata: Cultura eclesíastica y cultura laíca durante el virreinato*. Buenos Aires: Sudamericana.

———. 2007b. *Ciudades, provincias, estados: Orígenes de la nación Argentina, 1800–1846*, vol. 1, *Documentos*. Buenos Aires: Emecé.

Chorroarín, Luis José. 1911. *La enseñanza de la filosofía en la época colonial*. Spanish version of the first part of the "Institutiones philosophiae," 1–171. Notes dictated in Latin by Doctor L. J. Chorroarín in the Real Colegio de San Carlos in Buenos Aires in 1783. Spanish translation and introduction by Juan Chiabra. Buenos Aires: Coni Hermanos.

"Ciencias." 1822. *La abeja argentina*, no. 6 (Sept. 15): 242–248.

Classen, Constance. 2012. *The Deepest Sense: A Cultural History of Touch*. Urbana: University of Illinois Press.

Clayton, Michelle. 2011. *Poetry in Pieces: César Vallejo and Lyric Modernity*. Berkeley: University of California Press.

Cohen, Margaret. 1999. *The Sentimental Education of the Novel*. Princeton, NJ: Princeton University Press.

Comisión Nacional sobre la Desaparición de Personas. 1986. *Nunca Más: The Report of the Argentine National Commission on the Disappeared*. Introduction by Ronald Dworkin. New York: Farrar, Straus, and Giroux. First published 1984.

Connor, Steven. 2004a. "Intersensoriality." Lecture given at Conference on the Senses, Thames Valley University, Aug. 11. http://stevenconnor.com/intersensoriality.html.

———. 2004b. *The Book of Skin*. Ithaca, NY: Cornell University Press.

Contreras, Sandra. 2012. "*Facundo*: La forma de la narración." In Amante 2012, 67–93.

Coronado, Raul. 2014. *A World Not to Come*. Cambridge, MA: Harvard University Press.

Correas, Carlos. 2007. *La operación Masotta: Cuando la muerte también fracasa*. Buenos Aires: Interzona. First published 1991.

Cortázar, Julio. 2000. *Rayuela*. Madrid: Cátedra. First published 1963.

Crary, Jonathan. 1990. *Techniques of the Observer: On Vision and Modernity in the Nineteenth Century*. Cambridge, MA: MIT Press.

———. 1999. *Suspensions of Perception: Attention, Spectacle, and Modern Culture*. Cambridge, MA: MIT Press.

Croce, Marcela. 2005. *David Viñas: Crítica de la razón polémica*. Buenos Aires: Suricata.

Danto, Arthur C. 2013. "The Body in Philosophy and Art." In *What Art Is*, 76–98. New Haven, CT: Yale University Press.

Darwin, Charles. 1873. *The Expression of the Emotions in Man and Animals*. New York: Appleton. First published 1872.

Debord, Guy. 1990. *The Society of the Spectacle*. Translated by Donald Nicholson-Smith. New York: Swerve.

Delannoy, Luc. 2015. *Neuroartes, un laboratorio de ideas*. Santiago de Chile: Metales Pesados.

Delbanco, Andrew. 2005. *Melville: His World and Work*. New York: Knopf.

———. 2012. *The Abolitionist Imagination*. Cambridge, MA: Harvard University Press.

"Del discurso al Dr. Carta." 1827. *Crónica política y literaria de Buenos Aires*, no. 57 (July 20): n.p.

Deleuze, Gilles. 1992. *Expressionism in Philosophy: Spinoza*. Translated by Martin Joughin. New York: Zone Books.

Deleuze, Gilles, and Félix Guattari. 1987. *A Thousand Plateaus: Capitalism and Schizophrenia*. Translated by Brian Massumi. Minneapolis: University of Minnesota Press.

Desnoes, Edmundo. 1967. *Memorias del subdesarrollo*. Mexico City: Joaquin Mortiz.

Destutt de Tracy, Antoine. 1817. *A Treatise on Political Economy: To Which Is Prefixed a Supplement to a Preceding Work on the Understanding; or, Elements of Ideology*. Edited and with a prospectus by Thomas Jefferson. Georgetown, DC: Joseph Milligan.

de Torre, Guillermo. 1925. *Literaturas europeas de vanguardia*. Madrid: Caro Raggio.

———. 1965. *Historia de las literaturas de vanguardia*. Madrid: Guadarrama.

———. 2002. *Literaturas europeas de vanguardia*. Edited by José Luis Calvo Carilla. Mutilva Baja, Spain: Urgoiti.

Díaz Quiñones, Arcadio. 2006. "Fernando Ortiz (1881–1969) y Allan Kardec (1804–1869): Espiritismo y transculturación." In *Sobre los principios: Los intelectuales caribeños y la tradición*, 289–317. Buenos Aires: Universidad Nacional de Quilmes.

Didi-Huberman, Georges. 2008. *Images in Spite of All: Four Photographs from Auschwitz*. Translated by Shane B. Lillis. Chicago: University of Chicago Press.

Dinah. 2007. "Editorial: San Jorge." *Quilombo, cultura afro* (Buenos Aires), no. 22 (April). http://www.revistaquilombo.com.ar/revistas/22/q22.htm.

Donguy, Jacques. 2001. "Machine Head: Raoul Haussmann and the Optophone." *Leonardo Electronic Almanac* 34, no. 3: 217–220.

Dotti, Jorge. 1990. *Las vetas del texto: Una lectura filosófica de Alberdi, los positivistas, Juan B. Justo*. Buenos Aires: Puntosur.

Douglas, Ann. 1976. *The Feminization of American Culture*. New York: Knopf.

Eagleton, Terry. 1990. *The Ideology of the Aesthetic*. Oxford: Blackwell.

Echeverría, Esteban. 1870–1874. *Obras completas*. 5 vols. Edited by Juan María Gutiérrez. Buenos Aires: Carlos Casavalle.

———. 1991. *Obras escogidas*. Edited by Beatriz Sarlo and Carlos Altamirano. Caracas: Biblioteca Ayacucho.

Edwards, Erin E. 2009. "Extremities of the Body: The Anoptic Corporeality of *As I Lay Dying*." *Modern Fiction Studies* 55, no. 4 (Winter): 716–738.

Eiff, Leonardo. 2011. *Filosofía y política existencial: Merleau-Ponty, Sartre y los debates argentinos*. Buenos Aires: Universidad Nacional de General Sarmiento.

Ellis, Markman. 1996. *The Politics of Sensibility: Race, Gender, and Commerce in the Sentimental Novel*. New York: Cambridge University Press.

El telégrafo mercantil. 1801. Editorial. *El telégrafo mercantil* 1, no. 1 (Apr. 1): 3.

Eltit, Diamela. 2013. *Fuerzas especiales*. Santiago de Chile: Planeta.

Epplin, Craig. 2014. *Late Book Culture in Argentina*. New York: Bloomsbury.

Epstein, Jean. 1921. *La poésie d'aujourd'hui: Un nouvel état d'intelligence*. Paris: Editions de la Sirène.

———. 1988. "Magnification." In *French Film Theory and Criticism: A History/Anthology, 1907–1939*, vol. 1, edited by Richard Abel, 235–241. Princeton, NJ: Princeton University Press.

Evans, Brad, and Henry Giroux. 2015. *Disposable Futures: The Seduction of Violence in the Age of the Spectacle*. San Francisco: City Lights.

"Experimentos que pueden hacerse con el aparato de la radio." 1928. *El hogar*, July 27.

Fernández Moreno, César. 1967. *La realidad y los papeles*. Madrid: Aguilar.

Ferreira, Rocío. 2005. "La profesionalización de la periodista y escritora: Clorinda Matto de Turner obrera del pensamiento." In *Obras completas de Clorinda Matto de Turner*, edited by Antonio Cornejo Polar, 2:103–129. Lima: Latinoamericana Editores.

Fiering, Norman. 1981. *Moral Philosophy at Seventeenth-Century Harvard: A Discipline in Transition*. Chapel Hill: University of North Carolina Press.

Fijman, Jacobo. 1926. *Molino rojo*. Buenos Aires: El Inca.

Fliegelman, Jay. 1993. *Jefferson, Natural Language, and the Culture of Performance*. Stanford, CA: Stanford University Press.

Foucault, Michel. 1973. *The Order of Things: An Archaeology of the Human Sciences*. New York: Vintage. First published 1966.

———. 1995. *Discipline and Punish: The Birth of the Prison*. Translated by Alan Sheridan. New York: Vintage Books. First published 1979.

———. 2003. *"Society Must Be Defended": Lectures at the Collège de France, 1975–76*. Edited by Mauro Bertani and Alessandro Fontana and translated by David Macey. New York: Picador.

Franco, Jean. 2013. *Cruel Modernity*. Durham, NC: Duke University Press.

Fulkerson, Matthew. 2014. *The First Sense: A Philosophical Study of the Human Touch*. Cambridge, MA: MIT Press.

Gallagher, Catherine. 2006. *The Body Economic: Life, Death, and Sensation in Political Economy and the Victorian Novel*. Princeton, NJ: Princeton University Press.

Gallo, Klaus. 2006. *The Struggle for an Enlightened Republic: Buenos Aires and Rivadavia*. London: Institute for the Study of the Americas.

———. 2009. *El pensamiento de Esteban Echeverría*. Buenos Aires: El Ateneo.

Gammack, John G. 2002. "Synaesthesia and Knowing." In *Language, Vision, and Music*, edited by Paul McKevitt, Seán Ó Nualláin, and Conn Mulvihill, 157–170. Philadelphia, PA: John Benjamins.

Garramuño, Florencia. 2009. *La experiencia opaca: Literatura y desencanto*. Buenos Aires: Fondo de Cultura Económica.

———. 2015. *Mundos en común: Ensayos sobre la inespecificidad en el arte*. Buenos Aires: Fondo de Cultura Económica.

Gates, Henry Louis, Jr. 2007. "*Uncle Tom's Cabin* and 'The Man That Was a Thing.'" In *The Annotated "Uncle Tom's Cabin,"* by Harriet Beecher Stowe, edited by Henry Louis Gates Jr. and Hollis Robbins, xxxi–xlvii. New York: Norton.

Gay, Peter. 1984. *The Bourgeois Experience: Education of the Senses*. Vol. 1. New York: Oxford University Press.

Gikandi, Simon. 2011. *Slavery and the Culture of Taste*. Princeton, NJ: Princeton University Press.

Gilbert, Sandra M., and Susan Gubar. 1979. *The Madwoman in the Attic: The Woman Writer and the Nineteenth-Century Literary Imagination*. New Haven, CT: Yale University Press.

Giordano, Alberto. 2005. *Modos del ensayo: De Borges a Piglia*. Rosario: Beatriz Viterbo.

Giorgi, Gabriel. 2004. *Sueños de exterminio*. Rosario, Argentina: Beatriz Viterbo.

Girondo, Oliverio. 1999. *Obra completa*. Edited by Raúl Antelo. Nanterre: Colección Archivos.

Giunta, Andrea. 2001. *Vanguardia, internacionalismo y política: Arte argentino en los años sesenta*. Buenos Aires: Paidós.

———. 2004. "Rewriting Modernism: Jorge Romero Brest and the Legitimation of Argentine Art." In Katzenstein 2004, 78–92.

Goll, Ivan. 1922. *Les cinq continents: Anthologie mondiale de poésie contemporaine*. Paris: La Renaissance du Livre.

Gómez de Avellaneda, Gertrudis. 1993. *"Sab" and Autobiography*. Translated and edited by Nina M. Scott. Austin: University of Texas Press.

Gómez, Leila, and Sara Castro-Klarén, eds. 2012. *Entre Borges y Conrad: Estética y territorio en William Henry Hudson*. Madrid: Vervuert.

Gopnick, Adam. 2016. "Feel Me: What the New Science of Touch Says about Ourselves." *New Yorker* (May 16), 56–66.

Gorriti, Juana Manuela. 1977. *Cocina ecléctica*. Buenos Aires: Librería Sarmiento.

———. 2003. *Dreams and Realities: Selected Fiction*. Foreword by Francine Masiello. Translated by Sergio Waisman. New York: Oxford University Press.

———. 2004. *Cincuenta y tres cartas inéditas a Ricardo Palma*. Edited by Graciela Batticuore. Lima: San Martín de Porres.

Gradowczyk, Mario H. 1988. *Alejandro Xul Solar (1887–1963)*. Buenos Aires: Anzilotti.

Groussac, Paul. 1918. "El Doctor Diego Alcorta." In *Estudios de historia argentina*, 131–259. Buenos Aires: Jesús Menéndez.

Gumbrecht, Hans Urlich. 2014. *Our Broad Present: Time and Contemporary Culture*. New York: Columbia University Press.

Gunning, Tom. 2004. "An Aesthetic of Astonishment: Early Film and the (In)Credulous Spectator." In *Film Theory: Critical Concepts in Media and Cultural Studies*, edited by Philip Simpson, Andrew Utterson, and K. J. Shepherdson, 78–94. New York: Routledge.

Gutiérrez, Juan María. 1874. "Noticias biográficas sobre la vida de don Estéban Echeverría." In Echeverría 1870–1874, 5:i–ci.

Hallstead, Susan R., and Regina A. Root, eds. 2017. *Pasado de moda: Expresiones culturales y consumo en la Argentina*. Buenos Aires: Ampersand.

Halperin Donghi, Tulio. 1951. *El pensamiento de Esteban Echeverría*. Buenos Aires: Sudamericana.

———. 1988. *Tradición política española e ideología revolucionaria de mayo*. Buenos Aires: Centro Editor de América Latina.

———. 1998. "Prólogo: Sarmiento." In Sarmiento 1998, 9–53.

———. 2002. *Revolución y guerra: Formación de una élite dirigente en la Argentina criolloa.* Buenos Aires: Siglo XXI.

———. 2014. *El enigma Belgrano: Un héroe para nuestro tiempo.* Buenos Aires: Siglo XXI.

Halperin Donghi, Tulio, Ivan Jaksic, Gwen Kirkpatrick, and Francine Masiello, eds. 1994. *Sarmiento: Author of a Nation.* Berkeley: University of California Press.

Hansen, Mark. 2000. *Embodying Technesis: Technology Beyond Writing.* Ann Arbor: University of Michigan Press.

Hardt, Michael, and Antonio Negri. 2000. *Empire.* Cambridge, MA: Harvard University Press.

Harris, William W. 1835. "Virginia University Notebooks of William W. Harris of Nelson County, on Courses in Mental Philosophy under Professor George Tucker and in Chemistry under Professor John Patten Emmet." Accession no. 3780, Special Collections, University of Virginia Library, University of Virginia, Charlottesville.

Hartman, Saidiya. 1997. *Scenes of Subjection: Terror, Slavery, and Self-Making in the Nineteenth Century.* New York: Oxford University Press.

Hausmann, Raoul. n.d. "Optophonemes (1962)." UbuWeb. http://www.ubu.com/sound/hausmann.html.

Hayles, N. Katherine. 1999. *How We Became Posthuman: Virtual Bodies in Cybernetics, Literature, and Informatics.* Chicago: University of Chicago Press.

Heidegger, Martin. 1975. "What Are Poets For?" In *Poetry, Language, Thought,* 91–142. Translated by Albert Hofstadter. New York: Harper and Row. First published 1971.

Heller-Roazen, Daniel. 2007. *The Inner Touch: Archaeology of a Sensation.* New York: Zone Books.

Henríquez Ureña, Pedro. 1926. "La civilización manual." *Babel* 20 (August): n.p.

Herr, Richard. 1958. *The Eighteenth-Century Revolution in Spain.* Princeton, NJ: Princeton University Press.

Hirschman, Albert O. 1997. *The Passions and the Interests: Political Arguments for Capitalism before Its Triumph.* Princeton, NJ: Princeton University Press.

Howes, David, ed. 1991. *The Varieties of Sensory Experience: A Sourcebook in the Anthropology of the Senses.* Toronto: University of Toronto Press.

———, ed. 2005. *Empire of the Senses: The Sensual Cultural Reader.* New York: Berg.

Hubbard, Robert Thurston. 1828. "Notes in Moral Philosophy Class at University of Virginia and Initialled by George Tucker" (October 2). Accession no. 7093-1, Special Collections, University of Virginia Library, University of Virginia, Charlottesville.

Hudson, William Henry. 1949. *The Purple Land: Being the Narrative of One Richard Lamb's Adventures in the Banda Oriental in South America, As Told by Himself.* London: Gerald Duckworth. First published 1927.

———. 2006. *Idle Days in Patagonia.* Middlesex, UK: Echo. First published 1893.

Hugo, Victor. 1909. "Preface to Cromwell." In *Prefaces and Prologues,* 39:354–408. New York: P. F. Collier. First published 1827.

Huidobro, Vicente. 1942. *Cagliostro: Novela-film.* Santiago de Chile: Zig-Zag. First published 1923.

———. 1981. *Altazor; Temblor del cielo.* Introduction and notes by René de Costa. Madrid: Catédra.

"Ilustración de la mujer: Filosofía." 1854. *Album de señoritas,* no. 6 (Feb. 5): 42–43.

Jacoby, Roberto. 2011. *El deseo nace del derrumbe: Acciones, conceptos, escritos*. Edited by Ana Longoni. Barcelona: Ediciones de La Central–Museo Reina Sofía.

Jaksic, Ivan. 1989. *Academic Rebels in Chile: The Role of Philosophy in Higher Education and Politics*. Albany: State University of New York Press.

James, William. 1918. *The Principles of Psychology*. Vol. 1. New York: Dover. First published 1890.

———. 1985. *The Varieties of Religious Experience: A Study in Human Nature*. Introduction by John E. Smith. Cambridge, MA: Harvard University Press. First published 1902.

Jameson, Fredric. 1991. *Postmodernism; or, The Cultural Logic of Late Capitalism*. Durham, NC: Duke University Press.

———. 2013. *The Antinomies of Realism*. New York: Verso.

Jay, Martin. 1993. *Downcast Eyes: The Denigration of Vision in Twentieth-Century French Thought*. Berkeley: University of California Press.

———. 2003. "Somaesthetics and Democracy: John Dewey and Contemporary Body Art." In *Refractions of Violence*, 163–176. Abingdon, UK: Routledge.

———. 2005. *Songs of Experience: Modern American and European Variations on a Universal Theme*. Berkeley: University of California Press.

Jay, Martin, and Sumathi Ramaswamy, eds. 2014. *Empires of Vision: A Reader*. Durham, NC: Duke University Press.

Jiménez, Félix. 2013. *Audioeuforia: Fonografías e interferencias*. Carolina, Puerto Rico: Terranova Editores. Kindle edition.

Jitrik, Noé. 1967. *Esteban Echeverría*. Buenos Aires: Centro Editor.

———. 1971. *El fuego de la especie*. Buenos Aires: Siglo Veintiuno.

Joyce, James. 1986. *Ulysses*. Edited by Hans Walter Gabler. New York: Random House. First published 1922.

———. 1992. *A Portrait of the Artist as a Young Man*. Edited by Seamus Deane. New York: Penguin. First published 1916.

Jung, C. G. 1977. *Psychology and the Occult*. Translated by R. F. C. Hull. Princeton, NJ: Princeton University Press.

Jutte, Robert. 2005. *A History of the Senses: From Antiquity to Cyberspace*. Translated by James Lynn. Malden, MA: Polity.

Kac, Eduardo. 1996. "Ornitorrinco in the Sahara." *Leonardo Electronic Almanac* 4, no. 11 (November): 2–5.

———. 1998. "Transgenic Art." *Leonardo Electronic Almanac* 6, no. 11 (November): 4–5.

———. 2007. "Introduction: Art that Looks You in the Eye." In *Signs of Life: Bio Art and Beyond*, 1–27. Cambridge, MA: MIT Press.

———. n.d. "Holopoetry and Beyond." Vortice Argentina. http://vorticeargentina.com.ar/poesia_visual/escritos/holopoetry_and_beyond.html.

Kaes, Anton. 2009. *Shell Shock Cinema: Weimar Culture and the Wounds of War*. Princeton, NJ: Princeton University Press.

Kahn, Douglas. 1999. *Noise, Water, Meat: A History of Sound in the Arts*. Cambridge, MA: MIT Press.

Kaplan, Janet. 1998. *Viajes inesperados: El arte y la vida de Remedios Varo*. Translated by Amalia Martín-Gamero. Mexico City: Era.

Kaplan, Lawrence S. 1967. *Jefferson and France: An Essay on Politics and Political Ideas*. New Haven, CT: Yale University Press.

Katzenstein, Inés, ed. 2004. *Listen Here Now! Argentine Art of the 1960s*. New York: Museum of Modern Art.

King, John. 1985. *El Di Tella y el desarrollo cultural argentino en la década del sesenta*. Buenos Aires: Ediciones de Arte Gaglianone.

Klein, Naomi. 2007. *The Shock Doctrine: The Rise of Disaster Capitalism*. New York: Henry Holt.

Koch, Adrienne. 1943. *The Philosophy of Thomas Jefferson*. New York: Columbia University Press.

Korn, Alejandro. 1949. "Influencias filosóficas en la evolución nacional." In *Obras completas*, edited by Francisco Romero, 43–204. Buenos Aires: Claridad.

Kozak, Claudia, ed. 2012. *Tecnopoéticas argentinas: Archivo blando de arte y tecnología*. Buenos Aires: Caja Negra.

Kracauer, Siegfried. 1990. "Caligari." In Budd 1990, 241–255.

Kristeva, Julia. 1984. *Revolution in Poetic Language*. Introduction by Leon Roudiez. Translated by Margaret Waller. New York: Columbia University Press.

Kronfeld, Chana. 2016. *The Full Severity of Compassion: The Poetry of Yehuda Amichai*. Stanford, CA: Stanford University Press.

"La ciencia." 1877. *La alborada del Plata*, no. 2 (Nov. 25): 9–10.

Laera, Alejandra, and Martín Kohan, eds. 2006. "Introduction." In *Las brújulas del extraviado: Para una lectura integral de Esteban Echeverría*, 7–12. Rosario: Beatriz Viterbo.

Lanctot, Brendan. 2014. *Beyond Civilization and Barbarism: Culture and Politics in Postrevolutionary Argentina*. Lewisburg, PA: Bucknell University Press.

Lanning, John Tate. 1940. *Academic Culture in the Spanish Colonies*. New York: Oxford University Press.

"Las redactoras." 1852. *La camelia*, no. 8 (Apr. 27): 1.

Le Breton, David. 2010. *Cuerpo sensible*. Translated by Alejandro Madrid Zan. Santiago de Chile: Metales Pesados.

Lehrer, Jonathan. 2007. *Proust Was a Neuroscientist*. Boston: Houghton Mifflin.

Le Parc, Julio. 2004. "No More Mystifications!" In Katzenstein 2004, 56–58.

Lida, Raimundo. 1988. "Sarmiento y Herder." In *Estudios hispánicos: Estudios, esquemas*, 125–139. Mexico City: El Colegio de Mexico.

López, María Pía. 1997. *Mutantes: Trazos sobre los cuerpos*. Buenos Aires: Colihué.

Ludmer, Josefina. 1988. *El género gauchesco: Un tratado sobre la patria*. Buenos Aires: Sudamericana.

Mañé, Teresa. 1896. "Las enfermedades morales." *Búcaro americano* 1, no. 2 (Feb. 15): 31–33.

Manso de Noronha, Juana. 1854a. "Crónica de la quincena." *Album de señoritas* 3 (Jan. 15): 21–22.

———. 1854b. "Educacion de la muger." *Album de señoritas* 8 (Feb. 17): 58–59.

———. 1854c. "Mesas giratorias." *Album de señoritas* 2 (Jan. 8): 11–12.

———. 1854d. "Navegación a vapor." *Album de señoritas* 3 (Jan. 15): 24.

Marinetti, Filippo Tommaso. 1971. *Marinetti: Selected Writings*. Edited by R. W. Flint. Translated by R. W. Flint and Arthur A. Coppotelli. New York: Farrar, Straus, and Giroux.

Marks, Laura U. 2000. *The Skin of the Film: Intercultural Cinema and Embodiment*. Durham, NC: Duke University Press.

Martin. Terence. 1961. *The Instructed Vision: Scottish Common Sense Philosophy and the Origins of American Fiction*. Bloomington: Indiana University Press.

Martínez, Elia M. 1897. "Falsas doctrinas." *Búcaro americano* 2, no. 17 (Oct. 15): 287–289.

———. 1898. "Un problema vital." *Búcaro americano* 2, nos. 19–20 (Jan. 1): 217–330.

Martínez Estrada, Ezequiel. 1951. *El mundo maravilloso de Guillermo Enrique Hudson*. Mexico City: Fondo de Cultura Ecónomica.

Marx, Karl. 1964. *Economic and Philosophic Manuscripts of 1844*. Edited by Dirk J. Struik. Translated by Martin Milligan. New York: International.

Masiello, Francine. 1986. *Lenguaje e ideología: Las escuelas argentinas de vanguardia*. Buenos Aires: Hachette.

———. 1992. *Between Civilization and Barbarism: Women, Nation, and Literary Culture in Modern Argentina*. Lincoln: University of Nebraska Press.

———. 1994. *La mujer y el espacio público: El periodismo femenino en la Argentina del siglo XIX*. Buenos Aires: Feminaria.

———. 2001. *The Art of Transition: Latin American Culture and Neoliberal Crisis*. Durham, NC: Duke University Press.

———. 2004. "Joyce in Buenos Aires." *Diacritics* 34, nos. 3–4 (Fall–Winter): 55–72.

———. 2013. *El cuerpo de la voz (poesía, ética y cultura)*. Rosario, Argentina: Beatriz Viterbo.

Masotta, Oscar. 1965. *Sexo y traición en Roberto Arlt*. Buenos Aires: Jorge Álvarez.

———. 1968. *Conciencia y estructura*. Buenos Aires: Jorge Álvarez.

———. 1980. *El modelo pulsional*. Foreword by German Garcia. Buenos Aires: Altazor.

———. 2004. *Revolución en el arte: Pop-art, happenings y arte de los medios en la década del sesenta*. Foreword by Ana Longoni. Buenos Aires: Edhasa.

Massumi, Brian. 2002. *Parables for the Virtual: Movement, Affect, Sensation*. Durham, NC: Duke University Press.

Matta, Roberto. 1981. "El corazón está a la izquierda." Casa de las Américas. http://www.casa.cult.cu/matta/textos.htm.

Matto de Turner, Clorinda. 1896. "Economía doméstica." *Búcaro americano* 1, no. 2 (Feb. 15): 30–31.

———. 1898a. "La mujer y la ciencia." *Búcaro americano* 2, nos. 19–20 (Jan. 1): 318.

———. 1898b. "Redenciones." *Búcaro americano* 3, no. 21 (Feb. 8): 342–343.

———. 1901. "¿Otro año?" *Búcaro americano* 6: nos. 40–41 (Feb. 25): 590.

———. 1906. "Hojas sueltas." *Búcaro americano* 6, no. 43 (June 15): 638–639.

———. 1998. *Torn from the Nest*. Edited by Antonio Cornejo Polar. Translated by John Polt. New York: Oxford University Press. First published 1889.

Maurette, Pablo. 2015. *El sentido olvidado: Ensayos sobre el tacto*. Buenos Aires: Mardulce.

McLuhan, Marshall. 1962. *The Gutenberg Galaxy: The Making of Typographic Man*. Toronto: University of Toronto Press.

Melville, Herman. 2000. *Moby-Dick, Billy Budd, and Other Writings*. New York: Library of America.

Merleau-Ponty, Maurice. 1962. *Phenomenology of Perception*. Translated by Colin Smith. London: Routledge. First published 1945.

———. 1964a. *The Primacy of Perception*. Edited by James Edie. Evanston, IL: Northwestern University Press.

———. 1964b. *Sense and Non-Sense*. Edited and translated by Hubert L. Dreyfus and Patricia Allen Dreyfus. Evanston, IL: Northwestern University Press.

———. 1964c. "Einstein and the Crisis of Reason." In *Signs*, translated by Richard C. McCleary, 192–197. Evanston, IL: Northwestern University Press.

———. 1968. *The Visible and the Invisible*. Translated by Alphonsus Lingus. Evanston, IL: Northwestern University Press. First published in 1964.

McEnaney, Thomas. 2016. "Realismo sonoro y fidelidad literaria: Las obras de cinta de Eduardo Costa." *Revista de estudios hispánicos* 50, no. 2 (June): 371–386.

Meterlinck, Maurice. 1927. "La voz interior." *Caras y caretas*, no. 1520 (Nov. 19): n.p.

"Moda." 1852. *La camelia*, no. 6 (Apr. 22): 3.

Monder. Samuel. 2010. "Sujetos a Descartes." Unpublished SECOLAS conference proceeding, Mexico City.

Mora, José Joaquín de. 1849. *Curso de derechos del Liceo de Chile: Derecho natural y derecho de jentes*. La Paz de Ayacucho: Imprenta del Pueblo.

Moraña, Mabel. 2012. "Post-scriptum: El afecto en la caja de herramientas." In *El lenguaje de las emociones: Afecto y cultura en América Latina*, edited by Mabel Moraña and Ignacio Sánchez-Prado, 313–337. Madrid: Iberoamericana-Vervuert.

Moreno, María. 2016. *Black Out*. Buenos Aires: Random House. Kindle edition.

Munilla Lacasa, María Lía, and Marcelo Marino. 2016. "Cultura visual, moda y política durante la época de Rosas." In Hallstead and Root 2016, 76–93.

Nancy, Jean-Luc. 2007. *Listening*. Translated by Charlotte Mandell. New York: Fordham University Press.

———. 2008. *Corpus*. Translated by Richard Rand. New York: Fordham University Press.

Nelle, Florian. 1993. "Sarmiento excéntrico o del nacimiento de un sujeto a través de la sordera." *Dispositio* 18, no. 44: 65–77.

Neruda, Pablo. 1961. "Toward an Impure Poetry." In *Selected Poems*, edited and translated by Ben Belitt, 39–40. New York: Grove Press. First published 1935.

———. 2005. "Arte poética." In *Residencia en la tierra*, edited by Hernán Loyola, 133–135. Madrid: Catédra.

Nestrick, William. 1976. *The Cabinet of Dr. Caligari: The Abduction of Jane*. Mount Vernon, NY: Macmillan Films.

"Nuevas literarias: Fenómenos del galvanismo." 1822. *La abeja argentina*, no. 4 (July 15): 149–150.

"Nuevas literarias: Inhalaciones." 1822. *La abeja argentina*, no. 4 (July 15): 147.

Núñez, Guillermo. 2003. *La quinta del sordo*. Exhibition catalogue. Santiago de Chile: Centro Cultural Matucana.

———. 2014. *Dibujar con sangre en el ojo: Meses días horas (archivo cotidiano): El libro del dibujos*. Santiago de Chile: Das Kapital.

Olkowski, Dorothea, and Gail Weiss, eds. 2006. *Feminist Interpretations of Maurice Merleau-Ponty*. University Park, PA: Penn State University Press.

Olson, Charles. 1947. *Call Me Ishmael: A Study of Melville*. San Francisco: City Lights.

O'Neal, John C. 1996. *The Authority of Experience: Sensationist Theory in the French Enlightenment*. University Park, PA: Penn State University Press.

Ong, Walter. 1967. *The Presence of the Word*. New Haven, CT: Yale University Press.

O'Rourke, James. 1989. "Nothing More Unnatural: Mary Shelley's Revision of Rousseau." *English Literary History* 56, no. 3 (Autumn): 543–569.

Ortega y Gasset, José. 1923. "Tiempo, distancia y forma en el arte de Proust." *La nación* (Buenos Aires) (Jan. 14).

———. 1964. "La aparición del otro." In *El hombre y la gente*, 103–130. Madrid: Revista de Occidente. First published 1934.

———. 1975. *Phenomenology and Art*. Translation and introduction by Philip W. Silver. New York: Norton.

———. 2004. *Obras completas*, vol. 1 (1902–1915). Madrid: Taurus.

———. 2009. "La idea de principio en Leibniz y la evolución de la teoría deductiva." In *Obras completas*, vol. 9 (1933–1948), 927–1174. Madrid: Taurus.

Otter, Christopher. 2008. *The Victorian Eye: A Political History of Light and Vision in Britain, 1800–1910*. Chicago: University of Chicago Press.

Otter, Samuel, and Geoffrey Sanborn. 2011. *Melville and Aesthetics*. New York: Palgrave Macmillan.

Pacheco, Marcelo E. 2004. "From the Modern to the Contemporary: Shifts in Argentine Art, 1956–65." In Katzenstein 2004, 16–27.

Palti, Elías J. 2007. *El tiempo de la política: El siglo XIX reconsiderado*. Buenos Aires: Siglo XXI.

Panagia, Davide. 2009. *The Political Life of Sensation*. Durham, NC: Duke University Press.

Parada, Alejandro E. 1998. *El mundo del libro y de la lectura durante la época de Rivadavia: Una aproximación a través de los avisos de "La gaceta mercantil" (1823–28)*. Buenos Aires: Instituto de Investigaciones Bibliotecnológicas.

Pellegrini, Aldo. 2004. "Foundation for an Aesthetic of Destruction." In Katzenstein 2004, 32–36.

Pereira dos Santos, Nelson. 2007. "Nelson Pereira dos Santos: Resistência e esperança de um cinema." *Estudos Avançados* 21, no. 59: 324–352. http://www.scielo.br/pdf/ea/v21n59/a25v2159.pdf.

Piglia, Ricardo. 1980. "Notas sobre el Facundo." *Punto de vista* 3, no. 8 (March–June): 15–18.

———. 1986. *Crítica y ficción*. Santa Fe, Argentina: Universidad Nacional del Litoral.

———. 1993. "Echeverría y el lugar de la ficción." In *La Argentina en pedazos*, 8–11. Buenos Aires: Ediciones de la Urraca.

———. 2013. *El camino de Ida*. Barcelona: Anagrama.

Poe, Edgar Allen. 1914. *The Narrative of A. Gordon Pym*. In *The Works of Edgar Allen Poe*, vols. 9–10. Introduction by Chester Noyes Greenough. New York: Hearst. First published 1838.

"Por el mundo del misterio." 1925. *Caras y caretas*, no. 1391 (May 30).

Pratt, Mary Louise. 1992. *Imperial Eyes*. New York: Routledge.

Premat, Julio. 2002. *La dicha de Saturno: Escritura y melancolía en la obra de Juan José Saer*. Rosario, Argentina: Beatriz Viterbo.

"¿Qué es Calegari?" 1922. *Crítica* (June 9).

Quintana, Isabel. 2001. *Figuras de la experiencia en el fin de siglo*. Rosario, Argentina: Beatriz Viterbo.

Quiroga, Horacio. 1967a. "De sport." In *Obras inéditas y desonocidas: Época modernista*, vol. 8, edited by Angel Rama, 61–63. Montevideo: Arca.

———. 1967b. "El hombre artificial." In *Obras inéditas y desconocidas: Novelas cortas (1908–1910)*, vol. 1, edited by Angel Rama and with a foreword by Noé Jitrik, 95–132. Montevideo: Arca.

Ramírez, Mario Teodoro. 2011. *Humanismo para una nueva época*. Mexico City: Siglo XXI.

Ramos, Nuno. *O*. 2014. Translated by Florencia Garramuño. Rosario, Argentina: Beatriz Viterbo. First published 2008.

———. n.d. Website of the artist Nuno Ramos. http://www.nunoramos.com.br/portu/video.asp.

Rancière, Jacques. 2004. *The Politics of Aesthetics: The Distribution of the Sensible*. Translated by Gabriel Rockhill. New York: Continuum.

Rangel, Gabriela, ed. 2007. *Beginning with a BANG! From Confrontation to Intimacy: An*

Exhibition of Argentine Contemporary Artists, 1960–2007. New York: The Americas Society.

Reber, Dierdra. 2016. *Coming to Our Senses: Affect and an Order of Things for Global Culture*. New York: Columbia University Press.

Richard, Nelly. 1986. *Margins and Institutions: Art in Chile since 1973*. Melbourne: Art and Text.

Rinesi, Eduardo, and Rocco Carbone, eds. 2011. *David Viñas: Tonos de la crítica*. Buenos Aires: Los Polvorines.

Roca, Pilar. 2007. *Política y sociedad en la novelística de David Viñas*. Buenos Aires: Biblos.

Rodriguez, Fermín A. 2012. "Las operaciones de la crítica." In Amante 2012, 603–630.

Romero Brest, Jorge. 1969. *El arte en la Argentina*. Buenos Aires: Paidós.

———. 1992. *Arte visual en el Di Tella: Aventura memorable en los años 60*. Buenos Aires: Emecé.

———. 2004a. "Experiences 68." In Katzenstein 2004, 130–132.

———. 2004b. "Informal Art and Art of Today: A Very Updated Article and New Reflections." In Katzenstein 2004, 98–102.

Root, Regina. 2010. *Couture and Consensus: Fashion and Politics in Postcolonial Argentina*. Minneapolis: University of Minnesota Press.

Rosa, Nicolás. 1989. "Sexo, traición, Masotta y Roberto Arlt." In Rosa et al. 1989, 31–41.

Rosa, Nicolás, Adriana Astutti, Nora Avaro, Analía Capdevila, Sandra Contreras, and Alberto Giordano. 1989. *David Viñas y Oscar Masotta: Ensayo literario y crítica sociológica*. Rosario, Argentina: Ediciones Paradoxa.

Rosaldo, Renato. 1989. *Culture and Truth: The Remaking of Social Analysis*. Boston: Beacon.

Rousseau, Jean Jacques. 2010. *Emile; or, On Education*. In *Collected Writings of Rousseau*, vol. 13, edited and translated by Christopher Kelly and Allan Bloom. Hanover, NH: University Press of New England. First published 1762.

Rozitchner, León. 1955. "Comunicación y servidumbre: Mallea." *Contorno*, nos. 5–6 (September): 27–35.

———. 2007. *La cosa y la cruz: Cristianismo y capitalismo*. Buenos Aires: Losada. First published 1996.

———. 2011. *Acerca de la derrota y los vencidos*. Foreword by Horacio González. Buenos Aires: Editorial Quadrata.

———. 2013. *Persona y comunidad: Ensayo sobre la significación ética de la afectividad en Max Scheler*. Edited by Cristián Sucksdorf and Diego Sztulwark. Buenos Aires: Biblioteca Nacional. First published 1962.

Russolo, Luigi. 1986. *The Art of Noises*. Translated by Barclay Brown. New York: Pendragon.

Ruttenberg, Nancy. 1998. *Democratic Personality: Popular Voice and the Trial of American Authorship*. Stanford, CA: Stanford University Press.

Saer, Juan José. 1986. *Juan José Saer por Juan José Saer*, edited by María T. Gramuglio. Buenos Aires: Celtia.

———. 1993. *Nobody Nothing Never*. Translated by Helen Lane. New York: Serpent's Tail. First published 1980.

———. 1997. *El concepto de ficción*. Buenos Aires: Ariel.

Sánchez de Thompson, Mariquita. 2003. *Intimidad y política: Diario, cartas y recuerdos*. Edited by María Gabriela Mizraje. Buenos Aires: Adriana Hidalgo.

Sanín Cano, Baldomero. 1925. *La civilización manual y otros ensayos*. Buenos Aires: Babel.

Sarlo, Beatriz. 1980. "Narrar la percepción." *Punto de vista* 10 (November): 34–36.

———. 1992. *La imaginación técnica: Sueños modernos de la cultura argentina*. Buenos Aires: Nueva Visión.

———. 1993. "La condición mortal." *Punto de vista* 46 (August): 28–31.

———. 1994. *Escenas de la vida posmoderna*. Buenos Aires: Espasa Calpe.

———. 2016. *Zona Saer*. Santiago de Chile: Ediciones Universidad Diego Portales.

Sarlo, Beatriz, and Carlos Altamirano. 1991. "Prólogo." In Echeverría 1991, ix–li. Caracas: Biblioteca Ayacucho.

Sarmiento, Domingo Faustino. 1845. *Civilización i barbarie: Vida de Juan Facundo Quiroga*. Santiago de Chile: Imprenta del Progreso.

———. 1899. "Cable sub-marino." In *Obras completas*, 1885–1903, 21:374–376. Buenos Aires: Mariano Moreno.

———. 1993. *Viajes por Europa, Africa i América, 1845–1847*. Edited by Javier Fernández. Madrid: Archivos.

———. 1998. *Campaña en el ejército grande*. Introduction and notes by Tulio Halperin Donghi. Buenos Aires: Universidad Nacional de Quilmes. First published 1852.

———. 2003. *Facundo: Civilization and Barbarism*. Translated by Kathleen Ross. Berkeley: University of California Press. First published 1845.

———. 2005. *Recollections of a Provincial Past*. Translated by Elizabeth Garrels and Asa Zatz. New York: Oxford University Press. First published 1850.

Scholten, Hernán. 2001. *Oscar Masotta y la fenomenología*. Buenos Aires: Atuel.

Schrader, Ludwig. 1975. *Sensación y sinestesia: Estudios y materiales para la prehistoria de la sinestesia y para la valoración de los sentidos en las literaturas italiana, española y francesa*. Translated by Juan Conde. Madrid: Gredos.

Sedgwick, Eve Kosofsky. 2003. "Paranoid Reading and Reparative Reading." In *Touching Feeling: Affect, Pedagogy, Performativity*, 123–151. Durham, NC: Duke University Press.

Seibel, Beatriz. 2002. *Historia del teatro argentino: Desde los rituales hasta 1930*. Buenos Aires: Corregidor.

Sennett, Richard. 2008. *The Craftsman*. New Haven, CT: Yale University Press.

Seremetakis, C. Nadia. 1994. *The Senses Still: Perception and Memory as Material Culture in Modernity*. Boulder, CO: Westview.

Serres, Michel. 2008. *The Five Senses: A Philosophy of Mingled Bodies*. Translated by Margaret Sankey and Peter Cowley. New York: Continuum.

Shelley, Mary. 2007. *Frankenstein; or, The Modern Prometheus*. Edited and with notes by Maurice Hindle. New York: Penguin. First published 1818.

Shklovsky, Victor. 1975. "Art as Technique." In *Russian Formalist Criticism: Four Essays*, edited by Lee T. Lemon and Marion J. Reis, 3–24. Lincoln: University of Nebraska Press. First published 1925.

Sibilia, Paula. 2009. *El hombre postorgánico: Cuerpo, subjectividad y tecnologías digitales*. Buenos Aires: Fondo de Cultura Económica.

Silver, Philip. 1978. *Ortega as Phenomenologist: Meditations on Quixote*. New York: Columbia University Press.

Simmel, Georg. 1950. "The Metropolis and Mental Life." In *The Sociology of Georg Simmel*, translated by Kurt H. Wolff, 409–424. Glencoe: IL: Free Press. First published 1903.

———. 1997a. "A Few Words on Spiritualism." In *Simmel on Culture: Selected Writings*, edited by David Frisby and Mike Featherstone, 288–295. London: Sage. First published 1892.

———. 1997b. "Sociology of the Senses." In *Simmel on Culture. Selected Writings*, edited by David Frisby and Mike Featherstone, 109–120. London: Sage. First published 1907.

Skinner, Lee. 2016. *Gender and the Rhetoric of Modernity (1850–1910)*. Gainesville: University Press of Florida.

Smith, Mark. 2007. *Sensing the Past: Seeing, Hearing, Smelling, Tasting, and Touching*. Berkeley: University of California Press.

"Sofismas políticos: Culto de los antiguos, o argumentos a la chinesca." 1822. *La abeja argentina*, no. 8 (Jan. 15): 306–312.

Solar, Xul. 2006a. "Propuestas para más vida futura: Algo semitécnico sobre mejoras anatómicas y entes nuevos." In Artundo 2006, 146–151.

———. 2006b. "Vuelvilla." In Artundo 2006, 188–194.

Sommer, Doris. 1991. "Plagiarized Authenticity: Sarmiento's Cooper and Others." In *Foundational Fictions: The National Romances of Latin America*, 52–83. Berkeley: University of California Press.

Soros, Juan. 2011. "Del *Land Art* al campo íconotextual en la obra de Raúl Zurita." In *Zurita x 60*, edited by Paulina Wendt, 121–138. Santiago de Chile: Editorial Mago.

Sterne, Jonathan. 2003. *The Audible Past*. Durham, NC: Duke University Press.

Stewart, Susan. 2002. *Poetry and the Fate of the Senses*. Chicago: University of Chicago Press.

Stowe, Harriet Beecher. 1981. *Uncle Tom's Cabin; or, Life among the Lowly*. Edited by Ann Douglas. New York: Penguin.

Streeby, Shelley. 2002. *American Sensations: Class, Empire, and the Production of Popular Culture*. Berkeley: University of California Press.

Taylor, Charles. 2007. *A Secular Age*. Cambridge, MA: Harvard University Press.

"Telégrafos acústicos." 1827. *Crónica política y literaria de Buenos Aires*, no. 57 (July 20): n.p.

Terada, Ray. 2001. *Feeling in Theory: Emotion after the "Death of the Subject."* Cambridge, MA: Harvard University Press.

Ticineto Clough, Patricia, ed. 2007. "Introduction." In *The Affective Turn: Theorizing the Social*, 1–33. Durham, NC: Duke University Press.

Thompson, Kristen. 1990. "Dr. Caligari at the Folies-Bergère." In Budd 1990, 121–169.

Tompkins, Jane. 1986. *Sensational Designs: The Cultural Work of American Fiction, 1790–1860*. New York: Oxford University Press.

Toqueville, Alexis de. 1945. *Democracy in America*. 2 vols. Translated by Henry Reeve and edited by Francis Bowen. New York: Knopf. First published 1835, 1840.

Torchia Estrada, Juan Carlos. 1961. *La filosofía en la Argentina*. Washington, DC: Unión Panamericana.

Traisnel, Antoine. 2012. "Huntology: Ontological Pursuits and Still Lives." *Diacritics* 40, no. 2: 4–25.

Tsur, Reuven. 2007. "Issues in Literary Synaesthesia." *Style* 41, no. 1 (Spring): 30–52, 111–112.

Turcio, Froilán. 1927. "El sexto sentido." *Caras y caretas*, no. 1489 (Apr. 16).

Unruh, Vicky. 1994. *Latin American Vanguards: The Art of Contentious Encounters*. Berkeley: University of California Press.

Vallebona, Luigi. 2013. *Narrare il contatto col mondo: Percezione e memoria nell'opera narrativa di Claude Simon e di Juan José Saer*. Córdoba: Eduvim.

Vallejo, Antonio. 1926. "Criollismo y metafísica." *Martín Fierro* 2, no. 32: 197.

Vallejo, César. 1993. *Trilce*. Edited by Julio Ortega. Madrid: Catédra.

Valverde, Estela. 1989. *David Viñas: En busca de una síntesis de la historia argentina*. Buenos Aires: Plus Ultra.

Varchausky, Nicolás. n.d. "Resonances, Turbulences and Explosions." Website of Nicolás Varchausky. http://www.varchausky.com.ar/resonances-turbulences-and-explosions/.

Vegh, Beatriz, and Jean Phillippe Barnabé. 2005. *William Henry Hudson y la tierra purpúrea: Reflexiones desde Montevideo*. Montevideo: Linardi and Russo.

Vicuña, Manuel. 2006. *Voces de ultratumba: Historia del espiritismo en Chile*. Santiago de Chile: Aguilar.

Viñas, David. 1958. *Los dueños de la tierra*. Buenos Aires: Losada.

———. 1969. *Literatura argentina y realidad política*. Buenos Aires: Siglo XXI. First published 1967.

Vindel, Jaime. 2010. "Tretyakov in Argentina: Factography and Operativity in the Artistic Avant-Garde and the Political Vanguard of the Sixties." EIPCP. http://eipcp.net/transversal/0910/vindel/en.

Virno, Paolo. 2010. *E così via all'infinito: Logica e antropologia*. Turin, Italy: Bollati Boringhieri.

Wortham, Simon Morgan. 2015. *Modern Thought in Pain: Philosophy, Politics, Psychoanalysis*. Edinburgh, Scotland: Edinburgh University Press.

Zamudio Silva, Jorge R. 1940. *Juan Manuel Fernández de Agüero: Primer profesor de filosofía de la Universidad de Buenos Aires*. Buenos Aires: Facultad de Filosofía y Letras–Instituto de Filosofía.

Zurita, Raúl. 2003. *INRI*. Santiago de Chile: Fondo de Cultura Económica.

———. 2007. *Zurita/In Memoriam*. Santiago de Chile: Tacitas.

———. 2009a. *INRI*. Translated by William Rowe. Grosse Pointe Farms, MI: Marick Press.

———. 2009b. *Purgatory: A Bilingual Edition*. Translated and with an introduction by Anna Deeny Morales. Berkeley: University of California Press. First published 1979.

———. 2011. *Zurita*. Santiago de Chile: Ediciones Universidad Diego Portales.

———. 2016a. *Sky Below*. Translated and with an introduction by Anna Deeny Morales. Evanston, IL: Northwestern University Press.

———. 2016b. Public lecture delivered at the University of California at Berkeley, Apr. 22.

Index

Page numbers followed by f indicate figures; note: plates, identified here by plate number, follow page 000.